Dance Movement Therapy:
A Healing Art

highlighter noted 5/13 Aw

Senior Editorial Consultants/Authors:
Cathy Appel and Anne Mitcheltree

Contributing Authors/Editors:
Miriam Roskin Berger, Lou Cannon, Sharon Chaiklin, William C. Freeman, Terese Hall, Lenore Wadsworth Hervey, Susan Kleinman, Claire Schmais and Elissa Q. White

Sponsored by the
National Dance Association,
An association of the
American Alliance for Health, Physical Education, Recreation and Dance

On the cover: "Desperate Heart," dancer Valerie Bettis
(Photo courtesy Lloyd Morgan of the Barbara Morgan Archive)

Associate Editors: Mary Virginia Wilmerding, Ph.D., NDA Vice President of
Dance Science and Somatics; Dept. of Physical
Performance and Development, University of New Mexico
Colleen Porter Hearn, M.A., NDA Program Coordinator
Sheyi Ojofeitimi, M.P.T.
Carrie Nygard

Assistant Editors: Carolyn Craig, George Washington University
Juliana Mascelli, George Washington University
Jo Ann Schaefer, NDA Administrative Staff

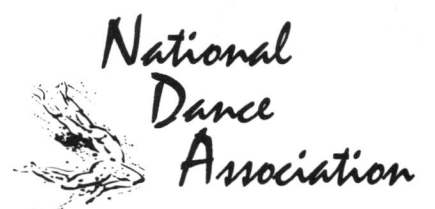
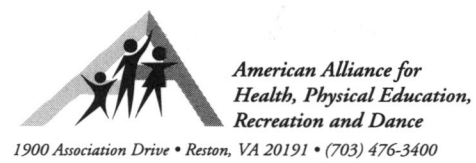

American Alliance for Health, Physical Education, Recreation and Dance
1900 Association Drive • Reston, VA 20191 • (703) 476-3400

The National Dance Association (NDA) encourages authors to freely express their professional judgment through their work. Therefore, materials and medical/technical terminology within this text represent the views of the author and do not necessarily reflect the position of NDA. The author's research, citations and reference structure herein do not completely follow AAHPERD publications guidelines. The author granted permission and provided all materials for publication. Copyright permission for any material that is not the original work of the author is the sole responsibility of the author and not the responsibility of NDA or AAHPERD.

2nd Revised edition copyright © 2005
1st Revised edition copyright © 1992
Copyright © 1988
National Dance Association
An Association of the
American Alliance for Health, Physical Education, Recreation and Dance (AAHPERD)

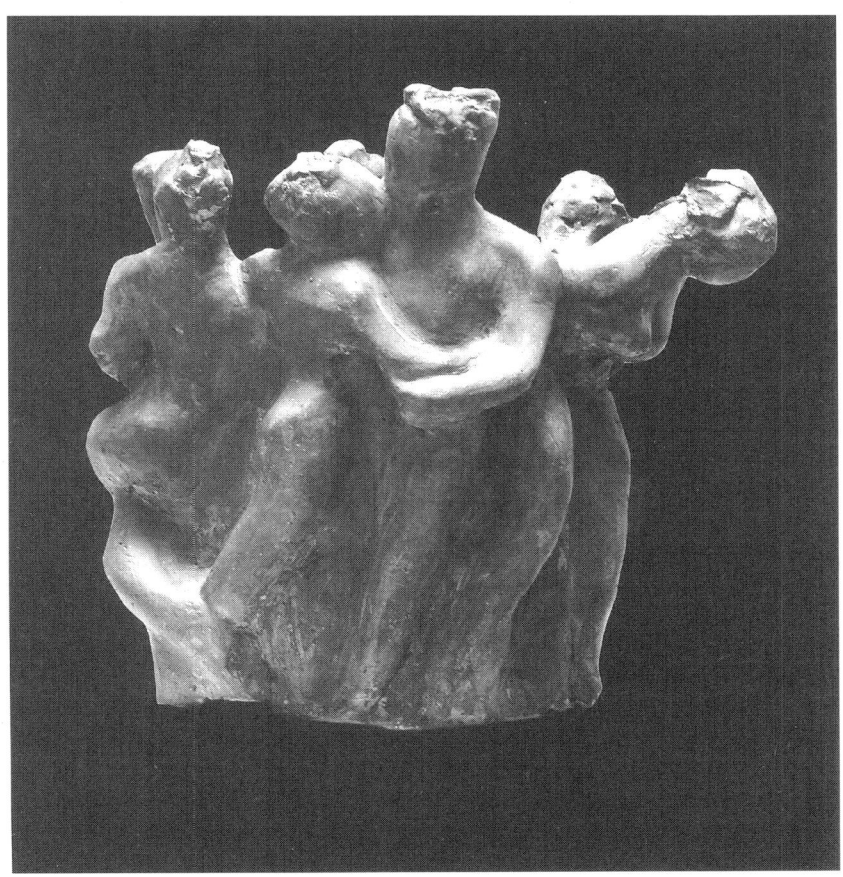

"Circle Dance" Sculpture by Lillian G. Levy (Photo by Leonard Forrest)

DANCE

To move
To be in the movement, when it is and where it is
To be there and nowhere else
To dance

Fran J. Levy
Goddard College
1966

Praise for
Dance Movement Therapy: A Healing Art

I highly recommend this book for practitioners of every level of experience. I've made use of it many times as a reference book. This revised and updated version can only serve to increase its value. The range and variety of information cannot be found elsewhere.—**Sharon Chaiklin**, ADTR; Past President, ADTA

Fran Levy's second edition is an important resource for the field in that it provides a survey of dance therapy history and evolution, offers different approaches to theory and practice and highlights the scope of populations served to date.—**Laurel Thompson**, MPS, ADTR, ATR-BC; Chair, Graduate Creative Arts Therapy Department, Pratt Institute

Fran Levy's extraordinary contribution encompasses the origins, theory and practice of dance therapy, tracing its development through the vital, creative, inspiring work of the pioneers and their descendents. She has produced an invaluable resource for all concerned with the healing power of the arts.—**Joan Chodorow**, Ph.D., ADTR; Author of *Dance Therapy and Depth Psychology* and *Active Imagination: Healing from Within*

Dr. Levy's core text has been required reading for students in Antioch New England's Dance Movement Therapy Graduate Program since it was first published and students and faculty alike are eager to absorb the new chapters and updates in this cutting-edge edition.—**Susan Loman**, MA, ADTR, NCC, KMP Analyst; Associate Chair, Department of Applied Psychology, Antioch New England Graduate School

Levy's updated and expanded edition is long overdue. Of particular import are new sections in Unit III...Chapters have been newly added dealing with children with special needs, victims of abuse; the physically challenged; work in the corporate settings and those with eating disorders. Important historical sections on dance therapy's influences, both geographically and theoretically, have been substantially updated and expanded. All those who teach and seriously study the theory and practice of movement therapy will need to acquire this new edition.—**Vicky J. Risner**, Music Division, Library of Congress

An inspirational book ..a must for all career counselors and for anyone else in the position of counseling, advising or educating others.—**Howard Figler**, Ph.D.; Author, *The Complete Job-Search Handbook*, 3rd Edition

This text is essential for anyone who is curious about Dance Movement Therapy. Dr. Levy has updated this most popular of DMT books with new chapters on exciting developments in the field and contributions from several reputable experts. This is the book we'll go to first for basic, accurate, thorough information about the field. We all, beginners and advanced therapists alike, will treasure Dr. Levy's comprehensive portrait of the field.—**Sherry W. Goodill**, Ph.D., ADTR, LPC; Associate Professor and Director, College of Nursing and Health Professions, Drexel University

Fran Levy has written a masterful treatise. It provides engrossing reading for anyone in the therapeutic fields or the theatrical professions or simply for anyone interested in the art of communication.—**Trudi Schoop** and **Peggy Mitchell**; Co-Authors, *Won't You Join the Dance*

Dedication

To my parents, Henry and Lillian Levy, who
shared with me, in countless ways, their love of life and
deep appreciation for personal and artistic expression.
To Rob, Marge, Len, Jocelyn, Mark, Sophia, and Julia
and to the Class family, Hector and Michelle,
and their classy kids: Michelle Lee,
Jennifer, Stephanie and Hector, Jr.,
with love and admiration.

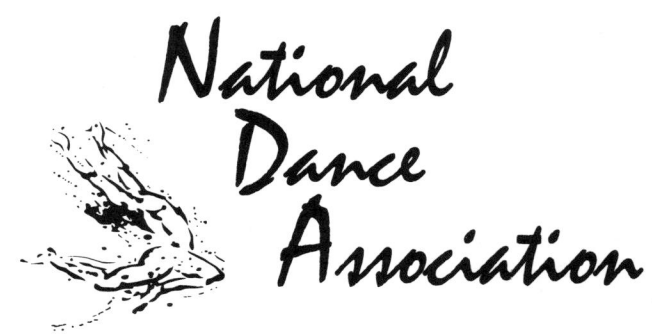

The mission of the National Dance Association (NDA) is to increase knowledge,
improve skills and encourage sound professional practices in dance education
while promoting and supporting creative and healthy lifestyles
through high quality dance programs.

Importance of Dance Movement Therapy

NDA leads the way in dance science and somatics and recognizes dance movement therapy as a crucial way for many to comprehend and express feelings, especially from the tumultuous events of the twenty-first century. With this commitment, NDA maintains its long-standing partnership with the American Dance Therapy Association (ADTA). In this beautifully crafted text, author Fran Levy demonstrates respect for past dance therapy leaders while examining the future of this vital profession.

Brief History

NDA is an association of the American Alliance for Health, Physical Education, Recreation and Dance (AAHPERD), with a spirit and purpose that were advocated by the early leaders. AAHPERD was established in 1885 and today serves almost 30,000 members. AAHPERD is comprised of six national, six district and fifty state organizations supporting the related fields. Modern dance icons like Margaret H. D'Houbler were instrumental in promoting dance education within AAHPERD and the nation. At the 1905 convention in New York City, then president Luther Halsey Gulick chose to highlight multicultural dance. Sculptor, athlete, scholar and physician, R. Tait McKenzie, captured the essence of movement in his artistic work, including the Luther Halsey Gulick Medal that is the highest AAHPERD honor. The dance section was established first in 1932 and in 1974, NDA became an association of AAHPERD.

Programs

For over 70 years, NDA has and continues to be the leader in dance education, as the founder of the first national dance honor society Nu Delta Alpha, *Dance for Health!* Project, *National Standards for Dance Education* and founding member of the National Consortium of Arts Education Associations. NDA's highest honor, the Heritage Award, has been presented to such distinguished dance educators as D'Houbler, Louis Horst, Ted Shawn, Katherine Dunham, Hanya Holm and Don McKayle. Other awards recognize both professionals and students for their achievements. NDA conducts workshops and conferences throughout the United States, publishes state-of-the-art materials and advocates for quality dance programs at all levels. The National Endowment for the Arts, Harkness Foundation for Dance, Capezio BalletMakers and the U.S. Departments of Education and Humanities have all supported NDA projects.

Contents

Acknowledgements i
Preface iv
Foreword by Elissa Q. White—With Testimonials ** vi
Introduction* The Shoulders on Which We Stand 1

UNIT I. EARLY DEVELOPMENT—THE PIONEERS OF DANCE MOVEMENT THERAPY 15

Section A. Major Pioneers on the East Coast 17
Chapter 1: Marian Chace: The "Grande Dame of Dance Therapy" 19
Chapter 2: Blanche Evan: Creative Movement Becomes Dance Therapy 29
Chapter 3: Liljan Espenak: Psychomotor Therapy 43

Section B. Major Pioneers on the West Coast 49
Chapter 4: Mary Whitehouse: Movement-in-Depth: A Jungian Approach to Dance Therapy 51
Chapter 5: Trudi Schoop: Dance, Drama, Mime and Performance 61
Chapter 6: Alma Hawkins: Humanistic Psychology, Imagery and Relaxation 73
Discussion: Similarities and Differences Among the Major Pioneers 77

Section C. Other Early Pioneers, Leaders and Contributors 81
Chapter 7: Dance Therapy Emerges in the Midwest 83
Chapter 8: Pioneering Literary Contributions 87
  Part A. Franziska Boas: Seminal Concepts 87
  Part B. Elizabeth Rosen: Trial and Error 94
  Part C. Dance Therapy Study 98
Discussion: Outline Depicting the State of the Art by 1960 101

UNIT II. SUBSEQUENT DEVELOPMENT OF DANCE MOVEMENT THERAPY 105

Section A. Laban Movement Analysis and Dance Therapy in the United States 107
Chapter 9: The Theoretical Contributions of Laban and Lamb 109
Chapter 10: Irmgard Bartenieff Brings LMA to America 113
Chapter 11: Zeitgeist at Bronx State Hospital 119
Chapter 12: Marion North: Personality Assessment and Treatment 123
Chapter 13: Judith Kestenberg: Movement Profile 127
Discussion: LMA: Varying Views 131

Section B. Further Expansion of Dance Therapy Theory and Practice* 133
Chapter 14: The Evolution of East Coast Influences 135
  Part A. Elaine Siegel: Psychoanalytic Approach with a Touch of Chace 135
  Part B. Zoë Avstreih: Psychoanalytic Perspective Integrating Chace and Whitehouse ... 138
Chapter 15: The Evolution of West Coast Influences 141
  Part A. Irma Dosamantes-Beaudry: Experiential Movement Psychotherapy 141
  Part B. Diane Fletcher: A Psychodynamic Orientation 144
  Part C. Janet Adler: The Witness/Mover Relationship 147
  Part D. Joan Chodorow: Whitehouse and Jung 147
Discussion: Comparing East and West Coast Trends 151
  Part E. Sharon Chaiklin Was There—1972 152

Chapter 16: Integration of Different Trends** 155
    Part A. Marcia Leventhal: Dance Therapy as Primary Treatment 155
    Part B. Penny Lewis: An Eclectic Approach 156
Chapter 17: Fran Levy's Multimodal Approach: Theory and Practice** 161

UNIT III. DANCE MOVEMENT THERAPY WITH DIFFERENT POPULATIONS 177

Section A. Children** 179
Chapter 18: Children with Special Needs** 181
    Part A. Young Children: Social, Emotional, Physical and Cognitive Goals 181
    Part B. Children at Risk: Violence Prevention 185
    Part C. Adolescents in the School System 187
    Part D. Movement Assessment in Schools 190
    Part E. Children with Severe Disturbance: Inpatient 190
    Part F. Children with Autism 192
    Part G. Children Who Have Been Sexually Abused 196

Section B. Adults* 201
Chapter 19: Individuals in Psychiatric Care* 203
Chapter 20: Victims of Physical, Sexual and Emotional Abuse and
Dissociative Identity Disorder (or Multiple Personality)** 213
Chapter 21: Women with Eating Disorders by Susan Kleinman and and Terese Hall** 221
Chapter 22: The Elderly* 229

Section C. Work with Individuals with Varying Physical Disabilities** 233
Chapter 23: Rehabilitation by Cathy Appel** 235

Section D. Other Applications of Dance Movement Therapy 247
Chapter 24: The Developmentally Disabled 249
Chapter 25: Additional Applications of Dance Movement Therapy 253
    Part A. Dance Movement Therapy in a Corporate Setting** 253
    Part B. Families* 254
    Part C. Blind and Visually Impaired 256
    Part D. Deaf and Hearing Impaired 258

UNIT IV. INTERNATIONAL GROWTH OF DANCE MOVEMENT THERAPY**
Introduction by Miriam Roskin Berger** 261
Chapter 26: International Growth of Dance Movement Therapy by Cathy Appel** 263

UNIT V. DANCE MOVEMENT THERAPY RESEARCH:
SURVEY RESULTS AND THE HERITAGE TREES 273
Chapter 27: Contemporary Thought on Research by Lenore Wadsworth Hervey** 275
Chapter 28: Review of Survey Findings—Past, Present and Future Trends 277
Chapter 29: Dance Therapy Heritage Trees—The Spread of Influence of the Major Pioneers* ... 283

Concluding Remarks 305
References 308
Index 319

* indicates partially revised
** indicates a new chapter in the book or a complete revision

Acknowledgements

I am deeply grateful to many leading dance therapists for their help and support in bringing back *Dance Movement Therapy: A Healing Art*. They believed in the importance of the book and were willing to contribute their valuable time and energy to see this third edition come to fruition.

A president of the American Dance Therapy Association, friend and colleague, with whom I collaborated for many years and whom I cannot thank enough is Elissa Q. White. Her conviction in this project's value, her expertise as a dance therapist and writer and her warmth and spirit have all been invaluable. Elissa believed in this book when it was just an idea. She helped me through the awkward stage when the manuscript was first written and mushroomed into a cumbersome 700-page dissertation. Finally, with Elissa's help, it evolved into a book in 1988 and revised here in 2005.

Also, for their love and continuous emotional support over the last several years, I feel profound gratitude to my sister, Marge Forrest and brother-in-law, Leonard Forrest.

1988 and 1992

Other outstanding dance therapy leaders read the first manuscript and graciously offered their excellent suggestions. Claire Schmais, Arlynne Stark, Sharon Chaiklin and Lou Cannon all helped to strengthen, tighten and deepen the text.

These clinicians and other notable dance therapists, many of whom are protégés of the major pioneers, generously shared their memories and experiences. Deborah Thomas, along with Sharon, Claire, Arlynne and Elissa, helped with the chapter on Marian Chace. Judith Bunney kindly located the Chace portrait. Janet Adler, Joan Chodorow, Judith Fried, Carolyn Fay, Jane Manning, Susan Wallock and Nancy Zenoff helped clarify the work of their mentor Mary Whitehouse. Feather King (Whitehouse's daughter) also enthusiastically read this chapter. Conversations with Blanche Evan and her protégés—Iris Rifkin-Gainer, Barbara Melson, Anne Krantz and Bonnie Bernstein—helped me develop the Evan chapter. Similarly, Trudi Schoop's input and that of her colleague and co-author Peggy Mitchell strengthened the Schoop chapter. I was fortunate to work with Alma Hawkins, Liljan Espenak, Irmgard Bartenieff and Franziska Boas on their chapters. In addition, Marcia Leventhal, a protégé of Hawkins, commented on the chapter about her mentor. Gertrud Michelson, Boas' daughter, clarified her mother's historical influences. To better understand the Midwest developments, Rhoda Winter Russell, Deborah Thomas, Miriam Roskin Berger, Joan Berkowitz and Joanna Harris were most helpful. Finally, the section on Rudolf Laban was written with the generous help of Martha Davis, Julianna Lau, Diana Levy, Mavis Lockwood, Susan Loman, Virginia Reed, Martha Soodak, Mark Sossin, Suzanne Youngerman and Jody Zacharias.

These personal communications bridged the gaps in dance therapy's history and added personal depth and vitality to these important chapters.

Other experts and leaders in related fields who contributed to the book's development and were instrumental in its completion included Zoë Avstreih, Felix Barosa, Dr. Howard Figler, Dr. Dominick Grundy, Stephanie Katz, Jon Klimo, Phyllis K. Jeswald, Penny Lewis, Elizabeth Meehan, Miriam Puder, Susan Sandel, Steve Sidorsky and Steve Wilson.

In addition, some special people gave me a great deal of encouragement in the early stages of my career. Noted psychologists Ellen Siroka and Robert W. Siroka believed strongly in my work and provided me with invaluable opportunities for professional growth. Others saw the special value of using dance and movement in psychotherapy with adults and supported my endeavors in this area. These colleagues and friends, Beth Anderson, George Biglin, Susan Davidoff, Janet Johnson, Sue Morfit, Jean Peterson, Dr. Howard Seaman, Katharine Sloan, Barbara Stein, Roy Teitz, Mary Watson and Joan Weinstock will remain dear to my heart.

Carolyn Braunstein, my editorial consultant for six years, gave of herself in such a generous and helpful way that words cannot thank her enough. Without her help, this book may never have happened.

Several others gave generously of their time and energy to what seemed like a job without end. Rise Rosenberg, Bettina Del Prett and daughter Christy, Staci Berger, Wahe Guru Kaur and Lillian Yacknowitz worked with me day and night on endless details. Anne Mitcheltree, assistant editor of *Movement and Growth*, reviewed this book "hot off the press." Also, my AAHPERD copy editor Anne Stuart and acquisitions editor Martin Connor were both a joy to work with and to know.

Every author needs knowledgeable and understanding friends and family who spur them on and share their frustrations. Therefore, I would like to thank these loving people: Nancy and Robert Schulman, Amy Schaffer, Ted and Ellen Newman, Phyllis Goodfriend, Steve Figler, Larry and Rita Levin, Joyce Wackenhut and my niece Jocelyn LaBianca.

During the course of my writing, I met dedicated, talented writers who shared their wealth of experience, including Nick Pappas, Jane Gerver, Dr. Michelle Gage, Dr. Ruth Resch, Dr. Anatole Dolgoff, Kathleen Barker and Leslie Pratt. Thea Schiller, a wonderful writer, teacher and person, reminded me of the power of writing. Jane Brody, the personal health columnist for *The New York Times*, has also been a great source of personal motivation.

I was also inspired by my association with many dance therapists, movement specialists and psychotherapists, including Harriet All, Jessica Calise, Lisa Dobbs, Irene Dowd, Jan Earl, Lee Goldberg, Judy Huffman, Carol Hutchinson, Wendy Kaiser, Berti Klein, Eileen Lawlor, Fern Leventhal, Jamie Lieberman, Susan Lovell and Billie Logan, as well as Regina Monti, Julie Miller, Lenore Powell, Lee Rubinfeld and Wendy Sobelman. I was moved by the clinical contributions of Maureen Costonis, Dianne Dulicai, Tina Erfer, Mary Frost, Robert Fuhlrodt, Joan Lavender, Helene Lefco, Harriet Powers, Paul Sevett, Marsha Weltman and Susan Kierr.

2004—Thank You for Holding the Flame

The dream of a third revision has become a reality—thank you for holding the flame.

First, I am grateful to my senior editorial consultants, Cathy Appel and Anne Mitcheltree. By acting as advisers and contributing new material, they broadened the knowledge base in the field. Cathy contributed two excellent chapters on people with physical disabilities and the international growth of dance therapy. Anne updated the heritage trees and combed the book for outdated language and information.

Others who contributed important new chapters are Susan Kleinman and Terese Hall, who wrote on eating disorders and Lenore Hervey, who summarized ideas from her new book on research and dance therapy.

Two pioneering dance therapists who, in their own words, shared their intimate knowledge of the history of dance therapy were Miriam Roskin Berger and Sharon Chaiklin.

In the discussion of the inspirational work of Norma Canner, thanks go to contributors Anne Brownell, Vivian Marcow-Speiser and William Freeman, as well as to Cathy Appel's creativity in skillfully pulling all of their contributions together. William Freeman also shared his expertise in work with children through his editorial contributions to the children's chapter.

I also would like to thank Lucy Neave, my editor, a Fulbright scholar from Australia who came to my rescue during the final stages of integrating new material with earlier work. Her skill as a writer and ability to gracefully handle stress and deadlines will be remembered.

In the chapter on my work, I thank my dear friend, Robert Cardonsky. He helped me look at this chapter in a fresh way and to completely update it. He generously shared his love of writing, enthusiasm and astute perceptions.

Many dear friends helped by being there when the going got rough; Judith Weiss, Amy Schaffer, Nancy and Robert Schulman, Patricia Stevens, Larry and Rita Levin, Joe and Elise Berman, Harriet Power, Robert Fuhlrodt, Conrad and Jane Wilson Cathcart, Jack Friedman, Selma Zimmerman, Fran Hamberg, Maria Kutiock, Hector and Michelle Class and their classy kids (Michelle, Jennifer, Stephanie and Hector Jr.), Susan Stratton, Jane Brody, Carol Crewdson, Marge McClure, Gail Scott Graf, Blair Glaser, Dennis Guttsman, Michael de Simone, Joyce and Andrew Daly, Sarah Falkner, Rose McKeon, Sally Rappaport, Evelyn Jennings, Svetlana Lazarev, Boris Gilzon, Eileen Lawlor and from Argentina, Diana Fischman and Laura Peralta.

There are too many people to list here but I was deeply touched by all of the correspondence I received from people who supported the book and wanted to see it back in print, from students and teachers alike.

Your words of support and love of the book spurred me on. This includes those at NDA/AAHPERD who worked in the publication of the third edition: Colleen Porter Hearn, program coordinator; past presidents

Fran Anthony Meyer and Kathleen Kinderfather; Virginia Wilmerding, dance science and somatics vice president; Carrie Nygard, JOPERD associate editor; Barbara Hernandez, publications unit director; Diane Wawrejko Cochran and the Fairfax County high school assistants, Ben Burkes, Chau Hoang and Laura Cerda. Interns Carolyn L. Craig and Juliana Mascelli, students of George Washington University, were diligent in their task of indexing and proofreading this book. Most importantly I wish to thank John C. Farrell, AAHPERD editor and Pamela James, a professional dancer and Yale graduate.

Finally, a special thanks goes to Shaw Bronner, a physical therapist, for introducing me to her colleague, Sheyi Ojofeitimi. Because of Sheyi's tireless and meticulous research in the final hours, when it seemed like we would never finish, we did. Also, a huge thank you goes to photographers Steve Clarke, Anthony Verebes, Leonard Forrest and Barbara Morgan for adding their artistic elegance, beauty and clarity to the pages of the book.

Preface

"Dancing shoes replace the therapist's couch. The underlying premise of dance movement therapy is, as Dr. Levy describes it, 'that body movement reflects inner emotional states and that changes in movement behavior can lead to changes in the psyche, thus promoting health and growth.' If you give...[people] room to move, their story can unfold...The trauma is in their bodies and movement helps them...express it."—Jane E. Brody, *The New York Times*, Oct. 18, 1995

In recent years there has been a resurgence of interest in the connection between mind and body and the use of the body to heal the mind and vice versa. We have long been aware of the profound benefits of motor activity on mind and body. Simultaneously, the need for individualized styles of self-expression and communication has received greater recognition. This is evidenced by the proliferation and integration of new forms of action and body-oriented therapies, as well as creative arts therapies.

This text is concerned with the need that many individuals have for nonverbal, physical forms of expression and how this need has fueled the development of dance movement therapy.

Most often referred to as dance therapy or dance movement therapy, the discipline has also adopted branch names, such as movement psychotherapy, psychoanalytic movement therapy, Jungian dance movement therapy, psychomotor therapy and so on. The American Dance Therapy Association (ADTA) has adopted the policy of referring to the discipline as dance movement therapy. The alternation in the field between the designations "dance" and "movement" stem largely from concern over preconceived ideas of what "dance" means. Some people feel inadequate or embarrassed when the word is used. Others fear that they will have to perform dance steps or display an aptitude for body movement, as opposed to simply expressing their thoughts and feelings. At times, in sessions, the witnessed psychomotor expression may not resemble dance in any formal or even informal sense. For example, an arm reaching out, a fist gesturing in rage, the symbolic rocking of a child or even the tilt of a head may all be elements of the expressive and exploratory process of dance therapy. While some will still joke about the "angry mambo," the "inspirational cha-cha," and "dancing one's troubles away," these stereotypes are quickly fading. Today, the field, broad in its application and diverse in its methodology and theoretical foundations, extends into every area of mental health.

Dance therapy is a form of psychotherapy. Differentiated from traditional psychotherapy, it utilizes psychomotor expression as its major mode of intervention and as the agent of change. The pages that follow explore the theory, practice and origins of dance therapy. The text begins with an explanation of how, in the early part of the century, the evolution of both the modern dance movement and the field of psychotherapy and psychoanalytic thinking laid the foundations for the emergence of dance and movement as a form of psychotherapy.

A brief review of these areas reveals several important overlapping trends. In the early part of the twentieth century, emphasis was placed on self-expression and self-exploration, a striving toward more honest communication and interaction, a growing acceptance of the inherent interaction between mind and body with recognition of the uniqueness of individual needs. These diverse areas of self-expression, one that originally focused on the mind (psychotherapy) or on the body (dance), broadened their parameters in the early 1900s and, in turn, merged dramatically in the 1940s and 1950s, giving birth to a new discipline—dance therapy.

Unit I identifies the major dance therapy pioneers who laid the groundwork for today's practice and influenced an entire generation of dance therapists. A thorough review of their theoretical and practical contributions is included. Unit I culminates in an outline depicting the state of dance therapy practice as it had emerged by 1960. This outline illustrates how far the field had come in its methodology and how the original leaders laid a complete and diversified foundation for today's practice—a foundation which, when understood, serves to clarify the state of the art today.

Unit II explores subsequent developments in the field. Section A reviews the influence of Laban Movement Analysis (LMA) and Effort/Shape on dance therapy and the various trends that grew out of this merger. These include the incorporation of psychoanalytic and developmental concepts interfaced with a comprehensive language and philosophy of movement.

Section B looks at how the original east and west coast dance therapy trends developed to influence an entire second and third generation of dance therapy leaders, some of whom began to integrate east and west coast trends in dance therapy and others who integrated theory and practice borrowed from related areas of study.

The contributions of several of these "new" leaders are identified and reviewed. This generation of dance therapists is best known for the creative integration of expressive methods drawn from many fields, as well as the exploration of a variety of theoretical frameworks that support the use of body movement and dance in psychotherapy. For example, aspects of Jungian analysis, ego psychology, object relations theory, psychodrama, Gestalt therapy and art therapy are discussed and incorporated into the theory and practice of dance therapy.

This section also provides extensive case material, which illustrates the integration of the expressive arts therapies into the theory and practice of dance therapy. In the final chapter of this section, special emphasis is placed on the use of the visual arts as an intermediary modality that can bridge verbal and nonverbal experience and the use of dramatic dialogue as a tool for organizing unconscious or chaotic material.

Dance therapy, once primarily strong in its practical applications and methodology, was developing theoretical and philosophical foundations in the late 1960s and 1970s. This growth has continued into the present and is reflected in this and the following unit.

Unit III discusses the clinical applications of dance therapy with specific patient populations. It has been significantly expanded and divided into sections. These include a new section on dance movement therapy with children (Section A), a section on dance movement therapy with different adult patient populations (Section B), which now includes chapters on victims of abuse and patients with eating disorders. Section C, by Cathy Appel, is also new and discusses dance therapy in rehabilitation. Section D, "Other Applications of Dance Movement Therapy," contains important work now being done in corporate settings. In addition to the areas mentioned above, individuals in psychiatric care, the elderly, people with developmental disabilities and the hearing and visually impaired are discussed. Like verbal psychotherapy, dance therapy techniques and theory vary tremendously to meet the needs of the individual.

Unit IV, also by Cathy Appel, is entirely new and discusses the growth of dance therapy around the world, viewed through the eyes of several generations of dance therapists in the U.S., who have traveled and taught abroad. The international growth of dance therapy has been unusually rapid. The challenge of bringing a nonverbal but universal medium, dance, to parts of the world where verbal translation is, at times, challenging and where cultural taboos and norms differ dramatically, has been deeply rewarding and enlightening to many.

Unit V discusses Dance Movement Therapy Research. Chapter 27 by Lenore Hervey explains a creative, aesthetic approach to research. A desire to honor the creative, body-oriented, artistic experience as therapy, without the "crutch" of relying on languages drawn from other psychological fields, is the topic of this section.

Chapter 28 includes a summary of the results of a 1985 survey conducted by the author on 101 leaders in the field, members of the Academy of Dance Therapists Registered. The major pioneers in Unit I were identified as a result of this survey along with the identification of major clinical, theoretical and dance movement trends that influenced contemporary thinking. The survey results were summarized and do not include the original charts.

Chapter 29 depicts the growth of dance therapy and the spread of influence among dance therapy leaders in the form of heritage trees. Anne Mitcheltree updated these trees.

This text is an attempt to trace, codify and synthesize the evolution of dance therapy, from its inception to its current scope and direction. The text provides detailed accounts of the theoretical and practical developments in the field and integrates important concepts borrowed from dance, psychology, the body-oriented therapies and nonverbal communication research. Case material can be found throughout. It is the hope of the author that this text will provide readers with an in-depth understanding of the dynamic discipline of dance therapy and the power of dance movement to heal. The names and identifying information of all patients discussed throughout this book have been changed to protect their privacy.

Fran J. Levy

Foreword

It's back! Fran Levy's book has been sorely missed. This valuable book, now considered a classic, "the definitive text," has been thoroughly updated and expanded.

Dr. Levy has paid particular attention to detail. She has compiled a very thoughtful, thoroughly researched and comprehensive book. The Introduction traces the avenues in dance, psychology and nonverbal communication that are interwoven and form the basis for our unique profession.

Dr. Levy treats the reader to an all-encompassing view of the field. The first unit gives a historical and chronological description of the profession, a compilation of published and privately circulated literature and personal communications concerning the six major pioneers in the field and their followers and protégés. Levy delineates in rich detail not only the theory and practice of the pioneers, but also what ties this broad and powerful field together—the love of dance and belief in its transformational value. All of the leaders in the field have been dancers and have experienced some epiphany through movement. Levy demonstrates how pioneers used a broad spectrum of psychological theories to affirm what they already intuitively knew regarding the power of dance.

Levy is a strong proponent of the integration of the arts into dance and psychotherapy practice. She has expanded her original chapter on multi-modal work, adding extensive and vivid case examples.

Levy has also greatly expanded the patient populations section to include new groups such as eating disorders, physical and sexual abuse, multiple personality disorder/dissociate identity disorder, rehabilitation (contributed by Cathy Appel) and dance movement therapy in corporations. These sections include rich case material, which demonstrate the depth and breadth of dance therapy today.

Another new section on the international growth of dance therapy and its leaders is thought provoking and sensitively written by Cathy Appel. The fact that dance therapy continues to spread around the world, even during this very tense time, attests to the universal nature of dance and the commonality of movement expression.

The power of dance therapy is in the here and now experience of the body in motion and it is difficult to capture in words. Marian Chace called this "basic dance." Sharon Chaiklin states, "Basic dance is the externalization of those inner feelings which cannot be expressed in rational speech but can only be shared in rhythmic and symbolic action" (1993, p. 257). Basic dance is not to be confused with dance as entertainment, but is dance as communication and self-expression. This basic dance makes research extremely challenging, but necessary. Research into the efficacy of dance movement therapy is beginning to emerge (*Chapter 27*).

I strongly support Levy's emphasis on the importance of simplifying language to describe the work that dance therapists do. One of the major contributions of this book is her careful distillation and delineation of complex material.

Invaluable to all in the profession is the re-emergence of original work, currently out of print and even forgotten. *Dance Movement Therapy* will serve all levels of practitioners, students and academics, as well as those in the performing arts.

Finally, Levy thoughtfully and optimistically speculates at the end of the book on the power of movement to heal both individual and world problems. She recognizes that this is a dream, but "a dream worth contemplating."

Elissa Queyquep White, ADTR, CMA
President and Charter Member of the American Dance Therapy Association
Founder, First Masters Degree Program in Dance Therapy, Hunter College

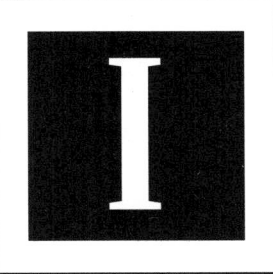ntroduction

The Shoulders on Which We Stand

Dance therapy, the use of dance movement as a psychotherapeutic or healing tool, is rooted in the idea that the body and the mind are inseparable. Its basic premise is that body movement reflects inner emotional states and that changes in movement behavior can lead to changes in the psyche, thus promoting health and growth. Helping individuals—those who are generally healthy, as well as those with mental illnesses and physical or mental disabilities—to regain a sense of wholeness by experiencing the fundamental unity of body, mind and spirit is the ultimate goal of dance movement therapy.

The use of body movement, particularly dance, as a cathartic and therapeutic tool is perhaps as old as dance itself. In many primitive societies, dance was as essential as eating and sleeping. It provided a means of expression, to communicate feelings to others and to commune with nature. Dance rituals frequently accompanied major life changes, thus serving to promote personal integration as well as the fundamental integration of the individual with society.

> The dance of medicine man, priest or shaman belongs to the oldest form of medicine and psychotherapy in which the common exaltation and release of tensions was able to change man's physical and mental suffering into a new option on health. We may say that at the dawn of civilization dancing, religion, music and medicine were inseparable. (Meerloo, 1960, pp. 24-25)

In contrast, the complexity and stress of modern living have led many people to feel alienated, out of touch with themselves, with others and with nature. Much of the turn-of-the-century Western thought subscribed to the credo of dualism, or the distinct separation of body and mind. Formal dance developed as a performing art, emphasizing technique, with little attention to how it affected the dancer. Medicine and psychotherapy became treatment, with the former focusing on the body and the latter on the mind. Psychotherapeutic treatment approaches were almost entirely verbal and not active.

During the first half of the 20th century, a trend began within many fields to break away from the limitations of these traditions. The modern dance movement sought to replace rigid and impersonal art forms with more natural, expressive movements emphasizing spontaneity and creativity. In the area of psychotherapy, there was a growing interest in the nonverbal and expressive aspects of personality. Out of this changing intellectual climate, dance therapy emerged in the 1940s and 1950s.

The Modern Dance Movement and Dance Therapy

Dance therapy can trace its earliest roots to modern dance in the early 1900s. Almost all of the major dance therapy pioneers began their careers as accomplished modern dancers. It was their experiences as performers and teachers that led them to realize the potential benefits of using dance and movement as a form of psychotherapy.

The modern dance movement was a reaction to the social and intellectual climate, as well as a rebellion against the established forms of the art. In politics, the arts and society at large, there was a movement afoot to liberate the person in order to examine the full range of human behavior and the motivation behind it.

In early 20th-century America, two types of dance were generally, though not exclusively, performed—ballet (in limited quantity) and show dancing. The most prevalent form was the latter—what Ted Shawn described as "chorus girls kicking sixteen to the right, sixteen to the left, turning a cartwheel and kicking the back of their heads" (Mazo, 1977, p. 18). Show dance, while popular, lacked content and was not considered a serious art form. Ballet, although recognized as art, had deteriorated, some believed, into empty technical display by the late 19th century.

The stage was set for the birth of a new art form, one that would help audiences organize and integrate their current experience. It was no accident that modern dance pioneers turned for inspiration to classical Greek theater, which had been designed for audiences to experience emotional catharsis (Mazo, 1977).

It was not enough, however, to simply add emotional content to the movement, but to connect the personal expression of the dancer to more universal insight about the human condition. It is the universality that holds the audience and makes an artwork meaningful rather than self-involved.

> Even if we are ... merely the spectators of the dance, we are still ... feeling ourselves in the dancer who is manifesting and expressing the latent impulses of our own being. (Ellis, in Steinberg, 1980, p. 254)

The early pioneers of modern dance turned inward as they sought new forms of creative self-expression that communicated not only their own personal experience and inner emotional content, but also universal themes.

> Modern dance replaced the fading content of Western dance with certain key notions: spontaneity, authenticity of individual expression, awareness of the body, themes that stressed a whole range of feelings and relationships. The great pioneers of its early years personified themes of human conflict, despair, frustration and social crisis. Frequently the choreography of the modern dancer crystallized into the age-old form of ritual. Such key innovations led directly to the essence of dance therapy. (Bartenieff, 1975, p. 246)

The revolution in dance was not an isolated event, but rather part of and consistent with revolutionary changes taking place in the overall intellectual climate of the late 19th and early 20th centuries. This was a time when new ideas and innovations were spilling over from various fields into others, creating a general environment of mutual influence, support and inspiration.

One innovator who had significant impact on the modern dance movement and on dance therapy was Francois Delsarte (1811-1871), "... a quite extraordinary and fascinating Frenchman ... who lurked behind quite a great deal of modern dance" (Fonteyn, 1979, p. 102). Delsarte had begun his career as an opera singer but lost his voice. He then devoted himself to researching and organizing a system of naturally expressive gestures for actors and singers to replace the superficial gestures and postures that dominated the theater during this period. His study of natural human movement led him to observe people in various walks of life doing everyday things. From his observations, Delsarte formulated laws he believed governed people's unconscious, expressive movement and employed these laws to interpret behavior. His work profoundly influenced his former profession, opera, as well as dancers and other performing artists.

Among the dancers who were influenced by Delsarte was Isadora Duncan (1878-1927). Building upon Delsarte's work, Duncan turned to the expressive gestures used in ancient Greek theater to build a new dance vocabulary. Isadora Duncan is referred to by some as the original pioneer of modern dance in the United States. According to Claire Schmais, a major dance therapy leader, it was Duncan who

> ... was the first to break away from the stultifying structure of classical ballet and champion dance as the emanation of emotions in harmony with external forces of the natural world. She saw dance as man's most fundamental response to the universe; reviving man's capacity to dance was the means through which his ability to live fully and freely could be renewed. (Schmais, 1974, pp. 7-8)

The work of Sir James George Frazer in the field of anthropology also had a major impact on the modern dance movement. The publication in 1890 of his book *Golden Bough*, which examined the role of ritual dance in primitive cultures, created an anthropological revolution that added more fuel to the dance revolution and hence to the emergence of dance therapy. Primitive ritual became a source of inspiration for modern dance, as the older concept of dance as an expression of magic, religion and spirituality was revived.

Chief among dancers who explored this spirituality was Ruth St. Denis. St. Denis, an American performer, looked to Eastern cultures for the spiritual ideas she could not find in the United States. Eastern dance styles provided her with themes, costumes and characters through which to structure and objectify her personal search. St. Denis, along with Ted Shawn, formed the Denishawn School of Dance that promulgated the developing concepts and techniques of modern dance. Many future stars began at Denishawn, including Martha Graham, Doris Humphrey and Charles Weidman. Moreover, Marian Chace, the major pioneering dance therapist in the United States, was a Denishawn disciple.

During the same time that modern dance was emerging in the United States, a similar dance revolution was fermenting in Europe. Led by Mary Wigman (1886-1973), the revolution centered in Germany. Perhaps driven by the need to give form through movement to the events of the time, Wigman pioneered a dance style that was strong, direct and austere in its communication with the audience. Margot Fonteyn (1979) describes Wigman's performances as "intense, concentrated, bare presentations, so pared down to the pure essence of personal expression that they appealed only to a very serious and dedicated audience" (p. 110). Among this "serious and dedicated audience" were several of the original dance therapy pioneers: Mary Whitehouse, Franziska Boas and Liljan Espenak in particular, as well as Trudi Schoop, Elizabeth Polk and later, Irmgard Bartenieff and Rhoda Winter Russell.

John Martin (1972), movement critic, historian and author of *The Modern Dance* (1933), says the following about Wigman:

> At its highest point of development we find the so-called expressionistic dancing with Mary Wigman as an outstanding practitioner. This class of dance is in effect the modern dance in its purist manifestation. The basis of each composition ... lies in a vision of something in human experience which touches the sublime. Its externalization ... comes not by intellectual planning but by feeling through with a sensitive body. The ... result ... is the appearance of entirely authentic movements which are as closely allied to the emotional experience as an instinctive recoil is to an experience of fear. (pp. 56-60)

This picture of Wigman's dance as authentic movement in its purest form was picked up on by Mary Whitehouse and has become the insignia for a large portion of dance therapy on the west coast. This concept, as Martin points out, was the essence of the entire modern dance movement spawned by Wigman in the early 1900s and carried to its therapeutic potential in the discipline of dance therapy.

Mary Wigman was a colleague and student of the movement philosopher Rudolf Laban. Laban's contribution was both theoretical and analytical, offering structure and analysis of movement in an unstylized teaching technique. Wigman also studied eurythmics (i.e., the representation of musical rhythms in movement) with Swiss musician Emile Jaques-Dalcroze and was, like Duncan, a student of Delsarte. She incorporated these progressive teachings, all of which had in common natural expressive movement and created her own style of teaching dance. Its major requirement was that the student finds his or her own unique style, once given the elements of dance upon which to build. That is, Wigman's movement medium was expressive/improvisational. Her technique provided a strong foundation for exploring human emotion, both personal and universal.

In the 1920s, Wigman's counterpart in improvisational and expressive movement in America was Bird Larson. Larson's major contributions to modern dance are not well known today due to her premature death in the 1930s. However, she profoundly influenced those who studied with her (see Evan, *Chapter 2* and Boas, *Chapter 8*). Early on at Barnard College and Columbia Teachers College in New York she referred to her work as "Natural Dance" and later, when she opened her own studio, it was called the "Larson School of Natural Rhythmic Expression." Her improvisational work was closely related to that of Wigman. Moreover, after hearing about Wigman in the late 1920s, Larson decided to visit her school in Germany. From this visit Larson brought back Wigman's use of percussion instruments as a facilitator for her already developed natural rhythmic dance techniques. The similarities between the improvisational dance technique of Wigman and those of Larson are especially significant in light of the fact that each left a profound and lasting impression on major dance therapy pioneers. The expressive opportunities which both Larson and Wigman afforded their students in the 1920s can be viewed as some of the earliest forms of dance therapy in the 20th century.

Dance therapists and modern dancers have sometimes referred to this focus on individual self-expression and exploration as contacting one's "inner dance." Encouraging the development of the inner dance was likened by many to encouraging the uncovering of the unconscious through body movement.

The overall intellectual climate of this early period revolved around the acceptance of the unconscious in

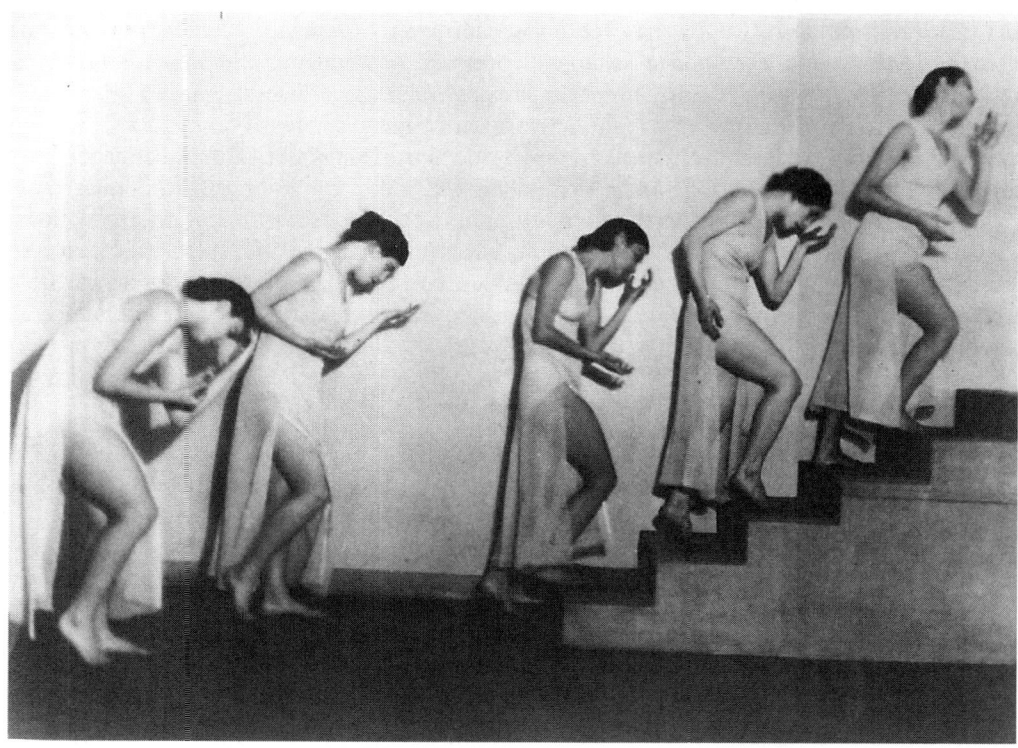

Bird Larson's students in performance (Photo courtesy Jerome Robbins Dance Division, The New York Public Library for the Performing Arts)

man as a potent source for deepening self-realization and reflection. The revolutionary work of Sigmund Freud in psychology, first introduced in the late 19th century, made a great impact on modern dance and dance therapy. Freud's work prompted an examination of the motivation behind human action, in contrast to the 19th century attitude that intense emotions were to be concealed. The innovative belief in the open expression of feeling gave dance both fresh subject matter and structure.

By the 1930s and 1940s, at about the same time psychoanalytic thought (the work of Freud, Adler, Jung and others) was gaining wider acceptance, the concept of the inner dance was becoming popular among modern dancers. While psychoanalysts were encouraging the expression of the unconscious through verbalization, dancers began to use body movement as the vehicle for similar forms of expression.

The writings of the early modern dancers in America clearly reveal the deep attention paid to the unconscious and the dream self. Some, like Martha Graham, attended to thoughts, feelings and insights from the unconscious and included these in their teachings and choreography. Others, like Mary Whitehouse and Marian Chace, were so moved by the interaction of psyche and soma through dance movement that they left the performance and choreography aspects of dance and focused exclusively on the psychotherapeutic aspect of dance. The environment was ripe for the translation of self-expression into psychotherapy through dance.

When dance therapy began in the 1940s, its practice was limited primarily to the back wards of mental hospitals. By the 1950s, another branch of dance therapy was beginning to emerge. As a result of the natural integration of dance with self-expression, some former dance performers and educators found themselves practicing dance therapy in their private studios. A few of these private practitioners began functioning as primary therapists utilizing dance therapy with what they termed as normal and neurotic individuals.

The dance therapy pioneers brought with them from their earlier modern dance experience a nonjudgmental attitude toward individual movement preferences, stressing the development of one's own expressive style and an emphasis on personal expression through uninterrupted improvisation. This legacy from the modern dance movement formed the foundation upon which each pioneer built her dance therapy practice in accordance with the needs of the population she treated and the setting in which she worked. By the end of the 1950s, dance therapy was already utilizing a broad spectrum of intervention styles. In addition, the rudiments of dance therapy theory began to emerge during this period.

As the dance therapy pioneers continued to explore the power of dance movement as a form of psychotherapy, they began to seek further understanding of the nature of personality and the effects that dance had on personality. This led them to investigate existing theoretical frameworks, particularly in the field of psychology, which gave expression to their own intuitive knowledge and supported their dance therapy practice. Thus, the discipline of dance therapy evolved in the 1940s and 1950s out of the merger of the modern dance movement with existing theories of group and individual psychology and psychotherapy.

Influences on Dance Therapy from Other Fields

The overall focus in the field of psychology during the first half of the century was on the use of verbalization as a medium for the expression of the unconscious. Nonverbal treatment approaches, including dance therapy, were not yet generally accepted. Nevertheless, included in the overall work of many psychological theorists and clinicians during this period were concepts and techniques that helped to lay the foundation for the later development and recognition of nonverbal treatment approaches. The following is a brief

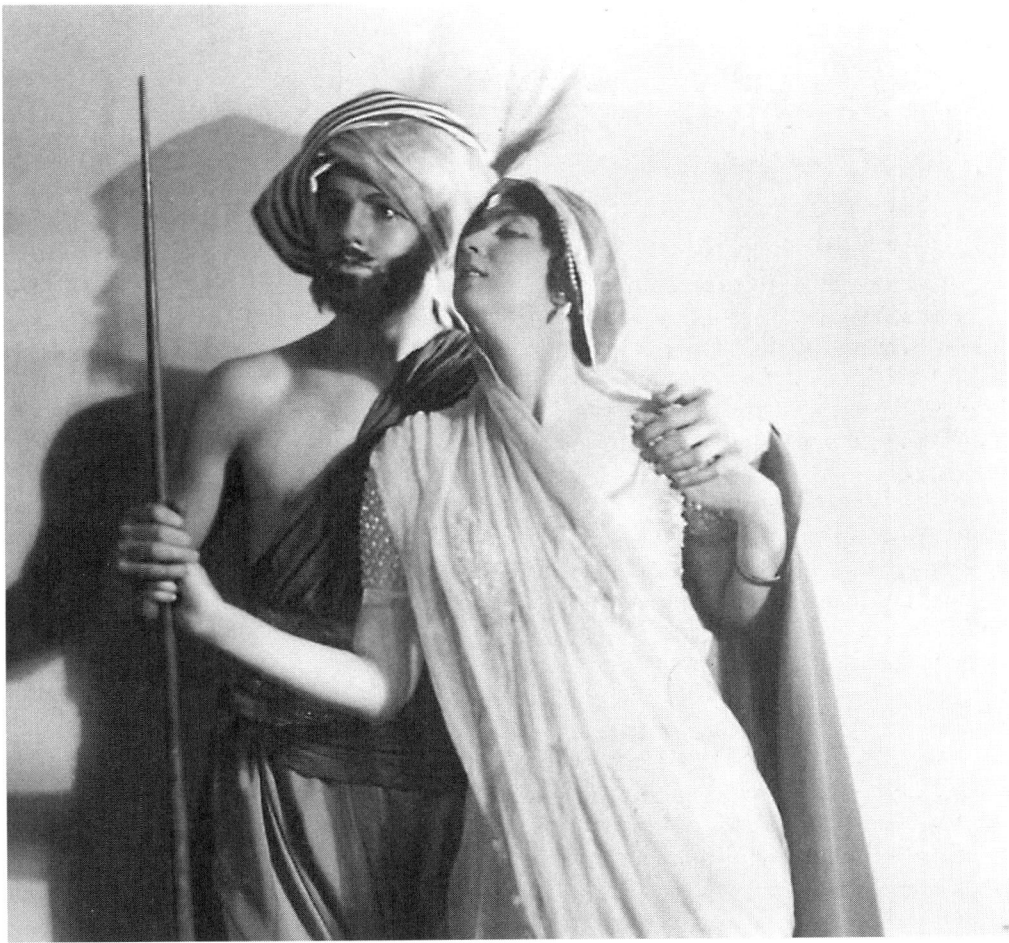

Ted Shawn and Ruth St. Denis, 1920's (Photo courtesy Jerome Robbins Dance Division, The New York Public Library for the Performing Arts)

review of the major theoretical frameworks that influenced the work of the dance therapy pioneers and that continue to have an impact on today's dance therapy.

Although Freud did not stress nonverbal expression as a treatment method, he did recognize the connection between the body and emotions, as well as the relationship between psychoanalytic thought and nonverbal communication:

> He that has eyes to see and ears to hear may convince himself that no mortal can keep a secret. If the lips are silent, he chatters with his fingertips; betrayal oozes out of him at every pore. And thus the task of making conscious the most hidden recesses of the mind is one which is quite possible to accomplish. (Freud, 1905, pp. 77-78)

In addition, Freud believed that conflict, with its resulting mechanisms of defense and repression, is the responsibility of the ego, which is "... first and foremost a body-ego" (Freud, 1923, p. 31).

Wilhelm Reich, an Austrian psychiatrist and psychoanalyst, was one of the first clinicians with a nonverbal orientation. In the 1920s, he began intensive studies of his patients' psychosomatic expressions in an effort to clarify the connections between the somatic and psychic realms. Reich discovered that while some patients were capable of verbalizing thoughts and feelings, others developed defenses or "armor," which were rooted in the body in the form of muscular tension. "Every increase of muscular tonus in the direction of rigidity indicates that a vegetative excitation, anxiety or sexuality, has become bound up...." (Reich, 1949, p. 342)

Reich introduced the use of muscular manipulation to overcome armoring and thus facilitate the release of repressed psychological material. His use of the body in therapy was controversial at that time, but was later popularized by Alexander Lowen in the 1960s.

Carl Jung's theory of active imagination brought attention to the therapeutic value of the creative act. He believed that fantasies and feelings from the primitive unconscious could be evoked and symbolically manifested in artistic experiences. This concept supports the work of dance therapists, who use dance movement—particularly the creative act of dance movement improvisation—to help individuals express the unconscious. Mary Whitehouse, a major pioneering dance therapist who integrated Jungian concepts into her work, ushered in the branch of dance therapy often referred to as "movement-in-depth—a Jungian approach to dance therapy."

The work of American psychiatrist Harry Stack Sullivan has also been significant for dance therapists. His interpersonal theory of personality evolved from the need to understand pathology within its cultural and interactional context. He believed that individuals develop personality characteristics and a sense of self through their interactions with their surroundings and through their perceptions of those interactions.

Sullivan (1962) is also known for developing a therapeutic methodology for people with schizophrenia that focused on accepting them at their own developmental level and interacting with them at this level. Most of all, he accepted them as equal human beings who could benefit from genuine communication with others. Sullivan's influence on dance therapy can be seen in the work of Marian Chace, who viewed dance therapy as a vehicle for direct communication with patients. Through the "therapeutic movement relationship" she was able to engage severely withdrawn psychotic patients in verbal and nonverbal interactions. It was this form of heightened communication and interaction that Chace excelled in and taught to her dance therapy disciples.

Alfred Adler's chief contribution to psychology was his belief that the aggressive drive is as important an influence on feelings, thoughts and behavior as the libidinal drive. He emphasized that children and adults need to feel a sense of strength, competence and mastery of their environment if they are to become an integral part of society and to master inherent childhood feelings of inferiority. Blanche Evan and Liljan Espenak, two major dance therapy pioneers, believed that Adler's work supported the use of body movement in treatment. Individuals who could learn to use their bodies in assertive, confident and competent ways, expressing feelings of independence and autonomy, would be able to more easily express such self-reliant behaviors and attitudes in other aspects of their lives.

Paul Schilder's (1950) important study of the body image examined the relationship between movement and the impressions of the senses within a psychoanalytic framework. He believed that the mental image or topography of the postural model of the body, which is instantly being constructed and destroyed, forms the basis of emotional attitudes toward the body. According to Schilder, all movement activities serve to build a stronger body image.

> There is so close an interrelation between the muscular sequence and the psychic attitude that not only does the psychic sequence connect up with the muscular states, but also every sequence of tensions and relaxations provokes a specific attitude. When there is a specific motor sequence it changes the inner situation and attitudes and even provokes a phantasy situation which fits the muscular sequence. (Schilder, 1950, p. 208)

Schilder was part of a group of clinicians and researchers who were experimenting with verbal and nonverbal uses of projective methods at Bellevue Hospital in the 1940s. Members of the group included Lauretta Bender in psychology, Franziska Boas in dance therapy, Margaret Naumberg in art therapy and Adolf Wollman in puppetry. Other pioneers in this area included Sidney Levy, Karen Machover, Henry Murray and Bruno Klopfer. Levy worked at Northport Hospital, Long Island and at the Veteran's Administration Mental Hygiene Service in New York. Specializing in the symbolism of animal drawings, Levy

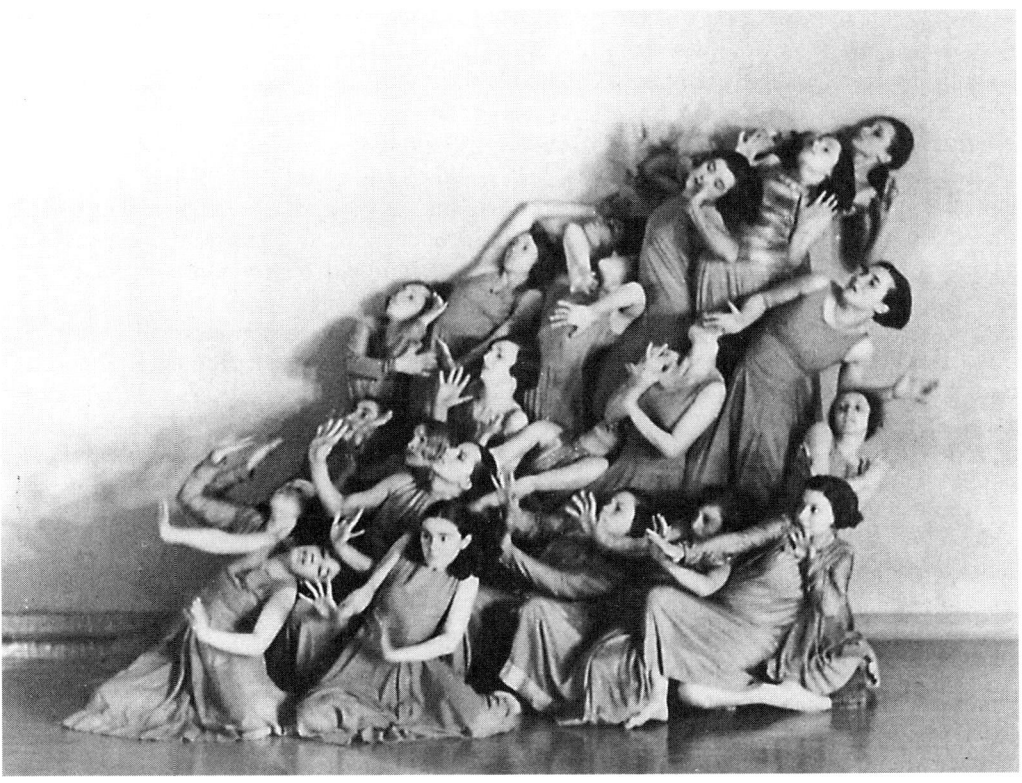

A movement choir directed by Mary Wigman, 1920's (Photo courtesy Jerome Robbins Dance Division, The New York Public Library for the Performing Arts)

taught projective technique in New York University's clinical psychology program from the 1940s through the 1960s. At Kings County Hospital, Machover specialized in figure drawing as a projective technique. Murray developed the Thematic Apperception Test in his work at Harvard University. Klopfer, known as the "Father of the Rorschach," wrote the first textbook in America on the Rorschach test. The kind of courses being taught and the ideas being explored at that time are typified in the title of one of Sidney Levy's courses at New York University: "The meaning of animals as symbols in dreams and drawing, literature and legend, ritual and religion, art and projective techniques."

The projective technique, a creative and exploratory style of intervention, was an integral part of the creative dance movement (a branch of modern dance) and was commonly used by the pioneering dance therapists to facilitate expression and insight. For the dance therapist, the projective method is a natural extension of the dance experience.[1]

In addition to existing psychological theories and techniques that influenced and encouraged the early development of dance therapy, there were other sources of support as well. Research concerning the nature of nonverbal communication and the relationship between the body and the mind added validity to the use of dance movement as a psychotherapeutic tool.

The first comprehensive study of nonverbal behavior, unparalleled in its human and animal insights, was Charles Darwin's *The Expression of the Emotions in Man and Animals* (1872), which defined the evolutionary aspects of facial and body expression. This inquiry into form, significance and action patterns led Darwin to postulate that expressive behavior, like physical structures, had survival value for the species. His research revealed that body movements not only had biological significance, as previously believed, but also had a correspondence with emotional expression.

Some researchers in the field of psychology further explored the link between the mind and the body. Their research focused mainly on gesture and posture and their associated emotional content.[2]

Despite this early interest and research in nonverbal communication, treatment that stressed nonverbal approaches did not gain wide acceptance until the 1960s and 1970s. This change in attitude came about gradually, perhaps due in part to the loosening of post-World War II societal restrictions, the continuing growth of modern dance and psychoanalytic thought and the dissemination of Eastern philosophies emphasizing the unity of body and mind. In addition, after a long hiatus, there was a new wave of interest in the nonverbal domain in the 1960s and 1970s, bringing attention back to earlier research in the area and inspiring new research.

The flourishing of nonverbal communication research during this period benefited dance therapy significantly. It brought new recognition to the importance of body movement in psychotherapy. It also provided a recognized methodology and terminology for researching and observing the meaning of movement behavior and the interconnection between movement and emotional expression.

Ray Birdwhistell (1952, 1970), an anthropologist and renowned nonverbal communication researcher, is credited with establishing a new discipline, kinesics, which is the study of structural units of movement in relation to social processes. His work spawned a new wave of scientific and therapeutic research that studied movement within a cultural context, linking movement patterns to speech patterns and interactional systems.

Albert Scheflin (1963, 1973), a psychiatrist, related the study of kinesic units to psychotherapy research. Using a communications model similar to Birdwhistell's, including both verbal and nonverbal components, Scheflin analyzed the variety and complexity of body movements that take place in a therapeutic session.

The work of William Condon and his associates (1963, 1964, 1966, 1967a, 1967b, 1968, 1969, 1974) focused on interactional synchrony and self-synchrony, detailing the order and rhythm of human behavior. His research has influenced dance therapy among children with autism. Adam Kendon (1970) also researched interactional synchrony and documented the organizational hierarchy of gesture and speech.

It was not uncommon for nonverbal communication researchers to use dance metaphors when describing the rhythmic flow inherent in human interactions. For example, Kendon made the following observation:

> The listener dances with the speaker to show he is with him, receiving him. He then gets the speaker to dance with him as a way of heightening the synchronization [communication and rapport] between them...(Costonis, 1978, p. 23)

Complementing the resurgence of nonverbal communication studies in the 1960s and 1970s was the flourishing of different, more experimental forms of therapeutic treatment. Among these were the hu-

---

[1] The projective method "seeks to gain information indirectly through the use of ... techniques ... designed to provide oppportunity for self-expression without verbal accounting" (Campbell, 1981, pp. 386-387). These techniques are purposely unstructured and often evocative. The individual is encouraged to express the complexities of his own personality through various idioms.
[2] See, for example, Ferenczi (1916), Deutsch (1922, 1947, 1951, 1952), Fenichel (1928, 1934), Krout (1931, 1937) and Malmo et al. (1950, 1951, 1956, 1957).

manistic psychological approaches, the action-oriented psychotherapies (e.g., dance therapy) and the body therapies, all of which have had varying degrees of theoretical and practical influence on dance therapy.[3]

The humanistic movement spearheaded by Carl Rogers (1951, 1961) and Abraham Maslow (1962, 1970) took a nonanalytical, nonjudgmental and antidiagnostic approach to personality and posed questions that transcended the traditional stress on psychological adaptation. Rogers and Maslow inquired into the processes that motivate people to aspire, excel, create and fulfill human potential. Their major contribution is an emphasis on the uniqueness of the individual and on methods of releasing creative and expressive potential. In essence, this so-called "third-force" in psychology seeks out the healthy aspects of the personality rather than pathology and weakness and in so doing opens the doors of expression to many different idioms—dance, drama, music, art and so on. Alma Hawkins, a major dance therapy pioneer, is among those dance therapists who have incorporated humanistic theory into their work.

Another form of psychotherapy that has achieved prominence during this time is the action-oriented psychotherapies. These include the creative arts therapies (dance, drama, music, art, poetry, etc.), psychodrama, gestalt therapy, psychomotor therapy and bioenergetic therapy.

The action-oriented psychotherapists acknowledge that thoughts and feelings are expressed and processed on many levels and that not everyone can benefit from formal psychoanalytic or strictly verbal methods. Therefore, they provide a milieu in which the individual is able to explore emotions through a combination of verbal and psychomotor methods (F. Levy, 1995).

One of the goals of the action-oriented psychotherapies is to integrate the body and the mind through the use of action techniques and projective psychological methods. One concept that unites these therapies is the belief that involving the body in the therapeutic process evokes unconscious psychological material and deeply held emotions. The action-oriented psychotherapist then structures the newly released material via drama, dance, art and/or writing to bring about deeper psychophysical awareness, catharsis and possibly insight.

One of the earliest of the action-oriented psychotherapies was psychodrama, developed by J. L. Moreno. Working within a group therapy structure, Moreno utilized the group process and group interaction to create and guide dramatic dialogues centered on the verbal and nonverbal acting out of feelings on the psychodramatic stage. He emphasized the use of therapeutic role-playing and role reversal, techniques which he originated.[4]

Some of the acting-out and role-playing techniques of psychodrama were incorporated into the work of Frederick S. Perls (1947, 1971, 1972), the founder of Gestalt therapy, and Albert Pesso (1969, 1973), who developed his own form of psychomotor therapy. Perls, in contrast to Moreno, placed more emphasis on the individual within the group than on the group's interaction. In addition to role-playing techniques, Perls also used other methods such as visualization, imagery and attending silently to the body. In contrast, one of Pesso's contributions was his utilization of the rhythmic expression of emotions within structured dramatic formats. As a former dancer, he understood the power of rhythmic activity and movement expression.

Alexander Lowen (1967, 1975) founder of bioenergetic therapy and disciple of Wilhelm Reich, differed from the other action-oriented psychotherapists in that he placed less stress on artistic structure (e.g., complex dramatic enactments and sublimation through shape and form) and instead emphasized the use of specific physical exercises based on Reich's theories. These exercises, he believed, released emotions and thus facilitated more meaningful verbalization.

Dance therapists incorporate some of the same techniques and theories as the action-oriented psychotherapists described above. What differentiates dance therapy is its emphasis on the use of the dance move-

---

[3]While some of these first emerged at this time, not all were new. Like dance therapy, some had developed earlier but did not gain popularity and acceptance until this period.

[4]It is interesting to note that Moreno brought psychodrama to St. Elizabeth's Hospital in the 1940s, at the same time that Marian Chace began her pioneering work there as a dance therapist. Though it is not known whether they worked together or influenced each other, there were remarkable similarities between these two pioneers. Each broke away from traditional, purely verbal treatment approaches and gave birth to a new approach to treatment. Each utilized the performing arts, incorporating body movement, verbalization and interaction, to deepen self-awareness and self-realization. Chace and Moreno were both uniquely gifted in their ability to conduct group therapy, using the group's dynamics to enhance and integrate the individual's experience of self.

form, integrated with verbalization, as the primary expressive modality. More specifically, some dance therapists see the attributes and dynamics of dance and movement as uniquely suited for the expression of the unconscious along with id, ego and superego expression, in addition to providing a framework for relationship building and body image and personality development.

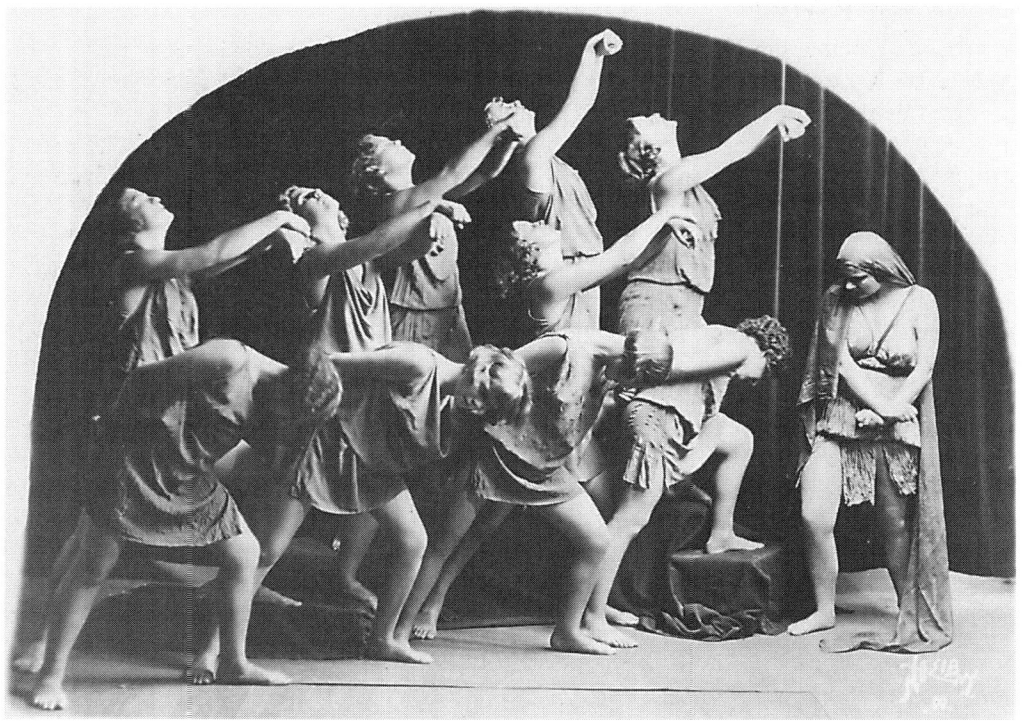

Isadora Duncan, her dancers (Photo courtesy Jerome Robbins Dance Division, The New York Public Library for the Performing Arts)

The various body therapies that have become popular since the 1960s also utilize methodologies, which overlap with dance therapy technique. The title "body therapy" encompasses various forms of movement work aimed at achieving efficient physical functioning on a muscular and skeletal level. Muscular balance and skeletal alignment together provide the individual with a greater ability to relax and to use body energy with increased flexibility, awareness and satisfaction.

The body therapies utilize methodologies of postural restructuring such as those developed by F. Mathias Alexander (The Alexander Technique) and Moishe Feldenkrais (1972, 1973), which stress self-awareness during movement and those developed by Mabel Todd (1937, 1953) and Lulu Sweigard (1974), which emphasize the use of imagery and visualization. Relaxation methods, such as those originated by Edmund Jacobson (1929) and techniques of deep muscular massage, such as those originated by Ida P. Rolf (n.d.), focus on the release of psychophysical tensions in the musculature.

At various times these techniques have been incorporated into dance therapy theory and practice. Unlike dance therapists, however, body therapists take more of a teaching or directive role. Generally, they do not focus on or develop the psychological or artistic aspects of expressive movement.

The flourishing of the various body therapies, action oriented psychotherapies and humanistic psychological approaches made available to individuals many different forms of therapeutic treatment. Their popularity, along with the new wave of nonverbal communication research during this period, added to the growing acceptance within the mental health community of action oriented and creative treatment approaches. This growing acceptance, however, was not in itself enough to bring dance therapy into the full light of professional recognition; it was up to dance therapists themselves to achieve this. Finally, while dance therapy borrows from, adds to and synthesizes many aspects of the theories and practices described above, it is distinguished by its dedication to using the elements of dance for safe personal expression and communication.

The Professional and Institutional Development of Dance Therapy

As dance therapy entered the 1960s, it was still being viewed as a unique skill possessed by a few rare and gifted individuals rather than as an established profession. Although the dance therapy pioneers had made many inroads into the field of mental health and had built a solid foundation of dance therapy practice, they were, for the most part, functioning more as individuals than as members of a professional community. Having moved gradually and naturally from dance into dance therapy, many still thought of themselves as dance teachers and some were unaware of the existence of the many others who were doing work similar to their own.

While there was some dance therapy literature during this early period, the actual articulation of theoretical concepts was still sparse and was more often spread through verbal exchanges with these pioneers rather than through their writings. Little work had been done in the area of empirical studies and in the establishment of a theoretical framework, which would serve to integrate the various aspects of practice.

Furthermore, there were no standardized requirements for the professional training of dance therapists and only limited training opportunities. Since academic institutions did not yet offer programs in dance therapy, students sought training through private apprenticeships with established dance therapists. In the late 1950s, independent training programs were offered by Marian Chace and Blanche Evan in New York and Trudi Schoop and Mary Whitehouse in California. Stark (1980), referring to the training offered by Chace, Whitehouse and Schoop, stated:

> Early training focused on the clinical application of dance therapy technique with little attention to the underlying principles or theories. In order to supplement their training, many students took courses in the social and behavioral sciences or enrolled in graduate programs ... in the field of human behavior. (p. 14)

Professional training through private apprenticeships continued in the 1960s. Schoop and Whitehouse continued their work in California and in New York; Evan, Chace, Espenak, Bartenieff and Rosen offered independent training programs.

During the 1960s, as various action oriented treatment approaches, including dance therapy, were becoming more widely accepted, dance therapists came to realize the need to professionalize the field. With the establishment in 1966 of the American Dance Therapy Association, dance therapy took its first steps toward becoming a recognized and organized profession.

At its inception, the ADTA was headed by Marian Chace and had 73 charter members. In that year, a committee of the ADTA formalized the definition of dance therapy: "the planned use of any aspect of dance to aid in the physical and psychic integration of the individual" (ADTA, 1966). This was later revised to read: "Dance therapy is the psychotherapeutic use of movement as a process which furthers the emotional, physical and cognitive integration of the individual." This change in definition reflects the change that the image of dance therapy had undergone since its early development in the 1940s. By the 1970s, more dance therapists were viewing their work as the equivalent of traditional verbal psychotherapy, differentiated only by the fact that it incorporated dance and movement techniques along with verbalization.

In the late 1960s, professional training emerged through the establishment of undergraduate level courses in dance therapy at various universities and colleges. In addition to providing new training opportunities for dance therapists, this had the effect of educating the public as to the presence and function of dance therapy. However, it also further diffused standards of professional training and exacerbated the need to organize and synthesize a curriculum of theory and practice that could be passed on to the following generations of dance therapists.

In the 1970s, graduate level courses in dance therapy began to emerge. Individuals could earn a Master's degree in dance therapy by organizing their own independent study programs at several universities and colleges. During this time, formal Master's programs in dance therapy also began to appear. The first, offered at Hunter College in 1971, was founded by Claire Schmais, Elissa White and Martha Davis and was funded by a grant from the National Institute of Mental Health.

The fact that graduate degree programs did not emerge until the early 1970s reflects the wide gap that separated the clinical practice of dance therapy, which had grown rapidly since the 1940s and the theoretical development of the field, which had lagged behind. In 1974, Sharon Chaiklin, a former president of ADTA, wrote:

> Dance and movement therapy is still building its theoretical foundations. There is, however, enough knowledge to demonstrate that there now exists that specialized base which a profession requires. The development of a high quality curriculum is presently an urgent need of the dance therapy profession. (1974, p. 63)

The ADTA has encouraged the development of such a curriculum through its efforts to establish standards in graduate education programs in dance therapy. In 1973, the board appointed Claire Schmais to the Ad Hoc Committee on Approval, which was responsible for establishing "Guidelines for Graduate Dance Therapy Programs" (Stark, 1980, p. 16). These guidelines were then used to establish standards of curriculum for graduate degree programs.

In addition to academic standards, professional standards of practice were being explored and formalized. In 1970, the first ADTA Registry Committee was established, consisting of three elected members: Elissa White (Chairperson), Susan Sandel and Irmgard Bartenieff. The general purpose of the Registry Committee was: a) to establish criteria for determining levels of professional competence, hence facilitating the hiring of dance therapists; b) to establish the ADTA as a professional organization with professional levels and standards and c) to validate dance therapists' professional identity.

Another area in which dance therapy has significantly expanded its interests, concerns and parameters, especially in the last decade, has been government affairs. The ADTA Government Affairs Committee has closely monitored government legislation and regulations relating to the profession and has initiated many actions and projects in this area.

In the last few decades, the ADTA's Board of Directors, along with committee chairs and regional and chapter leaders, have worked to bring dance therapy to a higher professional, educational and organizational level.[5]

In 2000, the National Board of Certified Counselors (NBCC) and the ADTA announced that the NBCC would recognize dance therapy as a form of counseling. Since 1995, the NBCC and ADTA have worked towards this goal. As part of the process, NBCC representatives reviewed dance therapy graduate programs, registry requirements and procedures, dance therapy research and publications and ADTA documents and records. A comparison of ADTA dance therapy graduate program requirements with the Council for Accreditation of Counseling and Related Educational Programs requirements for counseling programs found dance therapy graduate programs to be similar and comparable to graduate programs in counseling.

Only those dance therapists with Masters of Arts degrees in dance therapy or related mental health disciplines are eligible to sit for the counseling examinations.

The agreement between the NBCC and the ADTA designated the Academy of Dance Therapists Registered (ADTR) credential as the appropriate counseling credential offered by ADTA. This agreement has benefited consumers by making dance therapy treatment more accessible. The opportunity for collaboration between traditional counselors and dance therapists has increased opportunities for joint research, publications and educational opportunities, as well as stimulated dialogue between more conventional treatment modalities and the field of dance therapy.

Susan Eubanks, the associate executive director of the NBCC, remarked positively on the collaboration in the NBCC newsletter, saying that the collaboration would provide an additional avenue for counselors in practice and would unify the profession, as well as maximize the benefits for consumers and clients.

Dance therapists have also begun to seek licensure through legislation at the state level. The purpose of the legislation has been both to protect consumers from untrained people claiming to practice dance movement therapy and to ensure that dance movement therapists can legally practice psychotherapy in

---

[5]Space does not permit a comprehensive description of all the contributions made by the ADTA and its members. Further information about the Association and its activities can be obtained by writing to the ADTA at 2000 Century Plaza, Columbia, Maryland 21044 or accessing their website: www.adta.org.

states that regulate such practice.

In April 2002, New York became the first state in the country to pass legislation to license creative arts therapists using the title "Creative Arts Therapist." This legislation was the culmination of over 20 years of effort on the part of the New York Coalition of Creative Arts Therapies (NYCCAT). NYCCAT was formed to address the issue of licensing, as New York began to look for a way to regulate the practice of psychotherapy. The state legislature wished to create legislation that would cover all professions to be licensed to practice psychotherapy.

NYCCAT had to work hard to educate state legislators about creative arts therapy and to convince them that creative arts therapy should be a part of this legislation. Central to the success of this effort was the work of Joan Wittig. Wittig served over 10 years in the position of liaison from NYCCAT to the Joint Council for Mental Health Services Legislative Coalition, the larger body with whom NYCCAT collaboratively sought licensure. The bill in New York is scheduled to go into effect in 2005.

In the meantime, on November 1, 2002, Wisconsin became the first state in the country to actually complete and enact legislation to license creative arts therapists. Over the past few years as the state took steps to regulate the practice of psychotherapy, creative arts therapists sought to be included in a bill that would otherwise have made it illegal for them to continue to practice. When the bill reached its final version, the legislature included creative arts therapists in the body of the legislation and created a license for creative arts therapists.

A number of other states already allow dance therapists to apply for a license as counselors. In several other states that do not yet recognize creative arts therapy, such as California and Ohio, dance therapists have begun the necessary work that will result in a license.

The professional development of dance therapy has gone hand in hand with a rapid expansion of the field since the 1960s. Dance therapy is being used in medical and mental hospitals, clinics, rehabilitation centers, schools and in private practice. Today's dance therapists function as primary therapists, as ancillary therapists and as family and couples counselors. They serve a wide spectrum of patients of all ages, from individuals with severe emotional and physical problems and handicaps to healthy individuals seeking in-depth self-exploration through expressive movement. In short, dance therapy is moving into countless areas of mental health and even some corporate settings and continues to expand its educational, practical and organizational affiliations.

UNIT I

Early Development: The Pioneers of Dance Movement Therapy

Foundations of the theory and practice of dance therapy were laid in large part by six major pioneers in the United States. Marian Chace, Blanche Evan, Liljan Espenak, Mary Whitehouse, Trudi Schoop and Alma Hawkins developed a broad spectrum of clinical styles that contemporary dance therapists still use today.

This unit includes a comprehensive review of the work of these early pioneers. Section A discusses the work of Chace, Evan and Espenak and the development of their work on the east coast. Section B reviews the west coast pioneers: Whitehouse, Schoop and Hawkins. The geographical delineation is not, however, an arbitrary one; distinct forms of treatment were being developed on each coast in the 1940s and 1950s and these differences have become the content for ongoing discussion and exploration of dance therapy practice and its effects on various populations. Section C discusses the emergence of dance therapy in the Midwest and reviews the literary contributions of Franziska Boas and Elizabeth Rosen. The first comprehensive dance therapy study, completed in 1957, is also discussed in this section. Unit I concludes with an outline depicting the state of the art of dance therapy by 1960, summarizing the breadth of practice initiated by the major pioneers.

SECTION A

Major Pioneers on the East Coast

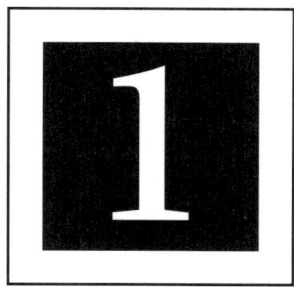 Marian Chace: The "Grande Dame of Dance Therapy"

Marian Chace (1896-1970) is the "Grande Dame" of dance therapy. In addition to her pioneering work with psychiatric patients, Chace made a major contribution through her teaching, serving as mentor to a large number of dance therapists, many of whom were instrumental in establishing the American Dance Therapy Association along with Chace. Many of today's leading dance therapists originally were trained by Chace and continue to espouse her methods. As a result, the Chace influence is still having a tremendous impact on the field (see Dance Therapy Tree and Survey Results).

Chace began her dynamic career as a dancer, choreographer and performer. She studied dance in New York in the 1920s with Ted Shawn and Ruth St. Denis at the Denishawn School of Dance and performed with their company.

> The broad and eclectic approach of ... Denishawn at that time enabled the pupils to find their own way of moving and developed their own abilities as choreographers and teachers as well as performing dancers. One was never taught a particular way of moving without having it related to the folk culture from which it came. The combination of modified ballet forms, contemporary dance, Dalcroze and other technical forms ... were to be developed. (H. Chaiklin, 1975, p. 2)

In 1930, Chace moved to Washington, DC, and began her own Denishawn School, where she continued to teach the ideas and methods she so respected.

Although Chace was originally dedicated primarily to performing, her interest in teaching dance broadened over time. She found that many of the students who came to her were not at all interested in dance as a performing art. They were often awkward and slow in class yet were persistent in their attendance. Chace was at first thwarted by their learning difficulties and puzzled by their enduring interest in the art of dance.

> Out of observing the nonverbal communication of individuals taking their first classes, I began to understand and meet the needs for which they were asking help. Instead of feeling frustration when they lagged behind the more adequate pupils, I tried to empathize with them as people.
>
> Obviously, my teaching was undergoing change. Unconsciously, my centering for all pupils became a support of them as people as well as dancers. While the students at the school found satisfaction in various ways, I think of the whole period of the 1930's for me as one of intense absorption in learning about nonverbal communication. (H. Chaiklin, 1975, pp. 15-16)

In the 1940s, Chace began experimenting with dance therapy, though this formal title was not yet used. She worked as both a therapist and a trainer, teaching her techniques to the staff where she worked, a school for rejected children and later a training school for girls. In 1942, she started working as a volunteer at St. Elizabeth's Hospital in a program then called "dance for communication" (H. Chaiklin, 1975, p. 12). A year later she began work on salary with the Red Cross using dance action with servicemen. Throughout this period, Chace continued in dual roles, as a therapist and as a performer. She was once quoted that, "When I was at the hospital, I felt needed at the studio and when I was at the studio, I felt needed at the hospital" (H. Chaiklin, 1975, p. 13).

Also during this period, Chace experimented with the effects of music on patients. Some called her a "music therapist" as well as a "dance therapist." Perhaps this derived from her Denishawn training, where music was emphasized. St. Denis had developed "music visualization," a process by which the specific qualities of the music were communicated through the movement, as well as the technique in which each dancer represented an instrument of the orchestra and moved when that instrument played.

One can see the Denishawn influence in several other aspects of Chace's work. For example, her background in folk dance steps and structures (such as the circle) was used by Chace to promote social interaction among her patients. In addition, her Denishawn training in production and performance was utilized in "The Hotel St. Elizabeth" (H. Chaiklin, 1975, p. 87), a theater piece written and produced by her patients at the hospital.

The words of Dr. Jay Hoffman, a physician at St. Elizabeth's Hospital, illustrate the power of Chace's work and presence with psychiatric patients.

> As one watches these patients—very sick psychotic patients—and Miss Chace dancing, one gains the impression that through this medium the patients have at last found it possible to step out of their constricted world and quoting one of them, "to reach outward." Their movements seem free, easy, comfortable; they undulate, flow and appear to express in motion or rhythm what they cannot express in words or in conventional social actions. That they can do this is a tribute to the unusual qualities of Miss Chace as a dance therapist but it is also a reminder to us that there are few, if any, really "inaccessible" patients. (H. Chaiklin, 1975, p. 81)

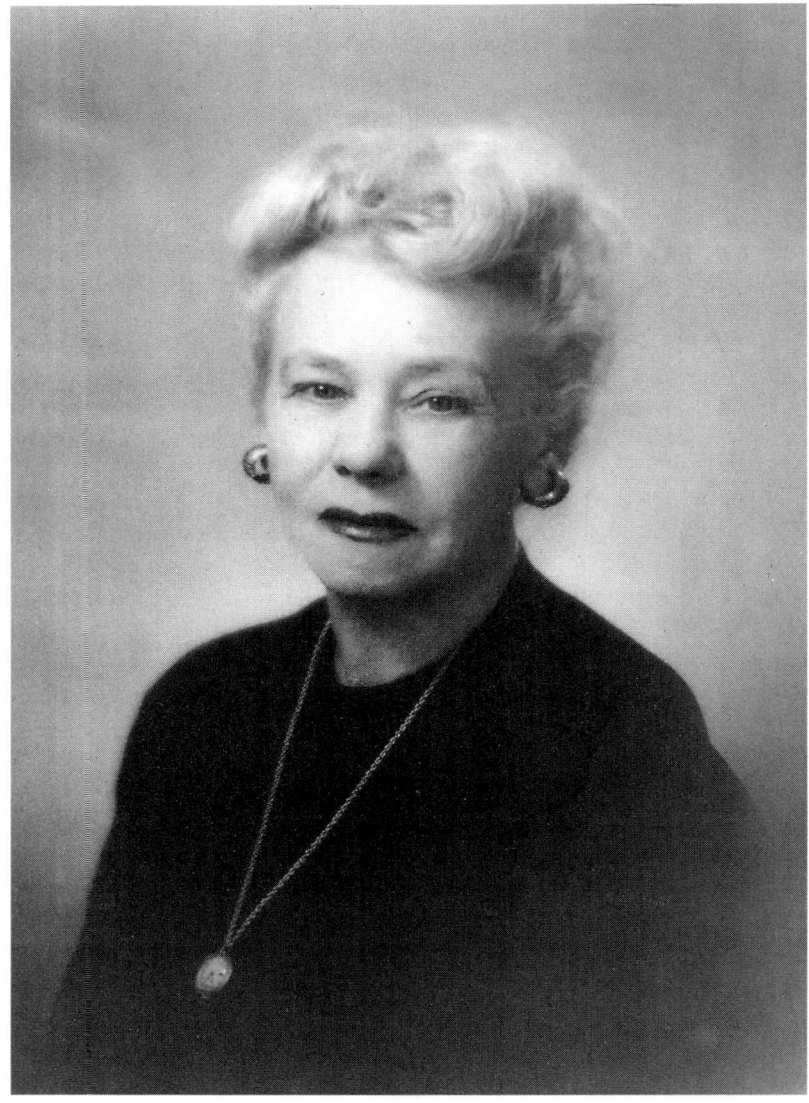

Marian Chace (Photo courtesy the Marian Chace Foundation, American Dance Therapy Association)

In the mid-1940s Chace began giving lectures and demonstrations of her work outside of the hospital. At one psychiatric facility, Chestnut Lodge, her presentation was so well received that she was hired to work there in 1946 and remained there for approximately 25 years. In the early 1960s, Chace started commuting to New York where she founded a landmark training program for dance therapists at the Turtle Bay Music School. Shortly afterward, she began spreading her ideas and methods in Israel in what proved to be a successful attempt at bringing her teachings abroad. In 1966, after helping to organize the American Dance Therapy Association, the "Grande Dame" of dance therapy became its first president.

Chace died in the summer of 1970. She left behind the art of using dance as a means of direct communication, expression and interaction with those whom others could not reach. She also left behind her unique group psychotherapy, a cohesive, complete and self-contained system of treatment, which creatively integrated verbal and nonverbal methods. Chace created great respect from her students, as well as some fear and trembling, because she was an intense and complex woman. Those who could get past the complexity and could find *themselves* in the technique are deeply indebted (S. Chaiklin & Schmais, 1979).

Theory

Chace's basic assumption was that "dance is communication and this fulfills a basic human need" (S. Chaiklin & Schmais, 1979, p. 16). She was deeply influenced by Sullivanian theories. Sullivan also pioneered in his work with schizophrenia. His major emphasis was on respecting the patient as a unique individual, worthy of empathic rapport and capable of genuine interpersonal interactions.

Chace also had a profound respect for the rights and needs of hospitalized patients. In addition, she had the intuition and skill to try various forms of verbal and nonverbal communication to reach patients. Others, who relied exclusively on verbalization to develop rapport, were often unable to establish contact with the patients assigned to Chace.

> In the psychotic, language loses much of its effectiveness as a means of relating to others, serving as a defensive barrier rather than a means of direct communication. The seriously ill mental patient relies to a large extent on nonverbal devices for the communication of his emotions. (H. Chaiklin, 1975, p. 71)

Believing that every patient had a desire to communicate, however buried that desire might be, Chace always sought after and engaged those parts of the patient's personality still available and wanting to "be heard and be well." In this respect, Chace was to the hospitalized patient in the 1940s what the humanistic psychologists Maslow (1968, 1978) and Rogers (1961) were to "healthy patients" in the 1960s. They all believed in, respected and engaged the healthy aspects of the individual.

Chace achieved this by closely observing and responding to the small idiosyncratic movements and gestures that constituted her patients' emotional expressions. Such direct movement expression, she believed, could break through verbal defenses. It is harder to disguise the physical expression of, or defense against, emotions than to hide their verbal counterparts. It was Chace's profound ability to use dance movement for self-expression and communication and her capacity to perceive, encounter, reflect and interact with the movement expressions of her patients that enabled her to draw them out of their psychotic isolation.

S. Chaiklin and Schmais (1979), protégés of Chace, organized her work into four major classifications: 1) Body Action, 2) Symbolism, 3) Therapeutic Movement Relationship and 4) Rhythmic Activity (to be referred to here as the Group Rhythmic Movement Relationship) (1979, p. 16).[1]

1. *Body Action.* The theory behind body action is well stated in this quote from Chace:

---

[1] The following description of the "Chace Method" builds primarily on two prior publications: the S. Chaiklin/Schmais (1979) article and the writings of Chace, which have been organized and published in an American Dance Therapy Association publication entitled *Marian Chace: Her Papers* (H. Chaiklin, 1975). Also see *Foundations of Dance Movement Therapy: The life and work of Marian Chace* (1993), edited by Susan Sandel, Sharon Chaiklin and Ann Lohn.

> Since muscular activity expressing emotion is the substratum of dance and since dance is a means of structuring and organizing such activity (i.e., the expression of emotion), it might be supposed that the dance could be a potent means of communication for the reintegration of the seriously ill mental patient. (H. Chaiklin, 1975, p. 71)

Although Chace rarely quoted theoretical ideas from Wilhelm Reich—and in fact would not have allied herself with Reichian technique—the theories inherent in her work presuppose the assumptions with which Reich was also experimenting in his own clinical work at that time (Reich, 1949). Chace and Reich paralleled each other historically and clinically, though Reich began in the 1920s. Both experimented with psychomotor therapeutic interventions as a way to unlock the thoughts, ideas and feelings that they believed were held in the musculature in the form of rigidity.

> Through dance action, the patient gains motility of the skeletal musculature. Recognizing the body parts, breathing patterns or tension levels which block emotional expression provides the therapist with clues to the sequence of physical actions that can develop readiness for emotional responsiveness; but it is not merely learning a movement which leads to change. The change occurs when the patient is ready to allow himself to experience the action in his body. (S. Chaiklin & Schmais, 1979, p. 17)

This parallels Reich's concept of the segmental arrangement of the body's armoring and his stress on the importance of the patient's readiness to experience his or her emotions (Reich, 1949). This quote also implies that the perceptively trained eye recognizes physical/emotional rigidities and blocks and certain structural changes occur in body movement behavior concomitant with personality changes. Again these concepts are seen in Reich's emphasis on what he called the identity of character and muscular armoring (Reich, 1949). In contrast, however, Reich did not use the dance form or stress an interactional approach—the mainstays of Chace's work.

2. *Symbolism.* The second classification, symbolism, describes the process of using imagery, fantasy, recollection and enactment through a combination of visualization, verbalization and dance action. Chace believed that problems could be worked through on a purely symbolic level and that interpretation or analysis was not always necessary. Through the power of movement, repressed and frightening emotions could be released in various forms; for example, patients interpreting images of animals as symbols of various thoughts, feelings and conflicts. Because the dance therapist accepts and empathizes with the unconscious and symbolic communications of the patient, the patient experiences a sense of trust and acceptance of his or her own expressive process. This, then, supports and encourages continued movement explorations.

This release can take place on different levels and through many different forms. After the release, a feeling of acceptance and trust of the dance therapist is established, allowing the content behind the symbolic forms and images to safely emerge into consciousness. (A deeper exploration of this process, with case examples, is found in Chapter 5 and 17.)

3. *Therapeutic Movement Relationship.* Chace had an unusual ability to kinesthetically perceive, reflect and react to her patients' emotional expressions through her own body movements and voice tone. This concept of the therapist's involving herself in a movement relationship or interaction with the patient as a way of reflecting a deep emotional acceptance and communication is Chace's revolutionary contribution to dance therapy. The theoretical assumption in this process of "mirroring" or "reflecting" is simple—and perhaps this is why it is so effective. By taking the patient's nonverbal and symbolic communications seriously and helping to broaden, expand and clarify them, Chace demonstrated her immediate desire and ability to meet the patient "where he/she is" emotionally and thus to understand and accept the patient on a deep and genuine level. In essence, Chace said to her patients through movement, "I understand you, I hear you and it's okay." In this sense she helped to validate the patient's immediate experience of him/herself.

4. *Group Rhythmic Movement Relationship.* The power of group rhythmic action was used by Chace to facilitate and support the expression of thoughts and feelings in an organized and controlled manner. The contagious aspect of rhythm could mobilize even severely withdrawn patients, with safe and simple rhythmic sequences providing a medium for the externalization of otherwise chaotic and confusing emotions.

Rhythm not only organizes the expression of thoughts and feelings into meaningful dance action, but also helps to modify extreme behaviors, such as hyperactivity/hypoactivity or a tendency toward the use of bizarre gestures and mannerisms. During the process of rhythmically exaggerating gestures and other nonverbal communications, Chace elicited and even suggested symbolism and content. This enhanced the patients' awareness of their body language and its symbolic meaning and gradually enabled them to modify extreme behavior and even verbalize some of the underlying conflicts.

In essence, the group rhythmic movement relationship provides a structure in which thoughts and feelings are shaped, organized and released within the secure confines of both the rhythmic action (which provides repetition and mastery) and the group structure and support.

Methodology

The Chace technique is a unique, complete and self-contained system of group therapy that utilizes dance movement as its predominant mode of interaction, communication and expression. It is a complete system in that it has a beginning (warm-up), middle (theme development) and end (closure). Each phase has its own style of intervention and purpose.

The Chace Technique

I. Warm-up

    A. Initial contacts
        1. Mirroring
        2. Clarifying and expanding the movement repertoire
        3. Movement elicitation/movement dialogue.
    B. Group development—gradual formation of circle
    C. Group rhythmic expression/physical warm-up

II. Theme Development

    A. Picking up on nonverbal clues
    B. Broadening, extending and clarifying actions (and intentions)
    C. Use of verbalization and imagery
    D. Various other theme-oriented possibilities (e.g., role playing, symbolic action, group themes)

III. Closure

    A. Circle
    B. Communal movement
    C. Possible discussion/sharing of feelings (H. Chaiklin, 1975)

The Chace warm-up is divided into three major parts: the initial contacts, the group development and the group rhythmic expression/physical warm-up.

Warm-up: Initial Contacts

This first stage of the warm-up was an intuitive and often spontaneous process. The patients would enter the dance therapy room where they could choose, if they wished, to play music from a selection of records. Meanwhile, Chace would watch, experience and interact with each patient, intuitively picking up the general tenor of the group. She had to move quickly in making contact with each patient, always keeping her senses available to the other patients, who might be moving alone or in small groups, so that they would never feel the lack of her presence. The goal was to establish direct communication and contact. She used this process to form the group structure as well as to keep it going.

The initial contacts took on certain specific intervention styles. The style Chace chose was determined by the emotional needs a specific patient projected at a given moment. For the purpose of clarification, the different intervention styles are here divided into three categories: 1. mirroring or empathic reflection; 2. clarifying, expanding and broadening the expressive movement potential and 3. movement elicitation/dialogue movements. Although differentiated here, these categories were not always clearly delineated in practice. The needs of the patient often required more than one style or an overlapping of several styles during a single interaction. For Chace, moving back and forth between these was as natural as the subtle shifts that took place in verbal dialogues. While these types of interaction were essential to the warm-up phase of the group, they also formed the core elements of the therapeutic movement relationship and thus were basic to all phases of the Chace technique.

1. *Mirroring or empathic reflection.* This involved Chace's ability to kinesthetically and visually experience that which the patient was experiencing and trying to communicate. In essence, Chace would "mirror" or reflect back via her own muscular activity and verbal narration what she perceived and experienced in the body action and the body of the patient. To an onlooker, this could have been interpreted as mimicry—but it was more than that. Mimicry is simply copying the form of the movement without incorporating its meaning. Mirroring of action and meaning, also referred to as kinesthetic empathy or empathic reflection, is a powerful tool and one of the major contributions that Chace made to dance therapy.

2. *Clarifying, expanding and broadening the expressive movement potential.* In this approach, Chace began where the patient was, expressing the initial contact with the patient by mirroring, but then gently extending a certain gesture to clarify its focus or aim. Chace basically helped the expression to evolve into a more complete movement statement, thus enhancing the patient's identification and commitment to his or her own personal expressions and communications.

The following is an example of a movement intervention Chace made with a psychotic patient. The intervention used both empathic reflection (mirroring) as well as a dance movement response to the patient's physical manifestations of feeling.

> One patient stands hunched forward, contracted through the abdomen, his whole posture that of a person in terror. The therapist feels the tension within her own abdomen and using this as a center of action, she develops a tension relaxation dance sequence. The original contraction she feels may be carried into an expansive movement or into some relaxed action neither of which can be construed as threatening. In either case, it must develop from or be closely related to the patient's own contracted movement. In his response to the therapist, the patient can carry his own contraction into a similar movement and thus help himself to break away from his fixed emotional muscular pattern. When action with the therapist has been established, this patient may be able to move away from his spot into the room. Later he may be able to dance by himself, with another patient or perhaps even during the same session, join the dance circle for short periods of time. (H. Chaiklin, 1975, p. 73)

In this example, Chace began at the point where the patient was, but then deciding that it was better not to stay in this fixed state, she gradually and delicately led the patient into other options, always watching and observing to see the effect of the intervention. This concept of leading the patient into new and more varied movement configurations, as well as more clearly focusing or exaggerating initial movement patterns, was the basis of clarifying, expanding and broadening the expressive movement potential. This powerful method was the core of Chace's gift to her patients and to the discipline of dance therapy.

3. *Movement elicitation/dialogue movements.* In this approach, Chace would interact with her patients, verbally and nonverbally, to elicit a movement response from them. For example, seeing a patient withdrawn in a corner, Chace might try to draw the individual out through initiation of a movement dialogue or role-playing. She might play the hurt child because the patient would not "come out and play," or make an evocative movement in an attempt to elicit or "demand" a response from the patient. An example of the latter might be a pantomime of playing with an imaginary ball and throwing it to the still patient. The decision to use specific forms of play, music and specific imagery to elicit movement dialogues was always based on the body expression of the patient.

The three styles of initial contact discussed above serve to summarize but do not cover all of the subtle styles of movement communication and interaction that Chace used. Chace described the initial contact phase of the warm-up process as follows:

> During this period, the therapist has the feeling of building multiple individual lines of communication, none of which may be neglected even momentarily and all of which will gradually be developed into a group activity, away from herself except as a catalyst.... At the moment when the patient indicates that he is conscious of dancing with another person, rather than merely accepting another dancer moving in a similar fashion, his eyes will suddenly focus on the therapist and he will touch her hands, usually grasping them hard. I always respond with a simple "Hello." Patients who have danced in this fashion often say to me, "You have known me from the beginning." (H. Chaiklin, 1975, pp. 74-75)

This early part of the group process is analogous to an image of the therapist as the center of a wheel from which spokes radiate. As Chace moved with the group, she would connect and mobilize the people on the periphery. Although she may have appeared to be involved with only one individual, she was in fact always attuned to the others, acting as the "hub" of the group, the emotional turning point of all activity.

Warm-up: Group Development

After the initial contacts were made, Chace began the group development phase of the warm-up process, assessing the group's readiness to form a circle. Being sensitive to individual differences, Chace was flexible regarding group structure, aware that some patients needed more distance than others. Timing was important. If she prematurely attempted to form the group structure, it would not succeed and if she waited too long, pandemonium could break out. It was understood that some patients might not be able to tolerate being part of the circle and so would participate from the sideline. Chace led from the circle itself as opposed to positioning herself in the center or outside.

> This section of the dance session starts gradually.... Small circles composed of varying individuals are forming, separating and reforming. Leadership passes back and forth from members of the group to the dance therapist and her assistants. Movements begin to lose their bizarre quality, returning to it as the circle again dissolves into individuals using movements of their own. (H. Chaiklin, 1975, p. 76)

Chace viewed this part of the session as a "testing period" (H. Chaiklin, 1975, p. 76). At this time, patients could feel their way into the group, testing whether or not they were able to maintain their individuality and still feel comfortable within the group. The emphasis at this stage was on developing individual and group rapport in order to build trust and openness in the group.

Gradually, more patients joined and became part of the group process. Verbalization was more prominent, complementing, clarifying and broadening the group movement and interaction. Almost simultaneously, the group's movements became more rhythmically synchronized. One could sense the patients beginning to relax with one another.

Warm-up: Group Rhythmic Expression/Physical Warm-up

At this point, the group was for the most part in a circle and some degree of group rapport had been established. Noticing certain physical tensions in the group, Chace might have initiated a simple rhythmic movement, such as a stamp, possibly to the beat of a familiar folk tune. She then gently guided the patients, through verbal narration and dance, into expressive movements, which incorporated the chest, abdomen and pelvic areas. In this way, she gradually moved the group forward on two levels simultaneously, developing group trust by initiating and facilitating activity that reflected group needs and developing full body movement by extending the dance action to include the entire body.

This extension of movement throughout the body helped to integrate the often fragmented sense of self in the severely disturbed individual. Guiding small movements into total body activity were simple rhythmic movements like swinging, pushing or shaking. The patient was encouraged to make a more complete commitment to and identification with his or her moving self. At this stage of the group process, Chace's movements were simple and easy, following rudimentary rules of movement so as not to confuse patients or scare them away from the group. This period also helped to bring in those members still outside of the group.

The warm-up served other purposes as well. The movements aroused in the patients a sense of enjoyment of body action. In addition, they helped to loosen the body and release excess tensions that could impede both the group process and the surfacing of emotional material. It is difficult to process emotions if the body is excessively tense.

Some preliminary emotional content often emerged during the latter stages of the warm-up. Chace noted that it was not uncommon to hear patients make statements that expressed self-realization, such as "This is me," "I can live" or "These are my hands and these are yours" (H. Chaiklin, 1975, p. 76). Chace also discussed patients expressing remorse at making personal discoveries long overdue—"This I should have known when I was a child," or awareness of despair and loneliness— "I never had a friend," "My mother never taught me to love" (H. Chaiklin, 1975, p. 76). These statements emerged spontaneously as part of the early group process. They were often spoken rhythmically, accompanying the group movements and frequently evoked supportive group responses in either verbal or nonverbal forms.

While emotional themes were crystallized during the warm-up process, they were not yet dealt with in depth. Instead, the focus was on developing the rapport, trust and physical readiness that enabled the group to support the deeper psychic material that might surface during the next phase of the group process.

Theme Development

Throughout the warm-up phase, Chace acted as a medium through which feelings in the group were picked up, processed and reflected back verbally and nonverbally to the individual and the group. During the theme development phase, when the group was a stronger and more cohesive unit, she continued to act as a medium but with increased focus and clarity. With her patients' nonverbal communications as a starting point, Chace used movement, verbalization, imagery and various theme-oriented actions to lead them into a deeper exploration of the affects, themes and conflicts that she noted during the warm-up.

For example, the group might be involved in a simple side-to-side swing, which one member appeared to be doing with an additional unconscious intention, as if he or she were saying in movement, "Get off my back." Perceiving this variation, Chace facilitated its development in a number of ways. She could start by simply intensifying this variation in her own body, bringing it to the attention of the others and then perhaps say a word or make a sound that would reflect the feeling she perceived. She then encouraged the group to relate to the emerging theme through continued use of rhythmic dance movement combined with the use of sounds and words.

In order to further focus and clarify the meaning behind this variation, she presented leading questions to the group, such as 'What is on your back?" "Do you imagine that you are talking to someone?" or "If there were something on your back, how would it feel or who would it be?" These questions often shed light on underlying conflicts and evoked material for further movement work.

At other times, Chace may have suggested a theme-oriented movement pattern. Observing certain rigidities in a patient's upper arms and back and realizing the patient's need to express anger via arm movements, she might have provided a symbolic action such as chopping. This would release emotional tension without overwhelming the patient's ego with a premature awareness of unconscious motivations.

Finally, Chace used verbalization as a form of narration, to reflect, guide and structure the group process. Through continual verbal narration, accompanied by dance movement and vocalization, she united the group and clarified its directions and intentions at all times.

Closure

Chace stressed the structuring of a supportive closure that allowed patients to leave with some sense of satisfaction and resolve. Sensing that the group interaction was about to reach a natural conclusion, she brought participants back into the circle structure. In order to put closure on the individual relationships, she found ways to acknowledge all group members and conclude the session by utilizing repetitive communal movements that provided the group with a feeling of connection, support, solidarity and well being.

A communal movement might have been holding hands and swinging or coming together in a large swoop down and then raising hands high together in the center. The repetitive format supported a gradual slowing down of the individual expressive process and encouraged participants to shift their focus back to the group.

Closure also frequently included patients spontaneously sharing feelings, memories and experiences verbally. Through this sharing, emotions were organized into meaningful verbal communication. Some patients had never before been able to experience such communication.

Summary

Chace was a brilliant pioneer and innovator in dance therapy. Although she worked at times individually, the power of her process was most clearly demonstrated in the group sessions. The group method that Chace presented was sound, simple and complete, with a natural progression from the individual to the group and from one stage to the next.

As other pioneers are discussed in the following pages, there is a certain amount of overlapping of theory and practice. For this reason, it is important to summarize the major and unique contributions that Chace made to dance therapy:

1. The therapeutic movement relationship;
2. The use of ongoing verbal narration as a form of reflecting on the group and individual process;
3. The use of rhythmic movement as an organizing and clarifying force and
4. The use of dance as a cohesive group process—a form of group psychotherapy.

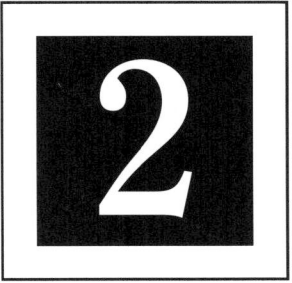

Blanche Evan: Creative Movement Becomes Dance Therapy

Blanche Evan (circa 1909-1982) began her career in dance as a dancer, choreographer and performer. For the last 30 years of her life, she was dedicated to the exploration of the use of dance as therapy. Evan was the originator of her own approach to dance therapy and was a pioneer in her emphasis on what she termed, the neurotic urban adult.

Evan's petite body and graceful, delicate movements belied her intense, persevering and outspoken nature. "She was a very complex and intense personality—very demanding, very giving, a fighter and an iconoclast—dissatisfied, yet hopeful, believing in basic human wholeness and possibility for each individual" (Melson & Krantz, personal communication, June 15, 1987).

Evan's career was profoundly influenced by her dance studies in the 1920s with Bird Larson, one of the early practitioners of "natural dance" and expressive improvisational dance. Evan believed that Larson "was the most and one of the very few objective teachers of that time, increasing skill yet preserving the health of the body and opening the way for the individual student to express her own creativity in dance" (Evan, personal communication, 1980). Devastated by Larson's premature death in the late 1930s, Evan became committed to carrying on and expanding upon her original teachings.

Evan was also influenced by the work of Dalcroze, Noverre, Stanislovski and Mensendieck. She studied Spanish and ethnic dance with Viola and La Meri (Evan, personal communication, 1980). However, her major interest was dance improvisation as a medium through which one's creative and emotional potential could be drawn out and actualized (Evan, personal communication, 1980).

In the late 1940s and early 1950s, Evan's area of specialization was creative dance with children. Between 1949 and 1951, she published ten articles on this subject.[1] While she did not call herself a dance therapist at this time, her writings revealed her dedication to helping children express a variety of thoughts and feelings through dance, including those that were forbidden and frightening.

Although she had extensive experience with children, and worked briefly with people with developmental disabilities and psychotic children at Bellevue in the 1950s, her major interest from the late 1950s until her death in 1982 was with an adult population that she labeled the "normal, functioning neurotic" (Evan, personal communication, 1980). One major concern that appeared first in her work with children and later in her work with the "normal, functioning neurotic," was with the suppressive adaptive patterns of the urban individual who, surrounded by the hardness of concrete and the time pressures of a mechanized society, had, she believed, lost contact with his or her body and emotions (Evan, 1964).

In the 1950s, Evan expressed concern over the fact that dance as therapy was being stressed for the psychotic individual but overlooked for the neurotic individual. Evan on the east coast and Mary Whitehouse on the west coast were the only dance therapists who stressed reaching this population. In addition, Evan and Whitehouse both stressed in-depth improvisation as the major intervening modality.

In 1956, Evan began to call her work "creative dance as therapy." In 1958, after studying at the Alfred Adler Institute of Individual Psychology and the New School for Social Research, she trained professionals and students in her approach.

---

[1]This collection of essays is now reprinted and available under the title, *The Child's World: Its Relation to Dance Pedagogy* (see References).

Although Evan gradually moved from a creative, educational emphasis to a psychotherapeutic emphasis, her later approach integrated much of her original teachings. This integration of creative and improvisational dance with the psychologies of Adler, Freud and others formed the foundation of her major contributions to the theory and practice of dance therapy.

In regard to the relationship between dance therapy and creative dance, Evan stated:

> Creative dance breaks the crust. Dance Therapy leads to unraveling the knots, to diagnosis and to active life, brain, habit change. The education of the emotions (an Adlerian term) is also possible. (Groninger, 1980, p. 17)

In her later years, as the field of dance therapy expanded, running the gamut from "movement psychotherapy" to "psychoanalytically oriented movement therapy," Evan remained firm and clear in her commitment to dance. She did not accept the word "movement" as an accurate substitute for the word "dance" (personal communication, 1980). She saw too much of dance therapy as being "antidance" and aspiring either to the verbal therapies, hence losing the inherent power of dance or to the "body/mind" therapies, which too often ignored the individual's emotions and diagnoses. Evan believed that "unlike many body/mind techniques which share some characteristics with dance therapy (breathing, posture and vocalization, for instance), dance therapy works at getting at the causes for the client's distress in the most primal, elementary way—self-directed movement" (Groninger, 1980, p. 17). Evan integrated the verbal and the dance into a full and primary psychotherapy, which she eventually called Dance Movement/Word Therapy.

Evan opened her first dance studio in 1934 in New York City and, in 1967, founded the Dance Therapy Center, also in New York. Later in life, due to health problems, she moved to Boulder, Colorado, where she continued to teach and see clients until her death in 1982. While in Colorado, she frequently traveled back to New York to teach. Four protégés who carry on her work today are Bonnie Bernstein and Anne Krantz on the west coast and Barbara Melson and Iris Rifkin-Gainer on the east coast. Also on the east coast, the author, who trained with Evan in the 1970s, incorporates this work into a multimodal approach to dance therapy and psychotherapy (Chapter 17).

Theory[2]

Evan stressed dance as the art form that utilizes the most direct and complete connection to the psyche, as differentiated from the visual arts or the use of a musical instrument.

> It is this need for psycho-physical union that Dance can so directly fulfill.... Its *instrument* of expression *is* the human body and its medium body movement. (1964, n.p.)

Creative Dance with Children

Evan believed that children could express in movement and metaphor what they were unable to express in words:

> *I could not find in language* the *equivalent* for the *violence* I have seen children express in dance. And I would have to be a poet to describe the sadness and the delicacy. (1964, n.p.)

It was Evan's conviction that in "true creative dance, the form springs from the source.... It comes and goes and there is not even a momentary reminder of that which has been expressed...." (1964, n.p.). Aside from these moments of breakthrough in dance, these intense feelings were frequently repressed. The major goal of Evan's work was to bridge the gap between psyche and soma, allowing that which became repressed or deadened to spring back to life through the resiliency of the body in the form of dance.

The challenge of the creative dance teacher as well as the therapist who utilized creative dance was to

---

[2]This discussion of Evan's theoretical base was derived from her very early publications on creative dance for children written in the late 1940s and 1950s, integrated with her more recent articles, ranging primarily from the late 1950s through the 1970s and organized chronologically in her "Packet of Pieces" (1945-1978).

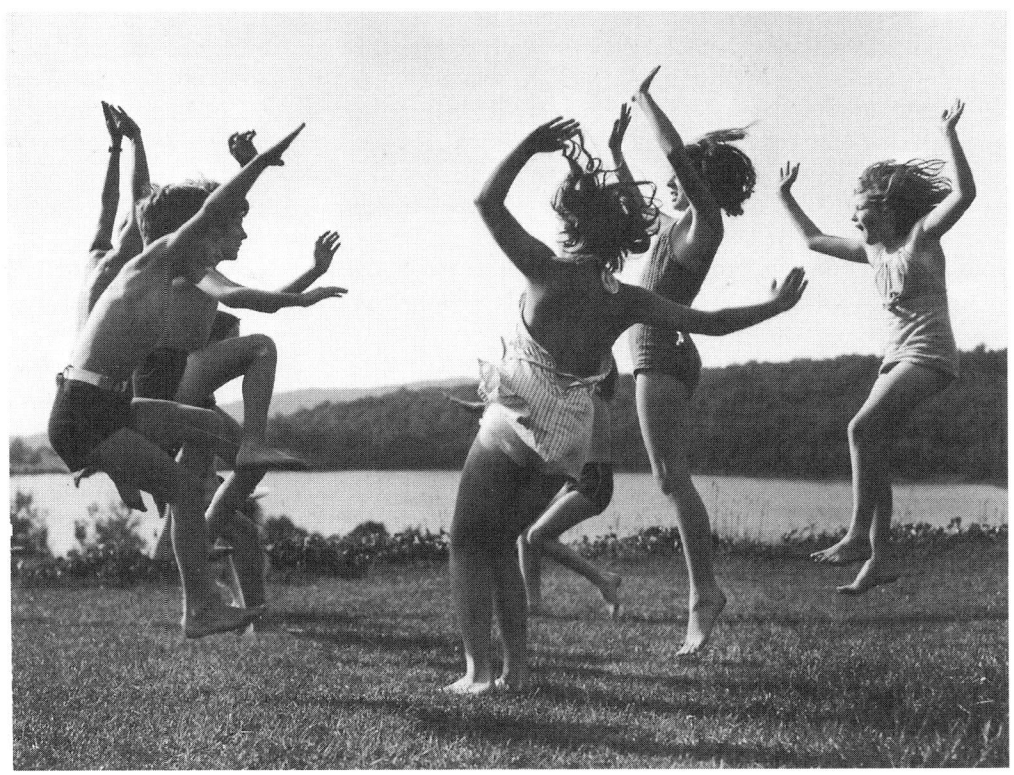

The unity of mind and body is expressed in the joy of these children dancing (Photo courtesy Lloyd Morgan of the Barbara Morgan Archive)

promote mind-body unification through expressive movement while still providing instruction in the basic skills of dance. Evan reminded us that the over-emphasis on teaching dance technique to children was peculiar to our culture. She cited other cultures in which dance was indigenous to life and was transmitted as part of the whole culture. She commented on the isolation of dance in Western society from everyday life experiences and realities. This was further complicated, she felt, by urban life and the mechanized society which forced us to adapt to tempos external to our own inner rhythms. In addition, she believed that urban children were too often thrown into physical and emotional isolation due to the lack of group-related activities, whether in play, religion or work.

Evan's theory was that the child, after being taught to move and sense his or her body correctly, was better equipped to organize and explore expressive movement sequences. She stressed that "… children actually do not feel any dichotomy between emotional 'expression' and 'technique' unless such separation is forced upon them" (Evan, 1964, n.p.). She gave the example of a child who was asked to beat a drum; in doing so, the child's entire body intensified with the dynamic rhythmic qualities the beat creates. In a similar fashion, a child who still experienced the integration of his mind and body, when asked to do a specific technique, permeated the action with his or her own affect. "Children will take any movement that even remotely lends itself [to dynamic expression] and transmute it through inner emotional response into a form fused with content" (Evan, 1964, n.p.).

Evan felt that modern dance and ballet too often geared themselves to the separation of mind and body, thus severing this dynamic quality, which Evan called "the life of Dance" (1964, n.p.). Hence, the challenge of integration became the major thrust of her work.

Dance Therapy with the Neurotic Urban Adult

In her work with urban adults, Evan frequently encountered complaints and excuses concerning issues of fatigue. She interpreted these issues as manifestations of inner drives toward repression, fear and dependency, causing clients to resist using their full physical potential. Evan cautioned the therapist against over-identifying with these repressive drives, which, she believed, was in constant struggle with and could be overcome by the opposing drives toward self-expression. Frequently, what the client needed was a push in the direction of feeling and experiencing the self (Evan, 1945-78, n.p.).

In accordance with Adlerian psychology, Evan believed that repressed aggression and anger were the major maladies of the neurotic. Because the neurotic's anger was repressed, so was his or her assertiveness and commitment to growing up. This was reflected clearly in the body musculature. "With action repressed, the energy is diverted to different kinds of tension: rigidity at one extreme, apathy at the other" (1945-1978, n.p.).

According to Evan, the hands, face and voice were often the last areas to be released. She spoke of the tendency for the neurotic to try to mask his or her feelings by constricting the facial muscles, which otherwise made the emotions visible. Regarding the voice, which she believed was the hardest to release, she stated, "Self-produced sounds seem to wake up the whole person in an immediate kind of way" (Groninger, 1980, p. 17). Through sound, the emotions were heard as well as seen. Evan reminded us that suppression in childhood was usually in sound more than in movement or that children were to be seen but not heard.

Another common problem of the neurotic was the exertion wasted in an attempt to maintain self-defeating attitudes (Evan, 1945-78, n.p.). If the body was trained for years in non-expression, the need to express may have eventually become lost. In severe cases, the resiliency of the muscles could be totally destroyed. "Body and spirit split and begin to atrophy; ego power shrinks to low self-esteem with an ineptness for both anger and love" (Evan, 1945-78, n.p.).

Evan's goal was to re-educate individuals to accept their bodily responses and needs which, she believed, existed prior to the repressive influences of family and society. This did not mean training individuals to be impulsive, but rather to use the expressive and creative aspects of the dance form as a vehicle for dramatic enactments of thoughts and feelings that might otherwise be repressed, destroyed or turned inward against the self.

Inherent in Evan's work was her stress on the use of the ego function of regression in the service of the ego.[3] Dance was viewed as an ego function. As such, it was directed and spontaneous use of rhythm, exertion and form, which helped individuals to experience and express repressed traumas and other forbidden and frightening thoughts and feelings. In short, for Evan, dance was a language very similar to words. But unlike words, dance represented a more direct communication and language of the self.

Finally, Evan worked with the whole person. That is, she emphasized the person in his or her world. She did not believe, as the traditional psychoanalysts did, that insight and the awareness of unconscious material alone constituted the goals of treatment. If an individual, after completion of psychotherapy, was not better equipped to cope with his or her life, both intrapersonally and interpersonally, Evan believed that the treatment was not successful (Melson, personal communication, 1987).

Methodology[4]

Overall Structure

Evan practiced for approximately 25 years both individually and in groups. Her methodology was composed of four major modes of intervention: the warm-up, "Evan's system of functional technique," improvisation/enactment and verbalization of thoughts and feelings. These basic intervention styles varied in order and were not all present in each session. The following discussion concentrates on the first three classifications, the role they play therapeutically and their interrelationship.

---

[3]While the terminology "regression in the service of the ego" was not actually used by Evan, it serves here to describe the movement process that Evan catalyzed.

[4]Most of the information in this section has been taken from the author's group dance therapy training with Evan in the early 1970s. This has been augmented by Evan's writings and by personal communications with Evan and Rifkin-Gainer in 1980 and with Rifkin-Gainer, Melson and Krantz in 1987.

Physical Warm-up

The warm-up was a process of releasing superficial/excess tension, helping the individual to achieve a state that mediated between relaxation and tension and thus paved the way for receptivity to bodily feelings, emotions and possible expressive actions. It was also used to move people out of apathetic and physically depressed states.

The warm-up was aimed at bringing people into contact with the reality of their psychophysical selves. Evan stressed that with clients using movement for the first time in an expressive manner, the warm-up was especially important. Its function was that of preparing the body both for corrective bodywork or functional technique and for the expression of thoughts and feelings often evoked later in the session through Evan's thematic improvisational work. It is important to stress that the warm-up was not designed to dissipate emotional conflict and its resulting tension, but to reduce the individual's excess tension, which Evan believed served to camouflage deeper problems.

Early in her career, Evan encouraged free swinging of the body in all directions for individuals who were very tense. She believed that the swing was usually the easiest, most accessible movement for everyone, providing a feeling of freedom, while at the same time offering security in its rhythm. Later, this emphasis on the swing moved to a more general emphasis on total joint mobilization through many different kinds of movements, for example, skipping, running, jumping, rotating and shaking out body parts (Rifkin-Gainer, 1986, p. 6). She often used drumbeats, which steadily increased in tempo so that individuals were led into faster and freer motions. She worked for a sense of ease and abandon in the body with the goal of eventually helping the individual to give in to the spontaneous creation of expressive form in improvisation.

The warm-ups were sometimes with or without music. Evan frequently asked if anyone wanted music and, if so, what kind. Often she let members do their own actions alone to warm-up and loosen the body; other times she had the group make a circle and each group member suggested or began a warm-up action, which the other members then picked up on. From here, group members could take turns at leadership.

Before completing the warm-up, Evan might have asked how the group felt and whether anyone needed more work on a particular part of the body. If someone did, more exercises were done. At times, Evan helped members release difficult tension areas by exaggerating their muscular rigidity and then releasing it. One loosening exercise was the isolation of body segments. For example, to a slow and then increasing drumbeat, she first had clients just release shoulders and then hips. Because her goal was always the integration of the whole body, Evan had clients do integration movements (e.g., large, rhythmic, total-body movements) before and after isolations. She believed most people were already tense and over-segmented.

It is important to note that there were times when Evan believed a warm-up was contraindicated. The warm-up, if used incorrectly or indiscriminately, could serve to prematurely dissipate important psychophysical energy that the client needed to mobilize him or herself in the direction of working through emotional conflicts and trauma (Melson & Rifkin-Gainer, personal communication, 1987). An experienced dance therapist can judge when the client arrives whether he or she is ready to move directly into pressing emotional material or if a warm-up is required first and what kind of warm-up is indicated.

Most often the warm-up was used. It was considered an essential part of the process, without which the body might not be able to fully process the unconscious material that frequently surfaced during the improvisational phase of the sessions.

The Evan System of Functional Technique[5]

Evan described the Evan system of functional technique in 1980 as:

---

[5]In the published material that Evan has written, there is little that describes in detail the Evan system of functional technique. However, in "Life is Movement, the Blanche Evan Dance Foundation" Evan has more than 100 pages of material on this technique. From her early articles (1964), Mensendieck's functional exercises, Todd, *The Thinking Body* (1937) and Scott, *Analysis of Human Motion* (1963) influenced her. The ideas presented in this section are abstracted from these articles and from the author's training with Evan in the early 1970s.

> Corrective exercise designed to retrain muscles to move in relation to nature's design in a rhythmic expansion and contraction.... Spontaneity and resilience ... are enhanced by the individual's discovery of his own rhythm and tempo. (Groninger, 1980, p. 17)

Evan's studies with Bird Larson laid the groundwork for her system of functional technique that rehabilitated and educated the body in an anatomically sound way (Rifkin-Gainer, et al., 1984, p. 14). Functional technique included postural work, coordination, placement of body parts and rhythmicity. This style of work was individualized, varied, adapting to the individual's unique anatomical needs. In Evan's words, functional techniques "... respects nature's plan of the body in action.... Changing the body tonus from destructive tension to resilience is vital" (Rifkin-Gainer, et al., 1984, p. 14).

Evan stressed the strengthening and alignment of the spine as the foundation of all action. She also commented on human verticality as our unique distinction from other species, believing that this distinction carried with it an emotional responsibility and physical task of supporting and balancing the body. Evan's concern with the spine centered on her belief that the functioning of the spine determined the overall ability to use the body as an "Instrument of Dance" (1964, n.p.) and therefore as an instrument of self-expression. She further believed that limitations in the overall strength and flexibility of the spine lead to insecurity and fear.

Some of the goals of functional technique are:

1. To rehabilitate the body;
2. To give the individual permission to take up and use space in a variety of ways that he or she would not feel free to try alone
3. To give the body the strength and range of motion that it will need for emotional expression, to provide the physical base upon which one can build one's own unique expressive movement vocabulary;
4. To help the individual to feel more secure about physical self-expression through the development of physical control;
5. To bring the individual into contact with parts of the body that were previously out of his or her conscious awareness and
6. To integrate functional contraction with functional release for the purpose of achieving more efficient and meaningful movement expression.

In regard to teaching functional technique, Evan stated:

> Technique need not be treated as an amputated limb of Dance. It is rather one of its functional organs. It can be presented so that its pursuit does not become a block to creative spontaneity.... The work in CREATIVE DANCE need not negate form. Ideally it should seek a new form that is the result of a union of unmannered technique with the creative use of [personal] content. (1964, n.p.)

Improvisation/Enactment[6]

Evan defined improvisation as:

> ... the spontaneous creation of form. Form and content ideally are one. Dance improvisation is the complete welding of yourself, as you are at the moment, with your theme, in terms of Dance. The beginning is the moment of merging; developing proceeds, climax is achieved and there is only one right moment for the end, when the theme, as it relates to you, has spun out its course. (1964, n.p.)

Here, Evan was referring to the inner sense of completion and what could be called the "internal clock," which unwound body movement in the spontaneous creation of form with an inherent sense of the beginning, middle and end. Evan placed equal stress on the physiological and psychological. She emphasized "... the need of the human being to experience the physical equivalent of the psyche in the body through action" (1964, n.p.).

---

[6]The following discussion comes from several sources, including Evan's article "I am the Sun" (1964), notes from Evan's "Intensive Dance Therapy Training" course, which the author took in the early 1970s, as well as Evan's write-up of the case of Pamela and a paper she published in 1970 in the *Journal of Pastoral Counseling*. The latter two are reprinted in her booklet entitled *Packet of Pieces* (1945-78). Ruth Benov did the most recent compilation of material on Evan in 1991 (See Bibliography).

Evan's improvisational work may be classified into three approaches: a) projective techniques, b) sensitization to and mobilization of potential body action and c) in-depth and/or complex improvisation. The first two categories represent what may have been called emotional warm-ups. They prepared the individual, through simple improvisational tasks, for the third category of more in-depth and/or complex improvisational work. The latter formed the major content of the dance therapy session and at times was likened to the free association process in psychoanalysis, but enacted on a motor level, i.e., psychomotor association.[7]

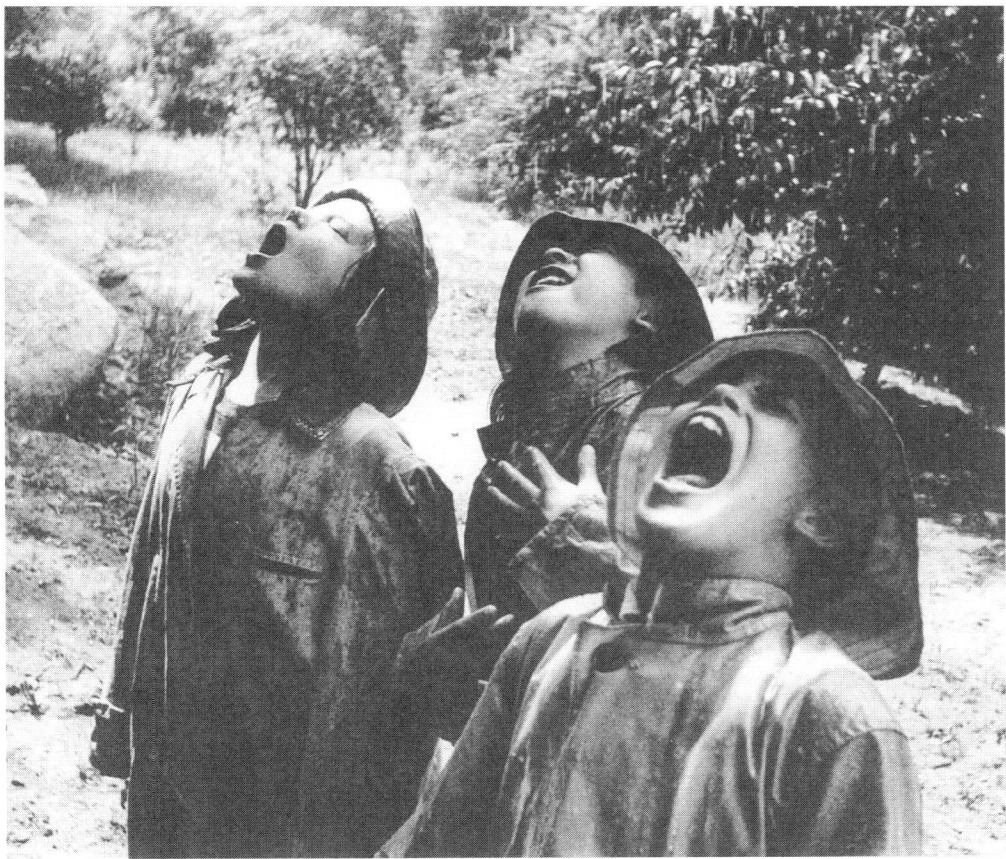

Children's faces and voices express their unity with nature (Photo courtesy Lloyd Morgan of the Barbara Morgan Archive)

Projective Technique

The use of the projective technique is a cornerstone of Evan's work, brought directly from her background in creative dance. Evan believed that adults could often benefit from being an animal, color or texture in movement. Evan used the projective technique both for self-expression and diagnostic purposes.

In utilizing creative themes, she made a choice as to how specific or general to be, which was determined by the client's needs. For example, in using themes from nature, she could either suggest categorical themes, like "be an animal" or "be an inanimate aspect of nature," or she could narrow the field slightly by asking the client to choose a four-legged animal or a reptile or a bird. Similarly, she might say, "choose a tree that most represents how you feel today." This latter example could also be done with water, wind, sky

---

[7]Many of the terms used here were selected in an attempt to describe and organize Evan's work. Evan herself did not use them in her teachings.

and so on. For example, if the client were asked to be water in any form, he or she had many choices: ice, vapor, the ocean, a brook, shower or storm. In this way, the client would fill in the blank with an image that was inevitably a projection of one part of his or her own feeling state. The client could feel turbulent like a storm, rough like the sea or gentle like a pond.

While exploring, for example, the turbulence of a storm, the individual might become aware of the feeling of anger, which, after a certain amount of unfocused release, might pave the way for a more structured release. For example, the anger might become focused at a specific person or event in the individual's life.

The projective technique in this case might be called an emotional warm-up or barometer in that it attunes the individual to a specific feeling that presses to express itself physically. After some discussion, the insights gained through Evan's observations and the client's self-reflection could be directed into a more complex improvisational structure where the client would focus his or her attention on the surfacing imagery or conflict and explore it in depth through body movement.[8]

Another style of the projective technique used by Evan was eliciting the fantasies of clients and, if not contraindicated, helping them to enact these fantasies in dance. For example, this could be a fantasy of their ideal self, of a place they would like to be or of something they would like to do or say to someone.

Finally, Evan used words, phrases and sentences to facilitate projection through body movement. She might have suggested as a warm-up to an in-depth improvisation that her client move spontaneously to the images that arose from several words, which Evan would toss out quickly and successively. These would be aimed at freeing the individual from inhibition and over-intellectualization, replacing these with spontaneity of associations and their corresponding movement responses. Evan also tossed out incomplete sentences, encouraging clients to complete them in movement, for example, "My body can _____," "I'm going to _____," "I feel _____," or "I want to be _____."

After such an exercise, discussion might take place on what occurred in the emotional warm-up process. From this, more intense themes may have emerged, which Evan and the client would then structure into more intense and comprehensive movement explorations.

Evan eventually moved away from the technique of offering imagery to her clients to utilizing images that emerged spontaneously from the therapeutic process. In the latter part of her career she noted certain risks in providing images to clients; she felt that a therapist could never know what clients' associations would be to externally prompted imagery (Rifkin-Gainer, personal communication, 1980; Melson, personal communication, 1987). This break from externally prompted themes was reflective of Evan's gradual move away from her creative dance background and toward more in depth psychotherapy through dance.

Sensitization to and Mobilization of Potential Body Action

Evan also used projective techniques in relationship to expanding the client's movement repertoire. The goal of sensitization to and mobilization of potential body action was to bring potential movement into actual movement through stimulating the elements of dance (i.e., time, space, intensity, rhythmic flow, content). This was accomplished by providing specific images, stimuli and movement directives. Evan may have played percussive instruments, varying the intensity, the rhythm and the instrument and thus providing varied stimuli to the body, such as fast/slow, staccato/legato, loud/soft, upbeat/downbeat and so on.

Another way to stimulate dynamic movement, as well as psychic and somatic projection, was through the use of props. Props usually demand action and specific qualities of movement. For example, a flowing scarf, though varied in its possibilities, may generally encourage different movements than a hoop or a ball. Also, scarves can vary greatly in their texture, weight and in the tactile sensations they stimulate, helping to determine the quality of movement for which they are most suited.

Words, especially verbs or adjectives, are also provocative in terms of exploring varieties of movement possibilities. For example, words used in opposition are especially evocative and meaningful: gather/scatter, open/close, strong/soft, round/angular, sunny/rainy, clear/foggy, morning/night, choppy/smooth and so on.

In these examples of verbal facilitation through contrasting movement themes, images have been pulled

---

[8]This progression from form to content, ushered in through projective techniques, is explored further in Chapter 17.

from several categories, such as time of day, tempo, texture, shape, weather and so on. Some of these contrasting images describe specifically the type of movement the dance therapist believes the individual needs to develop (e.g., round/angular). When the dance therapist uses or encourages the client to choose physically directive words such as round and angular, part of the projective aspect of the exercise is omitted and replaced with a "prescribed" movement pattern. The individual is directly encouraged to use the muscles the dance therapist believes he or she needs to develop for increased expressivity. On the other hand, words such as morning/night are subject to greater personal interpretation; they leave larger blanks for the individual to fill in with his or her own free associations. The latter is actually a projective technique that has the additional effect of broadening the movement repertoire.

Evan emphasized the importance of knowing why the therapist was asking an individual to do a specific movement exploration. Would one look (as in the latter example) for associations to the movement so as to provoke emotional content for future complex improvisations? Or, would one try (as in the former example) to build specific muscular strength, awareness and flexibility so that the body was ready for the unconscious thoughts and feelings that surface during these explorations? In either case, the individual was warming up to more intense and personal movement work.

Another technique for helping individuals to learn, experience and employ their full movement potential was to use the elements of dance directly, exploring the extremes and gradations of tempo, weight and space using action words, which guided the individual. For example, if an individual was working on a theme in a simple improvisation, Evan might have made movement suggestions to help the individual explore more fully certain movement qualities. She might have offered movement suggestions such as "Add weight," "Can you move faster?" or "Can you add rhythm to your movement?" This was more applicable to brief improvisations than to full complex improvisations, during which Evan usually just observed the process until the individual brought the improvisation to closure.

To encourage new movement qualities in interaction, Evan had individuals work in dyads with each taking turns in contrasting roles. This could take place through specific roles; for example, one person becoming a tree while the other was the wind. Again, this would encourage contrasting movement dynamics with room for projection of emotionally meaningful content, therefore acting as a warm-up for future in-depth work.

Finally, concrete images can broaden and expand the movement repertoire. Evan emphasized the importance of concrete and simple directions for beginners who were not accustomed to using their bodies to express feelings and ideas. Giving them a complicated or abstract direction too soon could encourage an over-intellectualization of the movement process and lose the emotional intent. As with the projective techniques, the possibilities for the use of concrete images were practically unlimited. Examples included pushing a wall, kicking a ball or wringing a towel. Any of these could be used for physical release, expanding the movement repertoire and stimulating projective material.

In summary, projective techniques and sensitization to and mobilization of potential body action at times overlap in function; they simply represent a different emphasis. The former emphasizes the surfacing of unconscious material, while the latter emphasizes broadening the movement repertoire. Because the muscles are the holder of emotions, any qualitative work on broadening the movement repertoire inevitably works to release the concomitant psychic associations and vice-versa: any work that loosens unconscious associations broadens expressive movement. In addition, both approaches facilitate the emotional warm-up through simple improvisational structures. These structures pave the way for the third aspect of Evan's work.

In-Depth Complex Improvisation—The Case of Pamela

Evan was prepared to structure an in-depth movement problem or theme out of any part of the dance therapy session. Movement directives evolved out of the physical warm-up, functional technique, the emotional warm-up (i.e., the projective techniques and mobilization of potential body movement) and/or the client's verbalizations. Evan frequently structured movement suggestions around thoughts and feelings the client had about his or her own body, including fears, fantasies, illusions and/or somatic identifications of oneself with others.

In the following case study of Pamela, Evan (1945-78) demonstrates the use of complex in-depth dance improvisation emphasizing dramatic enactment of past traumas.

In her work with Pamela, Evan began with the "movement interview," using specific exercises for the joint purpose of getting to know the physical strengths, weaknesses and potential of the client, as well as exploring how Pamela felt about and perceived her body. As Evan listened to and watched Pamela, she stayed alert for possible movement themes, which Pamela could later focus on.

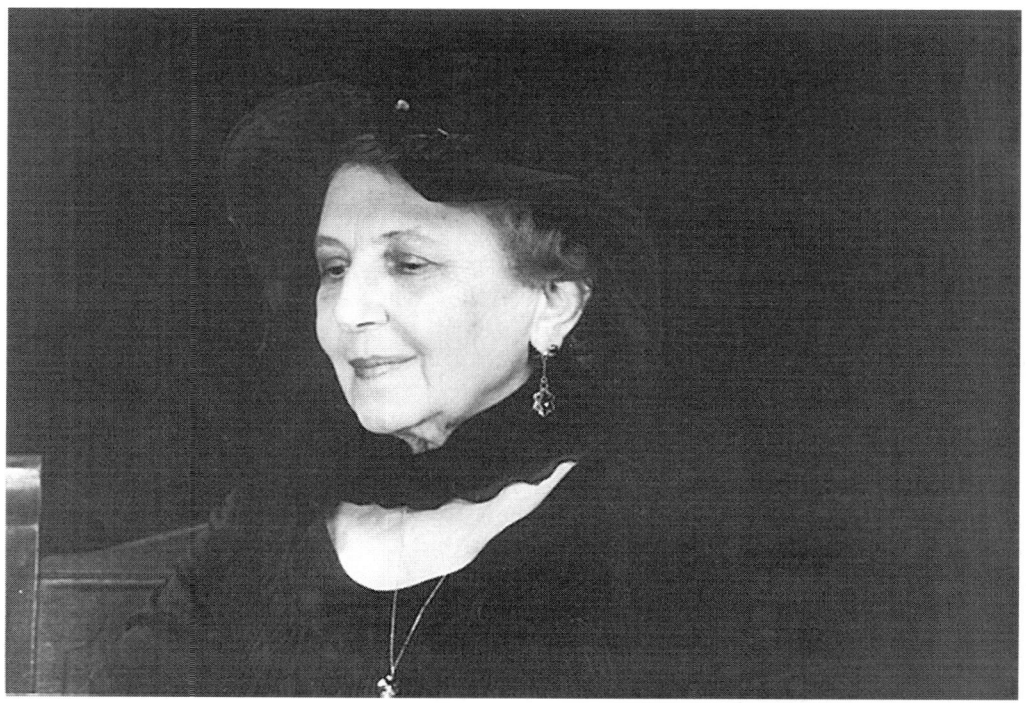

Blanche Evan (Photo courtesy The Blanche Evan Dance Foundation)

In her initial interviews, Pamela expressed many insecurities and doubts about her physical appearance. Evan decided to explore this further by asking Pamela to shut her eyes and describe her own body. Pamela gave a thorough description but said nothing of her arms and hands. When Evan questioned her about this, she replied that she felt the skin on her hands was like alligator skin. Evan did not pursue this further at this time. In regard to dancing, Pamela stated that she hated lying on the floor in dance class. She described her mother's body and walk, though it is not clear if Evan requested this information or if Pamela simply offered it. In her early discussion with Pamela, Pamela's preoccupation with her family's judgments of her body emerged. Evan believed that dance therapy could play an especially important role with individuals who have experienced severe family criticism and rejection of the parts of the body. Evan took note of Pamela's verbalizations in regard to family criticism and rejection as well as Pamela's initial omission of her hands and arms in her body description.

After gathering information, Evan asked Pamela to observe herself walking. Evan was surprised at the lack of reflection Pamela had concerning her own walk as compared to her detailed response to her body image. The only thing Pamela was very aware of was that she hated to stroll or walk slowly and that she would always feel an urgency to pass any slow walkers who were walking ahead of her. Next, Evan asked Pamela to run. Pamela said it was difficult to run without an image of why she was running. She also complained of a general lack of breath and endurance except when she had the image of running after someone. She was able to run without stopping for an hour. Along these same lines, Pamela also mentioned her extreme endurance when she was angry. Pamela was an actress and so she was aware of these peculiar variations in her patterns of endurance.

Further movement observation of Pamela revealed that when she ran, her feet, upon landing, did not make full impact with the ground. Evan spoke to Pamela about this and Pamela responded that she never put her full foot down because she disliked her feet, believing she was flat-footed and hence had ugly feet. Evan quickly intervened in this on a physical level, providing her with correct placement of her feet on the ground, which quickly corrected this problem.

In these early sessions, Evan asked Pamela to do several other exercises. In each, she noted Pamela's total use of her body. Some exercises went easily with little need for discussion. For example, Evan asked Pamela to lie down and place a drum on her abdomen to see what Pamela's breath capacity was and this Pamela did easily.

One theme that continually repeated itself in Evan's early observation was Pamela's frustration with people walking slowly in front of her. Because of the repetitiveness of this theme, Evan decided to pursue it. Hence, she asked Pamela for her associations to this image. In response, Pamela spoke of her mother who had two tendencies: one was to be very messy and take up a lot of space in the house and the other was to move slowly and in this way make Pamela late for appointments.

Evan, keenly aware of the importance of tempo and its effect on the body and emotional adjustment, explored how slowness affected Pamela in her own behavior. Pamela was able to recall periods of doing nothing when she had had plans to get things done. Also, when Pamela tried to lose weight, she frequently accompanied periods of not eating with not moving. Thus, while Pamela expressed resentment of her mother's patterns of slowness, her unhealthy attachment to her mother was evident in her own struggle with getting things done, her lack of endurance, her periods of doing nothing and coming late to therapy (a rare occurrence). In this case, Evan's major goal was that of helping Pamela to separate her own body image and behavior from that of her mother. The conflict between Pamela and her mother, centering around issues of timing, can be viewed from a nonverbal perspective in relation to Evan's definition of dance as it pertains to dance therapy: "space, time, body movement dynamics and content welded in unity" (1945-1978, n.p.). Thus, Evan's goal was to break through space, time, body movement dynamics and content for the purpose of unraveling this tight unit of behavior, which controlled Pamela on an unconscious level. The following describes the course of Evan's intervention with Pamela to help in achieving this goal of separation from the destructive relationship Pamela had with her mother.

After collecting pertinent information through exercises and discussion, Evan made her first major intervention. She asked Pamela to choose between two movement themes, which Evan posed. The first was to "assume the physical characteristics in movement of anyone who at any time had rejected her on the basis of bodily characteristics" (1945-1978, n.p.). The second was to "assume the physical characteristics in movement of her mother." Pamela chose the latter, though with initial resistance. In doing this Pamela began by becoming her mother, as she perceived her first in the present and then from the past. Evan explained to Pamela that she was "trying to take things out of her mind where they had been brewing and to begin to let them out through the channel of the body" (1945-1978, n.p.).

In Pamela's enactment of her mother from past memories she spontaneously dramatized three episodes of physical abuse. The enactment was composed of a rush of words, tears and movements. She suddenly became absorbed in the expressions of grief, anger, desperation and confusion as she switched in movement back and forth between the role of her mother violently assaulting her and her own frightened, angry and bewildered reactions, the reactions of a small child.

In the next session, Pamela returned saying she felt straighter in her posture and more able to tolerate and enjoy moving slowly. At this time, Evan emphasized that her goal was for Pamela to reclaim a positive identification with her own body and establish her own standards for personal evaluation, differentiated from the rejection and admonition of her mother. Evan took this opportunity to go over the functional technique exercises they had done so far and to encourage Pamela to do these exercises every day. Evan made the decision to emphasize rehabilitation of the body at this time when Pamela was feeling healthy and strong as a way to integrate and reinforce this good feeling. In this way the good feeling was solidified through its physical concomitant, good form.

Evan frequently integrated assignments outside of the therapy session with work in the session. Because of Pamela's feelings about her hands, Evan had her find pictures in artwork of hands. Her goal was to help Pamela find hands she responded positively to and to help her use these pictures to explore the conflicting feelings she had about her hands. Evan also provided her with exercises for her hands, but Pamela had an ambivalent response to these. When Evan saw that this work brought very disturbing memories back to

Pamela about her mother and also about having been pushed into dance classes as a child, Evan decided to temporarily suspend the exercise aspect of her work with Pamela.

During this period of intense ambivalence and blocking around the subject of hands, Evan stressed expressive movement activities employing dramatic enactments and other forms of body image work.

The following is an example of Evan's use of a dream to encourage exploration and insight through enactment and work on body image. Pamela had spoken of having several nightmares and waking up with partial paralysis. As Pamela described one of these dreams she was very agitated. Several sessions previously, Pamela had verbalized her problems quite persistently. Though Evan allowed this, realizing Pamela's desperate need to talk, Evan knew Pamela needed to return to movement in order to explore the subjective reality of the dream on a muscular level. When Evan saw Pamela becoming more agitated while discussing her dream, she finally interrupted, saying, "Stop talking and move" (1945-1978, n.p.). Evan felt that with this extra push for the nonverbal expression, Pamela would be much more able to probe her innermost associations, thoughts and feelings. This later became a theme in Evan's training of dance therapists, that is, an emphasis on bringing the expression back to its somatic reality (or source in the body) as opposed to encouraging verbal exploration and intellectualization.

Pamela complied with Evan's instruction and began to dance her dream. The movements prompted a cathartic release of tears along with more movement and verbalization, this time with deeper affect. In the dream enactment, Pamela externalized physically and verbally the sensation of women pursuing her aggressively and wanting something from her. In the dream Pamela was very small. She tried to hide but they came after her. She told Evan she wanted to be under the ground. When Evan threw her a blanket, she crouched under it and expressed ambivalence about touching her own body.

When Pamela finished the dream enactment, Evan asked her to look at her hands and describe what she saw. She then had her do the same with her face. Her response again indicated a negative and disturbed body image.

Evan then asked her when she remembered first not liking her body and she recalled it was when she was in a crib and ill. She recalled her arms being clamped down and not being able to breathe. Evan then asked Pamela to look at her hands again and in association to this she became aware of a sexual identity conflict, feeling neither male nor female but rather like an "oddity." Through her enactment of the dream along with the body image work (i.e., having Pamela talk about what she saw in different parts of her body) Pamela became aware of seeing her mother and grandmother as masculine and herself as very small in relation to them, as exemplified in her dreams.

The theme of being small, like the theme of moving slowly, returned regularly. Because of the persistence of this theme, Evan decided to explore Pamela's associations to "smallness." Evan approached this by telling Pamela she was going to give her a choice of three movement themes on which Pamela was asked to focus her movement work. Evan suggested that she begin with the theme "being little," but gave Pamela the option of beginning with one of the other themes if she preferred.

Pamela agreed to the first theme without hearing the others. When she began the movement work she crouched low to the ground. Evan insisted that she crouch even lower, becoming as little as possible. In doing this, Pamela became aware of a memory of falling in the bathroom while being bathed as a very small child and being laughed at by her mother and grandmother. She also recalled that this same feeling of smallness stayed with her in school as a child.

Summary

This approach appears to be that of exaggerating and, hence, externalizing the physical representation of the client's emotional state to fully experience her emotions. By encouraging the physical expression of the regression, the individual makes contact with early memories, as Pamela did (the fall in the bathroom). From this point, Evan and the client could probe this material that had been stored in the musculature, removing it from the individual's consciousness. In this way, Evan sought to take knowledge and insight out of the intellectualized, nonemotional state and into the reality of the individual's innermost emotions. Evan stressed regression (via body movement) in the service of the ego and for the purpose of total integration of the self.

Blanche Evan was a pioneer in the use of dance as therapy with the urban adult, who she perhaps humorously called the "normal neurotic." Evan believed that dance was man's natural tool for reuniting mind and body and that dance therapy was uniquely suited to reeducate neurotic urban adults to their natural expressive body rhythms, rendering them less vulnerable to external pressure. Evan's incorporation of creative dance improvisation (simple improvisation) with complex in-depth improvisation, complemented by her system of functional technique and her understanding of psychology, formed the foundation of Evan's dance therapy methodology.

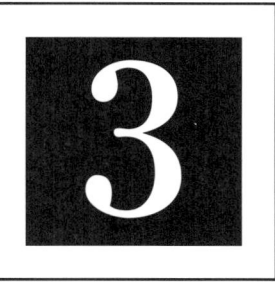 Liljan Espenak: Psychomotor Therapy

Liljan Espenak (1905-1988) was born in Bergen, Norway. In the late 1920s, she studied movement and dance in Dresden, Germany, with Mary Wigman at the Wigman Conservatory and toured with her as a member of her dance company for several years. Espenak received a diploma from the Wigman Conservatory and was a dance teacher at the Wigman School until 1934. She also attended the Berlin University and majored in physiology at the Hochschule fur Leibesubungen. During that time she had her own school of movement, which was accredited by the Prussian Board of Education. In addition to her education in dance and physiology, Espenak studied eurhythmics with Dalcroze and the gymnastic techniques of Mensendieck and Medau.

Fleeing Hitler's Germany, Espenak went first to England and then to the United States. In the 1940s, she taught dance in New York City at the YWCA and at the Wright Oral School for the Deaf. In the 1950s, she studied psychotherapy for three years at the Alfred Adler Institute and actively integrated her own knowledge of psychology with her already well-developed knowledge of the expressive, social and personal nature of dance. In 1961, Espenak became the Director of the Division of Creative Therapies, Institute for Mental Retardation, New York Medical College. Subsequently, she became assistant professor and coordinator of a postgraduate course in Psychomotor and Dance Therapy at New York Medical College's Mental Retardation Institute and a dance therapist at the Alfred Adler Mental Hygiene Clinic (Espenak, personal communication, 1980).

Espenak was responsible for influencing many second-generation dance therapists through her early course in dance therapy given at New York Medical College (1961-1981), the first of its kind offered on a postgraduate level. She was also well known for her work with people with developmental disabilities and for her work in private practice.

Like all of the early pioneers, Espenak did not consciously decide to become a dance therapist. Rather, her career moved naturally from modern dancing, to teaching creative dance, to dance therapy. Her original goal was to be an "ideal teacher," but she said, "… when groups became emotional later on …the process became dance therapy and I, a dance therapist" (1981, p. 10). Her first contact with dance therapy as a professional discipline was the early course she took with Marian Chace at the Turtle Bay Music School.

Espenak, like many others in the field, owed a great deal to Wigman and Laban. She believed that the combined contributions of Laban's theoretical and descriptive approach to dance and Wigman's creative improvisational approach formed the foundation upon which dance therapy is now structured.

> Unintentionally, this combination gave dance therapy its two most important facets, the free improvisation by the creative emotional self and the organizational structure needed to harness and project the emotions. (Espenak, 1979, p. 72)

Espenak's work combined the psychoanalytic theory of Adler with the mind/body theories of Lowen (1967, 1973) within the context of what she called "psychomotor therapy." She defined psychomotor therapy as an "extension of dance therapy through application of diagnostic tools for treatment on the medical model of observation, diagnosis, treatment" (Espenak, personal communication, 1985). This integration of Adlerian concepts into a psychomotor modality helped to strengthen and broaden the formulations on which dance therapists base their work.

Espenak wrote several excellent papers and the book *Dance Therapy: Theory and Application* (1981), in which her ideas were clearly outlined and discussed. She also developed a set of movement diagnostic tests and in the 1960s began training students at New York Medical College in psychomotor therapy.

Theory

Our discussion of Espenak's theoretical base focuses on her integration of Adlerian concepts into the discipline of dance therapy. Espenak noted that Adler began his professional career as a neurologist in Vienna and she believed his early training influenced his "holistic" (mind/body) approach to psychology (1979).

Espenak stressed three major Adlerian concepts as being integral to dance therapy: the aggression drive, inferiority feelings and social feelings (i.e., the need to be accepted by the community). Espenak also referred to a fourth classification of Adler's, that is, life style and first memory, which will be discussed in the following section on Espenak's methodology.

Adler's acknowledgement of the aggression drive and his belief that it was as important and significant in development as the sexual drive (libido) were revolutionary. Freud, at first, negated Adler's emphasis on the aggression drive and sibling rivalry, but toward the end of his life, stated openly his acceptance of Adler's major contribution and acknowledged his own short-sightedness in this area (Ansbacher, 1956).

Espenak believed that the aggression drive was natural and necessary to life and if repressed, the dynamic force and life-giving source in the personality would also be repressed (Ansbacher, 1956; Espenak, 1979).

> When aggression drive is seen as original life force, life energy, unconscious desire to live, it becomes an expression of health and natural dynamics for which we must be deeply grateful, if illness or early repressions have not extinguished it. Dealing with suppressed aggression drive through dealing with anger is a frequent and important goal of psychomotor therapy. (Espenak, 1979, p. 76)

In her discussion of the aggression drive, Espenak frequently referred to the Adlerian concept of childhood feelings of inferiority. Espenak integrated both Adler's aggression and inferiority theories with Freud's libidinal concept of the pleasure principle.

> Without the biological aggression drive and the pleasure principle, the inferiority feelings would not result in striving for superiority, but be accepted as unchangeable... Inferiority feelings then remain together with the developing recognition of the powerful surroundings and acceptance of their interaction. The aggressive drive, however, will lead to nonacceptance of this position and result in striving for superiority as a means of obtaining the pleasure principle. (Espenak, 1979, p. 76)

In other words, the human instinct toward aggression combines with the child's awareness of one's physically or emotionally inferior role in society. These two aspects of existence push the individual to find ways to master the environment and the self.

Espenak believed that working directly on the body, developing physical strength, grounding and an expressive movement vocabulary could counteract the original feelings of inferiority and dependency. For example, the acts of stretching, pulling, pushing, leaping, running and skipping all engendered feelings of taking charge, defying gravity, making one's self larger and better and generally enhancing feelings of wellbeing. Moreover, as the movement sequences in which the individual engages become more intricate, requiring greater control and mastering, a natural sense of one's potential ability to learn and conquer combats the original feeling of inferiority (Espenak, 1979).

Espenak's theoretical framework also incorporated Adler's emphasis on the importance of developing social feeling and cooperation. He believed that if the individual's abilities in this area were either unused because of actual physical isolation of some kind or repressed due to personal rejection or deprivation in early childhood, a sense of stability and effectiveness regarding relations and rapport with the broader community was unattainable. This then encouraged feelings of insecurity, anger and fear (Adler, 1927; Espenak, 1979).

Espenak incorporated Adler's stress on social rapport in connection with the use of dance therapy in groups. She noted that Adler began using verbal groups for their therapeutic value with children in Europe in the early 1900s. It was Espenak's belief that "dancing together and interrelating singly with a group, is an ideal form for discovering and developing social feeling" (Espenak, 1979, p. 77). In regard to specific theory concerning the therapeutic value of group dance therapy, she referred to the values familiar to most forms of group therapy, such as support, rapport, validation, breaking through isolation and receiving group feedback.

Espenak often used group work as the second phase of a patient's treatment program. The first phase, individual work with the patient, prepared him or her for the development of social feeling within a group dance therapy approach.

Methodology

Espenak integrated her thinking with her knowledge of the work of Alexander Lowen. Her work, which began in the late 1950s and early 1960s, reflected the spirit of the times as well as a similarity with other contemporary trends within the dance therapy discipline.

Espenak's approach to the use of movement in psychotherapy put emphasis on what she called laying "the groundwork for movement" (1979, p. 80). When the inhibitions and/or repressions of the individual did not allow for free movement of certain parts of the body or for spontaneous movement expression, Espenak facilitated the movement process through structuring movement sequences designed to strengthen certain parts of the body, loosen and relax constricted body parts and/or help the patient to experience body parts previously out of the patient's conscious awareness. This approach overlapped in some aspects with Lowen's bioenergetic work and with Blanche Evan's functional technique.

In Espenak's (1972) paper, "Body-Dynamics and Dance in Individual Psychotherapy," she described three cases in which she used the introduction of certain movement sequences for the purpose of building an expressive movement vocabulary and a tolerance for the expression of specific emotions. Espenak used her own set of movement diagnostic tests as a guide to identifying the strengths and weaknesses in the patient's psychophysical integration. This set of tests was administered at the start of treatment and at three-month intervals thereafter. She then formed a treatment plan based on her diagnostic findings.

One of these case studies (1972) provides a good example of her clinical practice. This is the case of a patient, "O.," referred by a psychiatrist because of his disassociation from his body. Because of O.'s lack of physical awareness and immobility in certain parts of his body, he was unsuccessful in his desire to be an actor.

> Upon testing, O. indicated numbness in the sacrum and at the base of the neck. His legs seemed to work independently of his torso and he carried his shoulders and head as a separate unit. The chest was immobile and sunken; the head forward as if in hopelessness. This demonstrates a lack of coordination in the body between the upper and lower parts, due to the inactivity and numbness of the sacrum. The first step in therapy was to stimulate and establish control in the sacrum. Therefore, the first sessions were devoted to learning the sensation of kicking the floor. His kicks had no force and manifested no improvement in coordination until his sacrum was unlocked by having him [correctly] push a heavy object, in this case, a piano, thus forcing action through the sacrum to the legs. (Espenak, 1972, p. 115)

In this brief sequence, Espenak demonstrated her use of the diagnostic movement test as her guide to the psychomotor needs of the patient. She saw tension in the musculature of the sacrum and splits in the integration and coordination of the patient's body parts, legs independent of torso and head and shoulders as a separate unit. From this body analysis she decided to start by stimulating sensation and control in the sacrum area. She had the patient kick the floor as a means of releasing tension in the constricted sacrum. However, when this was unsuccessful, she suggested another movement configuration, a push, which brought about immediate results. Then, after she worked with O. to release specific areas of tension and facilitate control of new areas of the body, O. brought a record to the session for improvisation. Upon moving to this record, he displayed his anger in a new and direct way. He revealed new areas of constriction in the upper chest and neck. Therefore, revitalization of these areas became the next step in treatment.

In her continued work with O., Espenak also used relaxation exercises, which helped to bring O. in touch with these constrictions in his body and the need to relax in these areas. Espenak noted that as a result of these structured movement sequences and relaxation exercises, there was an increase in the scope, both physically and imaginatively, of his improvisations.

Once this physical improvement in coordination with the subsequent increase in self worth was achieved, a creative approach to reach him emotionally was introduced. O. was encouraged to imagine and imitate the ruler of Egypt, the Pharaoh. In watching O. put this image into action, it was clear that he had found a new sense of power (Espenak, personal communication, 1987) and that this new feeling about himself could be further encouraged by the acting out of creative imagery. The sequence that emerged was:

1. Building strength, awareness and relaxation into specific areas of the body;
2. Suggesting certain movement sequences that affect the areas of the body where excess tension or numbness has occurred and
3. Using improvisation and music as an active way to integrate the body's newly released energy sources into creative, expressive dance movement.

In this brief sequence, Espenak started by teaching or initiating specific movement sequences, like kicking the floor and pushing the piano. She had a specific plan regarding which muscles needed usage and strengthening and which muscles needed release.

Movement Diagnostic Tests

Espenak developed a set of Movement Diagnostic Tests for use with all her clients with both developmental and emotional disabilities (1970). She described the background that led to the development of the tests as follows:

> Wigman's work was wholly of a creative nature built on Laban's theories, giving it structure. Using this in a medical setting, as in the Clinic for Mental Retardation, forced me to adapt the material to more scientific use—hence, the formula Observation-Diagnosis-Treatment, as in other therapeutic processes. This gave birth to the Diagnostic Tests. (Espenak, personal communication, 1985)

The Movement Diagnostic Tests are grouped into six basic categories that provide information about

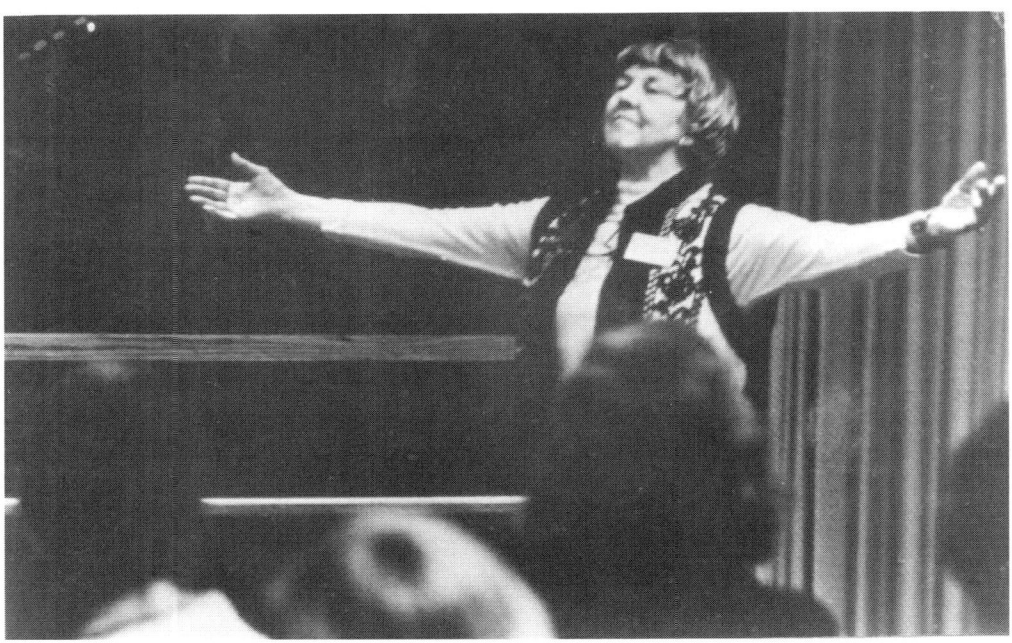

Liljan Espenak demonstrating one of her diagnostic tests (Photo courtesy Fran Levy)

"the positive and negative components of the patient's personality" (1970, p. 10).

The first category deals with emotional response and consists of two tests. Test 1A, "Body Image," is a muscular test in which the patient is asked to walk on his or her toes. The patient's posture during this activity reveals information about his or her ego strength and self-assertion. Test 1B, "Emotional Response (Spatial Relationships)," involves improvisation, either in the form of free interpretation of music or through the use of suggested themes, images and/or symbols, which relate to the patient's life. This provides information about "the life style and emotional climate of the patient" (1970, p. 10).

Test II, "Degree of Dynamic Drive (Force Adjustment)," demonstrates "the physical and motivational energy applied in performance of a task" (1970, p. 10). In this case, the task is pushing a heavy object. Espenak found that the degree of energy displayed by the patient could indicate the degree to which he can be challenged by the therapist.

Test III, "Control of Dynamic Drive (Rhythm, Time Concepts)," deals with the patient's sense of time.

> Control and organization of time reveals both the individual's inherent personal rhythm (as a sum total of his personality) as well as his ability to adjust to any given organization from outside (i.e., to cooperate). (Espenak, 1970, p. 11)

This test stresses breathing as the most natural rhythm in one's life and thus an indication of one's inner feelings. Breathing is closely interconnected with both physiological and emotional changes in the body.

Test IV, "Coordination (Body-Awareness and Locomotion)," is a test of the patient's movement-flow as indicated in walking.

> In normal locomotion, the sacrum performs a small wheel-like movement which allows a smooth and relaxed change of weight from one foot to another. In case of disturbance this wheel-like action will be hampered and the execution will be jerky or rigidly inactive. (Espenak, 1970, p. 12)

Espenak saw coordination as the physical expression of the individual's mental and emotional control. "The movement of walking is ... the best natural demonstration of ... the interaction of body and mind" (1970, p. 12).

Test V, "Endurance (Constancy)," measures the patient's "kinesthetic drive combined with mind control, endurance" (1970, p. 12). It utilizes various tolerance tests, including the use of repetitions of movement, to determine the patient's attention span, ability to concentrate and tolerance for frustration and stress.

Test VI, "Physical Courage (Anxiety States)," measures the patient's ability to perform movements that may seem somewhat threatening. These include "walking backwards, walking a spiral leaning more and more towards the center (experiencing force of gravity) and several floor exercises, rocking and rolling backwards" (1970, p. 12). Anxieties relating to movement, such as fear of falling or running downstairs, are closely linked to the fears the patient experiences in everyday life.

Summary

Liljan Espenak, a pioneer in the field of dance therapy, developed and directed the first dance movement therapy postgraduate training program in the early 1960s, both academic and practicum. The program was in existence until 1981, when she discontinued it in order to devote her time to reaching a broader group of students through weekend workshops in the United States and abroad.

In addition, Espenak organized conceptual formulations that integrated her findings from her Diagnostic Movement Tests into a complete psychomotor therapy treatment program. The goals of her work were to integrate and strengthen both the mind and body, believing that one deeply influences and is intricately connected to the other.

Finally, Espenak was particularly noted for her excellent integration of Adlerian psychological concepts into both a theory and therapy of mind and body.

SECTION B

Major Pioneers on the West Coast

Mary Whitehouse: Movement-in-Depth: A Jungian Approach to Dance Therapy

Mary Whitehouse (1911-1979) was a major dance therapy pioneer who worked and taught on the west coast. Her teachings have profoundly influenced many major contemporary leaders in the field. Whitehouse, whose early work began in the 1950s, wrote, "Odd, but I turned into a dance therapist without realizing it, simply because no such thing existed when I started" (1979, p. 51). She knew something was different in her teaching of dance, but didn't have a name for it. Later she came to call her work "movement-in-depth" (Wallock 1977, Pallaro 1999).

During this early period, Whitehouse read an article on dance therapy written by Marian Chace. Her response to the article was one of acknowledgment: she realized for the first time that she was not alone, that others were also using dance as a way to reach people on new levels. The individuals working with Chace, like those who came to Whitehouse, had little interest in dance as performance. They were seeking something more personal.

Whitehouse worked both one-on-one and in groups with individuals whom she considered to be fairly well functioning. She believed that the early pioneers in the field differed from each other greatly according to the population with whom and the setting in which they worked. Whitehouse frequently worked with dance students in her own studio.

Whitehouse believed that with students, a greater emphasis could be put on uncovering unconscious material, whereas with hospitalized patients, due to a more fragile ego structure, greater stress needed to be placed on emotional support and providing patients with more structured forms of expressive movement. While both populations relied on the strengths of the therapist during sessions, students generally, she contended, could tolerate less therapist direction and more psychic probing than hospitalized patients.

Many of Whitehouse's dance students were already involved in verbal psychotherapy and thus frequently possessed both a movement and psychoanalytic vocabulary prior to their work with her. This often assisted them in utilizing the Whitehouse method of self-discovery through movement (Whitehouse, 1963).

Two major areas of study influenced the work of Mary Whitehouse. The first was her intensive study of modern dance at the Mary Wigman School in Dresden, Germany. The second was her experiences in Jungian psychoanalysis. Of her Wigman training, she wrote:

> The Wigman training prepared me for a particular approach although I did not know it at the time; it made room for improvisation, placing value on the creativity of the people moving. It assumed that you would not be learning to dance if you had nothing to say. (Whitehouse, 1979, p. 52)

Although she also studied with and was greatly influenced by Martha Graham and others, it appears that her work with Wigman left the deepest imprint. She stated:

> I came home from Germany with improvisation so much a part of my training, so available to me as a teacher, that I was appalled to find that it was not accepted over here. Now it is the other way around, nobody wants to stand still for a plié because they are so busy being expressive. (Wallock, 1977, p. 69)

In the 1950s and early 1960s, Whitehouse went through a period when dance lost importance to her personally (Whitehouse, 1979). Later, as a result of her exposure to Jungian analysis, she came to view her own dance movement with increasing attention to symbolism and meaning. This revitalized her interest in dance as a form of self-expression, communication and revelation.

At the same time, Whitehouse was also reevaluating the word "dance" in terms of her teachings.

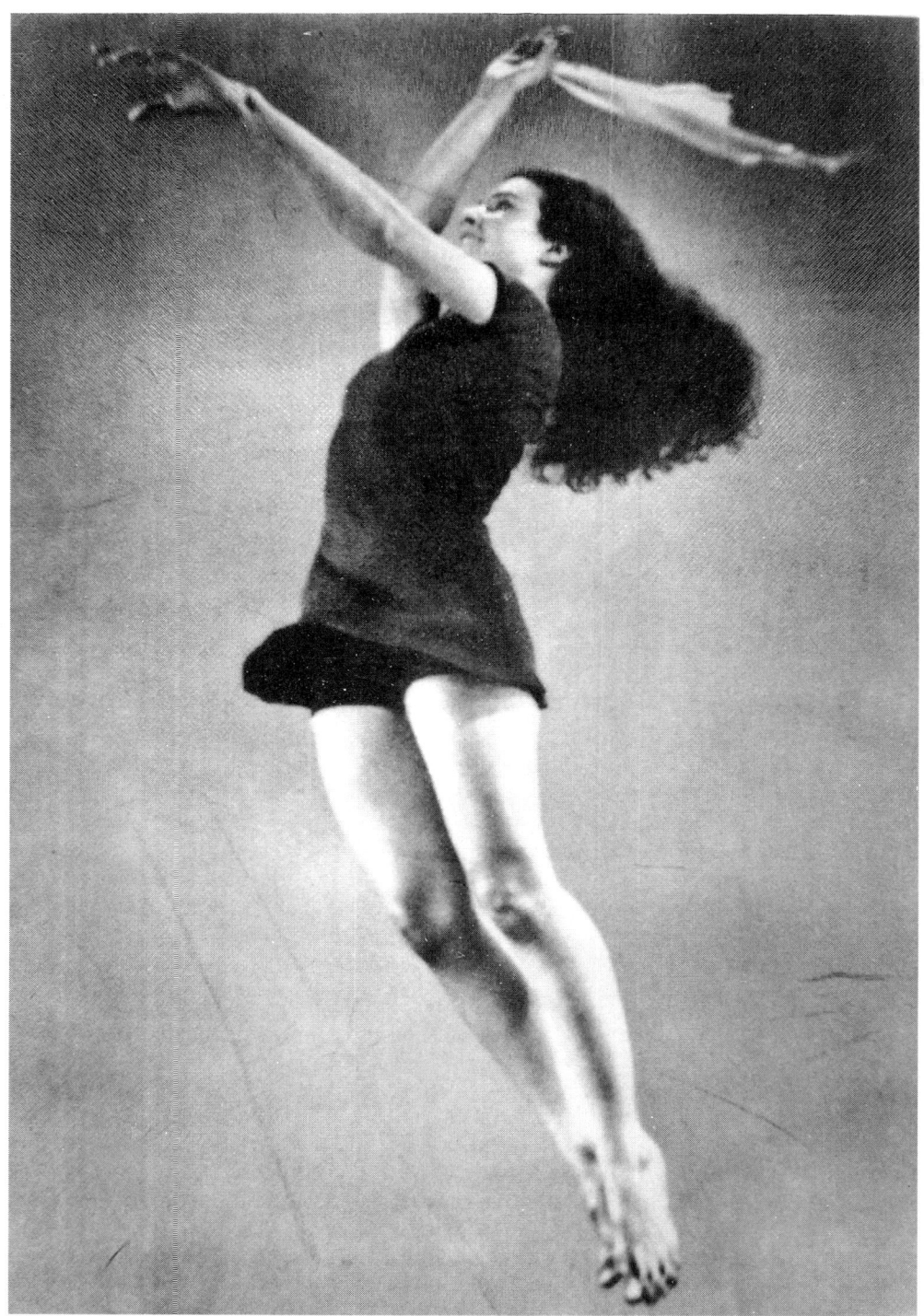

Mary Whitehouse in her youth as a dancer (Photo courtesy Feather King)

> Whatever it was, we were traveling away from dance. I had to call it movement. In order to find what it was that truly moved people, I needed to give up images in them and in myself of what it meant to dance. (1979, p. 53)

Whitehouse thought that the word "dance" denoted a finished product. She viewed the therapeutic use of dance as a process of delving unselfconsciously into the deeper layers of personality, the source of body movement (Wallock, 1977). Accordingly, she did not see this spontaneous type of movement expression as one that could be reproduced or repeated and still maintain the same depth of personal meaning. Hence, resulting from her own personal experiences with dance and movement, combined with her deeper insight into personality obtained through her exposure to Jungian analysis, she used the term "movement-in-depth" to describe this new level of dance movement expression.

In later life, Whitehouse underwent a long struggle with multiple sclerosis. Faced with decreasing motor ability, she nevertheless continued her work. Her final sessions and writings were conducted from a wheelchair. Today, the work of Mary Whitehouse continues to have a major impact on dance therapy.

Theory

When asked to describe her theoretical model of dance therapy, Whitehouse began by stating her philosophical view of a theoretical model:

> I have to be honest—presenting a polished theoretical model to students interested in dance therapy, without admitting that it is achieved in the first place alone, with pain and struggle, may not be true for a second generation, but needs to be known. If it is not, such a theoretical model can be easily learned without any reference to personal gifts or temperament. It can be adopted wholesale and imposed on patients, as clearly as any teacher of dance takes an acquired style and imposes it on her students. (Whitehouse, 1979, p. 53)

As mentioned earlier, Whitehouse was most strongly influenced by her work with Wigman in the modality of dance movement improvisation and her exposure to Jungian psychoanalysis. Through the integration of these, she developed a unique theoretical and practical approach to dance movement therapy. The major issues relevant to her approach are: 1) Kinesthetic Awareness, 2) Polarity, 3) Active Imagination, 4) Authentic Movement and 5) Therapeutic Relationship/Intuition.

Kinesthetic Awareness

Kinesthetic awareness is, Whitehouse believed, the individual's internal sense of his or her physical self. She believed that some individuals naturally had more kinesthetic sense than others but that in either case it could be awakened, developed and encouraged (1963).

> ... if kinesthetic sense is never developed or seldom used, it becomes unconscious and one is in the situation ... that I can only call living in the head, which fact the body faithfully reflects, since it must move, by acquiring a whole series of distortions, short circuits, strains and mannerisms accumulated from years and years of being assimilated to mental images of choice, necessity, value and appropriateness. (Whitehouse, 1963, p. 6)

Whitehouse discussed kinesthetic awareness as the individual's ability to make a "subjective connection" (1963, p. 11) with how it felt to move in a certain way. She contrasted kinesthetic sense with exercises, which encouraged muscular release but without the "corresponding experience of ... personal identity" (1963, p. 11). Whitehouse believed that it was not enough to work with the body mechanically, facilitating release as if the body were an object on which things occurred with no subjective responses. Instead, Whitehouse stressed the body as the subject/organism that personally reacts and responds to everything that happens.

Polarity

Whitehouse believed, along the lines of Jungian thought, that polarity was present in all aspects of life and emotions.

> Applied physically, it is astonishing that no action can be accomplished without the operation of two sets of muscles—one contracting and one extending. This is the presence of polarity inherent in the pattern of movement. (Whitehouse, 1979, p. 55)

Influenced by her Jungian training, Whitehouse put special emphasis on the concept of polarity and how it affects the functioning of the body and mind, as well as how one can observe polarized drives during the dance therapy process.

Whitehouse (1979) stressed that things are never black and white in life. That is, while we may be forced to choose one path in life over another or one form of expression over another, the one not chosen for conscious expression does not go away, it simply goes unrecognized. Moreover, in its disguised and unconscious state, it continues to exert pressure and create conflict.

Because dance inherently engages opposites, "... a dancer does not stop to think of curved/straight, closed/open, narrow/wide, up/down, heavy/light—these are a myriad pairs" (1979, p. 55), the dancer automatically engages in polarized expression. Hence, the modality of dance is perfect for the spontaneous release of opposing drives.

Active Imagination

Active imagination, the third aspect of the Whitehouse method, grew out of her concern for kinesthetic awareness and polarities. Whitehouse applied active imagination, a Jungian method of freeing one's associations to allow in all levels of conscious and unconscious experience, physically in the dance therapy process. Whitehouse stated:

> ... the inner sensation, allowing the impulse to take the form of physical action is active imagination in movement, just as following the visual image is active imagination in fantasy. It is here that the most dramatic psycho-physical connections are made available to consciousness. (Wallock, 1977, p. 48)

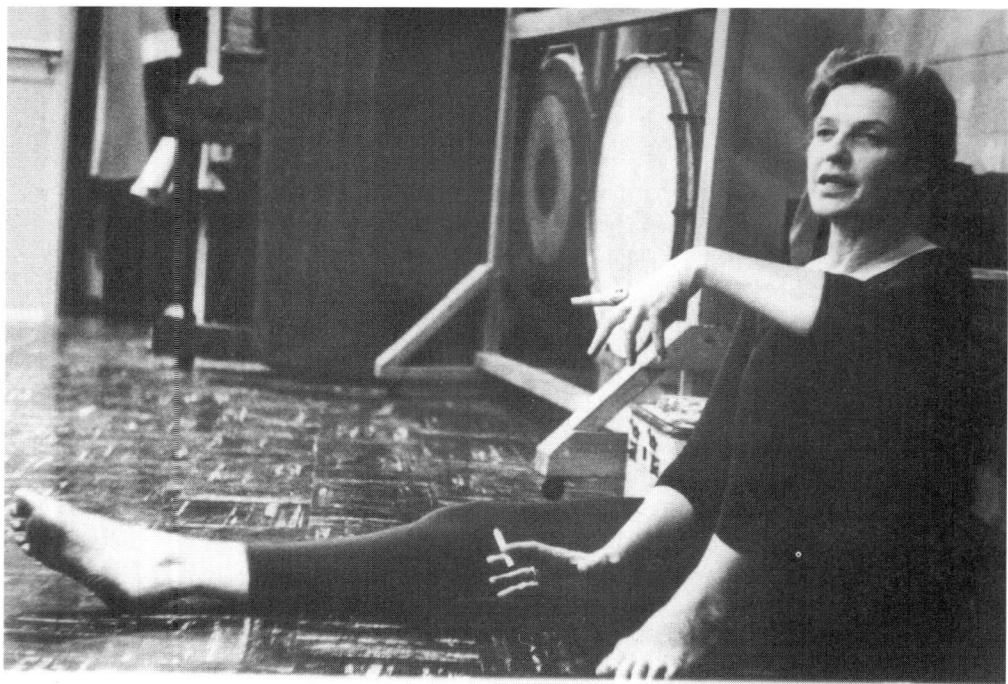

Mary Whitehouse, early 1960s, conducting a group in her California studio
(Photo courtesy Feather King)

Whitehouse's basic goal was to release unconscious emotions which she believed became "buried in the body, in tissues, muscles and joints ..." (Wallock, 1977, p. 50) that is, to make the unconscious conscious. She believed that this could occur if the individual was provided with the proper supportive environment, movement vocabulary and facilitation (see Methodology below). Active imagination facilitates this process as follows:

> While consciousness looks on, participating but not directing, cooperating but not choosing, the unconscious is allowed to speak whatever and however it likes. Its language appears in the form of painted or verbal images that may change rapidly, biblical speech, poetry (even doggerel), sculpture and dance. There is no limit and no guarantee of consistency. Images, inner voices, move suddenly from one thing to another. The levels they come from are not always personal levels; a universal human connection with something much deeper than the personal ego is represented. (1979, p. 58)

In this quote, Whitehouse described the psychoanalytic practice of releasing repressed unconscious material through the process of loosening and relaxing the ego's defenses against spontaneous expression. In addition, she supported Jung's concept of the personal unconscious being united with an unconscious that extends beyond the personal self to a universal or "collective" unconscious. Finally, she was pointing to the importance of the conscious self or ego, as the observer who watches and participates but does not censor or control the individual's physical expressions. In one sense, she was describing the process of building the powers of the observing ego through the mechanism of freeing associations by way of body movement. In another sense, she was describing a spiritual process of expressing universal forms, which would not normally be part of one's conscious movement repertoire.

Through the process of active imagination in movement, Whitehouse believed that one could experience what Jung called the "Self." The "Self," with an upper case "S," stood for the unconscious that goes beyond the immediate and personal concerns of the ego, that is the self, with a lower case "s". When Whitehouse spoke of the "Self," she was referring to a specific Jungian definition of the unconscious. However, Whitehouse did not develop a more clear or concise definition for this concept. Zenoff (personal communication, 1980), one of her protégés, said of Whitehouse's work:

> She resisted talking about theoretical concepts. "You don't have to understand it—it is the beauty of the unknown." When I tried to pin her down, I felt scattered, but she had a focus, even if I couldn't comprehend it.

Many of Whitehouse's students, now major leaders in the field, have studied Jungian psychology in depth and have attempted to broaden and clarify many of these concepts as they relate to the expressive movement process.

What is clear is that active imagination can become a movement experience only if it is expressed on a level of movement that is not consciously directed. This level of movement Whitehouse called "authentic movement." In 1933, John Martin was the first to use the term authentic movement to describe what he experienced while watching a performance by Mary Wigman. In light of Wigman's profound influence on Mary Whitehouse, it is not surprising that Whitehouse described her students' movements by the same term. Today when the term "authentic movement" is used in dance therapy, it often refers specifically to the Whitehouse approach.

Authentic Movement

Authentic movement is necessary if active imagination through the musculature is to take place. Whitehouse described authentic movement as being

> ... in and out of the Self at the moment it is done. Nothing is in it that is not inevitable, simple ... undiluted by any pretense.... It can be just one hand turning over or it can be the whole body [in motion]. (Fay, 1977, p. 69)

Whitehouse contrasted authentic movement with its opposite, "invisible movement" (Whitehouse, 1979, p. 57). Invisible movements are movements that lack a genuine emotional charge. The word "invisible" referred to the invisibility not of the muscular action but rather of the underlying emotions or thoughts, which the movement fails to express. Instead, a stylization of action or muscular rigidity is visible. Whitehouse believed that this basic difference in movement quality was, again, a demonstration of polarities, a tendency to express and a tendency to repress or hide.

In order to clarify the qualitative difference between these two levels of movement, Whitehouse (1979) used the term "I am moved" to describe the experience of authentic or visible movement and the expression "I move" to describe controlled or invisible movement. She explained, "'I move' is clear knowledge that I personally, am moving. I choose to move ..." (1979, p. 57), whereas "I am moved" is a moment when the individual relinquishes control and choice, allowing the "Self" precedence in moving the body freely. Whitehouse described this process as "surrender that cannot be explained, repeated exactly, sought for or tried out" (1979, p. 57).

It is interesting to note that in an unpublished article (prepared for the Analytic Psychology Club), Whitehouse made a statement not seen in her later publications but significant to understanding the development of her theoretical framework. She did not make a clear distinction between the movements of the conscious self and the movements of the unconscious self. She stated:

> The core of the movement experience is the sensation of moving and being moved.... Ideally, both are present in the same instant and it may be literally an instant. It is a moment of total awareness, the coming together of what I am doing and what is happening to me. It cannot be anticipated, explained, specifically worked for, nor repeated exactly. (1963, p. 4)

In this quote, Whitehouse described the experience of authentic movement, though this label was not yet used. Compare her statement here, "It cannot be anticipated, explained, specifically worked for, nor repeated exactly" with her later (1979) description of authentic movement as "surrender that cannot be explained, repeated exactly, sought for or tried out" (p. 57). Although these two descriptions are almost identical, there is an important difference.

In her 1963 paper, there was an emphasis on the spontaneous synthesis in movement of "what I am doing" (i.e., "I move") and "what is happening to me" (i.e., "I am moved"). Whitehouse appeared to be looking for and appreciating a total and unified movement experience (authentic movement) in which there is simultaneous awareness of both "I move" and "I am moved." In her later literary contribution, however, authentic movement referred not to the unified movement experience described in her earlier writing but to a pure "I am moved" experience. In the later work, there appeared to be more emphasis on the separation between "I move" and "I am moved," implying that any experience of the former would dilute the authenticity of the latter.

This difference seems to hinge on a changing definition of "I move." Originally, this term was used to describe an experience of "myself moving" that did not imply self-consciousness or external controls, but rather an observing part of self that looked on without directing or judging. Later, however, Whitehouse began using this concept to describe controlled "invisible" movements, which failed to express underlying (authentic) emotions and thoughts. Thus, "I move" took on a totally different meaning, making it impossible to coexist with visible (authentic) movement.

It can be argued that this change is simply a matter of semantics. On the other hand, Whitehouse may have become more extreme in her later life in response to the dramatic and tragic physical changes she experienced during her long struggle with multiple sclerosis. This must have had a profound influence on her perceptions and may have led her to emphasize the "I am moved" experience.

It is likely that Whitehouse viewed the movement process as a continuum ranging from one polarity (invisible movement of the conscious self) to the other (authentic movement of the unconscious self) and stressed varying degrees of each depending on the individual's needs at different times. It seems clear, however, that Whitehouse never wanted to *totally* remove consciousness from movement. Given her belief about polarities, that "there is no such thing as choosing only one end of the scale" (1979, p. 55), the author believes it is more likely that she wished to unite these opposites, to achieve a total awareness that encompassed both conscious and unconscious movement.

During improvisational work, Whitehouse did help individuals to temporarily relegate consciousness to a silent observing role, thus allowing the unconscious to express itself via authentic movement (active imagination in movement). However, this does not necessarily mean that the authentic movement process is totally unconscious. Although the unconscious is given free rein to express itself, the conscious mind is still present in a silent observing role, "participating, but not directing, cooperating but not choosing" (Whitehouse, 1979, p. 58). If the conscious mind is "participating" and "cooperating," there must be some element of "I move" present during the "I am moved" experience. It is possible, therefore, to conclude that Whitehouse did not aim to guide her clients to one extreme end of the movement continuum, but rather to help them find a point along the continuum or perhaps transcend it, where "I move" and "I am moved" coexist and can be simultaneously experienced.

Therapeutic Relationship/Intuition

The foundation of Whitehouse's approach to dance therapy was her stress on the therapeutic relationship and intuition. She believed that the therapist was at different times a teacher, a mediator and a leader (Wallock, 1977). Her approach to the therapeutic relationship was trusting her intuition first, then helping clients to trust their intuition and finally emphasizing the therapist's ability to begin at the level of readiness that the client presented.

> Starting where the client is can only mean willingness to be anonymous oneself in favor of observing, quickly and without barriers, what is available to that individual. (Whitehouse, 1979, p. 60)

Whitehouse stressed that this seemingly simple process was often quite difficult to accomplish. It required that the dance therapist put aside preconceptions of what the client should do and instead, take the role of not knowing what is correct for a particular individual, letting the individual find his or her own solution.

Whitehouse emphasized two concepts in her approach that may seem contradictory, yet with deeper examination prove complementary. The first is the skill of the therapist in exerting restraint while the client initiates his or her own movements and/or thoughts. The effort to start where the client is means waiting for the client to evolve and shape his or her own movements without imposition or direction from the therapist. The nondirection of movement sequences is translated to the client as room for internally prompted movement.

The second is for the therapist to trust his or her intuition in directing the client while being prepared to accept the client's own judgment as to whether these directive suggestions are helpful or not. Rooted in this approach is the therapist's own security and nondefensiveness, which allows the client to respond either positively or negatively to the suggestions and to the therapist.

What superficially appears to be opposing rules is actually the therapist's considerable skill in perceiving the point where therapeutic intervention is needed or a moment in which waiting patiently is more productive.

Methodology

The intervention styles of Whitehouse, similar to the other pioneers in dance therapy, were at times directive/externally prompted or nondirective/internally prompted or a combination of the two. This was determined by the client's readiness and needs. In her publications, Whitehouse emphasized the importance of the quality of the therapeutic relationship, without which, she believed, the therapeutic movement process would not unfold.

Whitehouse stressed the role of the therapist as the mediator and mirror. Although she did not give an exact definition of what she meant by mediator, she did give the following statement in her interview with Wallock (1977).

> It is as if there is a certain amount a person can do alone and beyond that they have to come to somebody else to really see what they are doing.... I often experienced my eyes as the eyes that were looking so that the person could shut his. Much of the movement was done with closed eyes, even when up on the feet.... Somehow, if I were looking, the person could afford to let go and let it happen because I was watching. (p. 72)

Whitehouse's contribution is in a style of intervention rather than an emphasis on particular techniques. She once stated, "I have an approach, not a method, much less a theory" (1963, p. 3). Whitehouse's major mode of intervention, which has become very influential among those contemporary dance therapists who work in private studios, was active imagination through the medium of movement. The various techniques she used to begin sessions all aimed to eventually lead her clients to improvisational work, through which the active imagination process could be expressed.

Whitehouse often started a session by offering a quick choice to the client, for example, "What would be most comfortable, easiest—lying, sitting, standing?" (1979, p. 60). She found that individuals differed in their choices of a starting position and that providing a choice gave the individual a chance to make an independent decision about how he or she was most comfortable and in what direction the session would go. In this respect, Whitehouse's approach was primarily a client-centered one.

Another way Whitehouse began sessions was by teaching dance technique and/or simple movement tasks or ideas. She drew primarily on Martha Graham's technique, but her style of imparting this technique was uniquely her own. Whitehouse stressed that teaching dance technique and providing simple movement tasks gave the client a feeling of self-confidence as well as greater kinesthetic awareness and thus facilitated the move to more difficult tasks or ideas. This theme appears again and again amongst the early pioneers.

Some of her protégés, such as Jane Manning and Judith Fried (personal communication, 1985), believe that Whitehouse's greatest gift was her ability to transform the learning of dance technique into a deeply personal and emotionally unifying experience. Their memories of Whitehouse focus on her use of dance technique and simple movements as a way of getting clients in touch with their inner feelings and thus preparing them for in-depth improvisational work.[1]

An example of starting sessions with simple movement tasks might be the use of warm-up structures. For example, she might suggest that clients work first only with specific body parts (arms, legs, face) or she might encourage using only the right side or left side of the body for a certain movement theme (Zenoff, personal communication, 1980)

Whatever the style of opening a session, the client at some point will usually need help deciding on the next step. Whitehouse acknowledged the responsibility the therapist faces in helping the client become sensitive to and able to express his or her own movement process. It is in this situation that the therapeutic relationship becomes essential, with intuition guiding the therapist in deciding whether or not intervention is needed and if so, what kind of intervention would be most helpful.

Whitehouse assessed the clients' ability to allow movements and ideas to flow freely. Sometimes she utilized music to encourage individuals to begin to dance. If she saw that a client was capable of allowing a free flow of thoughts and feelings in movement, she then provided an unstructured environment within which the client could make all of his or her own movement decisions.

When this was not possible, she provided movement themes or broad creative structures within which the client could project thoughts and feelings through movement. For example, to provoke imagery and associations she might suggest they were in a cocoon and then ask if it was large or small, stiff or soft, unyielding or flexible.

As discussed earlier the projective technique was commonly used by dance therapists to facilitate expression and insight, but was initiated in different ways. This creative and exploratory style of intervention was an integral part of the creative and modern dance movement from which dance therapy was built. It appears that, for the dance therapist, the use of the projective technique was as natural as the use of dance itself.

Whitehouse used metaphors and projective techniques in movement improvisation. In the following example, she gradually adds more personal levels of content to her initial use of imagery.

> ... work begins on the floor, focusing quickly on the opposites involved in up/down. Each is explored.... Everyone then goes on to discover the movement possibilities of the continuum on which up and down exist.... This brings a pair of opposites into contact with each other. The third stage ... introduces an image... "The earth is my mother. The sky is my father." (Whitehouse, 1979, p. 66)

---

[1] Not all of Whitehouse's protégés stress this concrete, body-oriented side of her work. Others, such as Joan Chodorow, Nisha Zenoff and Janet Adler, remember her as focusing primarily on improvisation and the integration of abstract Jungian concepts with body movement. Because of these two differing views of Whitehouse, when many of her former students get together and discuss her work it often seems as though they had studied with two different teachers. (Manning, personal communication, 1985)

Here, after the initial images of "up" and "down" had already begun, Whitehouse suggested the concept of earth/mother and sky/father. In this way she added possible personal symbolism or meaning to "up" and "down" for those who could make use of it.

Whitehouse rarely (if ever) spoke while a client was involved in a movement improvisation, but if a client stopped and Whitehouse believed the individual needed help she might ask certain facilitating questions such as, "What happened?" "Where did you go?" "What did you find out?" From the information she received she then made suggestions or asked questions to help the client deepen and/or focus his or her movement explorations (Zenoff, personal communication, 1980). One way was through observations of the individual's movement, such as "I saw at a specific moment when your feelings changed and looked free" or "What did you think when you moved your arm upward?" In other words, Whitehouse commented on what she saw in a way that was not an interpretation of the meaning of the movement but rather a comment on the movement sequence as she observed (Zenoff, personal communication, 1980). During these pauses in the movement improvisation, Whitehouse stressed the importance of talking in order to understand and integrate verbally the psychomotor events. She then frequently utilized the material that surfaced to structure a theme on which the next or continuing improvisation might focus. As Adler (personal communication, 1980), a protégé of Whitehouse, has said, "She encouraged talking to integrate what happened into the individual's consciousness; she was not impressed with catharsis alone."

Although Whitehouse did not actually dance with her clients, she did move toward them at moments when support was needed. Aside from these moments she basically stayed on the periphery, but according to Zenoff:

> I always felt she was right with me; I experienced her presence very deeply and it allowed me to go into myself and my movements. You could feel her empathy even toward the end of her life when she was in a wheelchair. Her presence was part of the healing process. (Zenoff, personal communication, 1980)

The following case example demonstrates the active imagination process through body movement. It also demonstrates Whitehouse's style of letting the patients begin in the fashion that they choose and then working with them patiently as their movements develop. Special emphasis is placed on the therapist's ability to wait and create a milieu that allows individuals to find their own unique style of expressive behavior at their own pace. Whitehouse recalled:

> I remember a dancer who came to the studio regularly. We had been working with the pull of gravity. One morning she sat on the floor with her arms on her bent knees and I put on very slow music.... I said, "Don't assume it's fast or slow, don't assume it's down or up, don't assume anything. Just begin where you are." (Wallock, 1977, p. 70)

The following describes in Whitehouse's words the client's reaction:

> To her amazement, very slowly, like an iceberg moving a glacier, she rocked to the right and to the left, back and forth and when it came to the point of falling, she fell and the energy rebounded in her body and she rolled, rolled, rolled across the floor. She sat up white-faced with surprise. The falling did not strike her as anything special but she was absolutely unprepared for the rolling. That's what I mean by catching me and the person by surprise because the process that is the movement has really moved them. Sometimes it happens, sometimes it doesn't. It is a kind of openness that is willing to allow something to happen as well as not to happen. (Wallock, 1977, p. 70)

It is this giving in to the spontaneous movement process that Whitehouse spoke of as a precursor to the surfacing of images from the unconscious layers of the psyche. In other words, the active imagination process implemented itself through the modality of authentic movement.

The next case example demonstrates one client's ambivalence toward this unfolding process as well as Whitehouse's conceptualization and interpretation of the client's imagery during the session:

> A young woman stood at the edge of the big studio. In front of her there seemed to be marshes—water lay everywhere but there was enough dry land to pass through [active imagination]. She crouched, carefully putting one foot in front of the other, proceeding out into space. The water seemed to come up around her; she felt as if it engulfed her and said to herself, "Oh, I must try to make friends with it." She sat down, allowing the water all around her body but not her head. No matter how she played, ... [her] head took no part ... At last she ... said, "No, no...." (Whitehouse, 1979, p. 58)

In this example of active imagination, Whitehouse pointed to the Jungian symbol of going into the water as dipping into the unconscious parts of the personality. This patient would only go so far. She protected symbolically the mental or rational part of herself by not relaxing her head, but rather straining to keep "her head above water." In this way she fought against allowing herself to become completely in her unconscious.

In Whitehouse's subsequent session with this woman, all of her images had stopped; no material was coming into consciousness. Whitehouse (1979) suggested, "we go back to the water and the marshes" (p. 58). In response, the client walked to the middle of the studio and immediately was able to re-experience the water. The events that followed demonstrated this individual's conflict about entering the unknown realms of her unconscious.

> She lay flat this time, playing in it with her hands. It was very shallow, barely covering the ground and not going anywhere ... again came the feeling of the head resistance ... suddenly she could not bear it; she got up and walked away. This time she found herself in a burning desert. There was absolutely nothing but the heat.... She said she was clawing in the sand to get at the water beneath the surface, longing to find it ... despairing because it had disappeared. (1979, pp. 58-59)

This case demonstrates what Whitehouse must have been referring to in her use of the word "mediator." As she stood observing and experiencing with her client, she acted as the mediator between this individual's opposing drives, that is, the drive to express versus the drive to repress thoughts and feelings. Although it was difficult to leave the client in this desperate state, Whitehouse believed in the process and the natural timing of the client and did not attempt to facilitate or control the client's response. Instead, Whitehouse empathized with her struggle and despair, encouraging her to meet the depths of the unconscious when she felt she was ready. At the same time, she permitted the client to maintain her defenses and conscious controls over potentially overwhelming body movements and emotions. In this way, through her empathic rapport, she mediated the client's opposing drives while simultaneously encouraging the client to make her own decision as to how far to go in either direction.

The two case examples cited above demonstrate Whitehouse's role as a patient, empathic observer. She encouraged and supported the therapeutic movement process in light of the individual's readiness for self-expression through this medium. Her role was one of being "with" the client as he or she encountered his or her own personal experience in both thought (imagery) and muscular (movement) themes.

Summary

Whitehouse was gifted in her ability to develop the Wigmanian improvisational approach to dance into an in-depth psychomotor therapy. She also had a deep respect for Jungian thought and was able to project her understanding of the power of movement into this framework. This merger of two powerful tools, expressive dance and Jung's active imagination, form the foundation of Whitehouse's contribution to dance therapy.

Trudi Schoop: Dance, Drama, Mime and Performance

A major pioneer from the west coast, Trudi Schoop (1903-1999), made many unique contributions to the practice of dance therapy (Schoop, 1978, 2000). As a result of her training and career as a mime, complemented by her wonderful sense of humor, she brought a personal versatility and flexibility to her interactions with patients. A book describing her work, *Won't You Join The Dance?*, was written with friend and colleague Peggy Mitchell and was published in 1974. Much of the discussion that follows has been abstracted from this work.

Schoop was born in Switzerland in 1903. At the age of 16, with no formal dance education, she held her first dance recital at the Schauspielhaus in Zurich. Though her debut was a tremendous success, she felt the need for technical training. In addition to her study of classical ballet, she familiarized herself with the pioneering dance forms that were prevalent in Europe at that time, including the methods of Wiesenthal, Duncan and Laban (Mitchell, personal communication, 1987).

> My stage career was the strongest influence because there I built characters on the stage. I had to find out how they felt, how they would move, how they would behave. On stage I could abstract and objectify. (Wallock, 1977, p. 62)

Schoop's own personal experience with mime was one of externalizing or "objectifying" her own conflicts on the stage. "If other people could laugh, then the conflicts were not so terrible" (Wallock, 1977, p. 62). The combined use of mime and humor for the expression of conflict later became the two primary cornerstones of her dance therapy practice and two of her major contributions to the field.

Schoop began practicing dance therapy as a volunteer at Camarillo Hospital in California in the 1940s and later became employed there. Schoop taught in France, Germany, Switzerland, Italy and the United States.

Theory

Schoop believes that who we are is reflected and manifested in our bodies. In addition, what happens in the mind has a concomitant reaction in the body and what happens in the body has a concomitant reaction in the mind. For this reason, postural attitudes and physical alignment are reflective of one's mental state. Furthermore, through the body and senses one formulates a mental picture of reality. It is the harmonious interaction between psyche and soma that promotes functioning without conflict (Schoop & Mitchell, 1979).

It was this harmony that Schoop found painfully lacking in her patients. She saw in their postures all of the stresses and tensions indicative of internal conflicts and stemming from opposing and repressed drives. Schoop believed that all individuals are pulled by opposites, "all individuals encompass the complete range of every feeling, action [and] thought …(Schoop & Mitchell, 1979, p. 37). But, due to societal taboos, one side of the individual must go "under cover."

> Hospitalized patients demonstrate clearly how devastating the toll [of this repression] can be. It's as if they have become one-sided, locked into a single feeling, all others consigned to oblivion. (Schoop & Mitchell, 1979, p. 38)

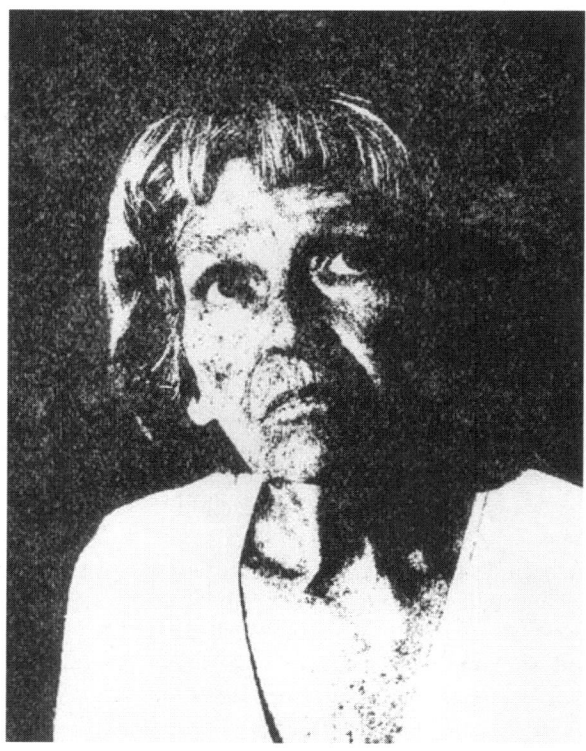

Trudi Schoop (Photo courtesy Anthony Verebes)

Schoop believed that in one form or another, the repression exerts pressure on the personality of the patient and in so doing undermines his or her integrity and performances. For this reason, one of her major goals was to bring the patient's repressed side to consciousness through expressive movement.

In this connection, Schoop (1979) reflected upon the "UR experience." She described this German word as follows:

> *Energy:* the vital force which keeps the whole universal complex on the move. From the microcosm of the atom to the magnitude of the great whirling bodies of matter in our heavens and beyond, there exists the ceaseless life-force of the UR Energy. (Schoop & Mitchell, 1979, p. 36)

Schoop also described UR as endless space and/or endless time that continues with no apparent reason. She contended that man forgets nothing and "that deep within each human lies a recognition of the UR experience" (Schoop & Mitchell, 1979, p. 36), that is, the totality. It was her feeling that we, as humans, live on two levels; one is the linear day to day and the other is the universal. She saw dance as one way in which we confirm both this finite (muscular level) and infinite (energy level) connection to life. In her lyrical and poetic manner, Schoop connected the rhythmic contractions and releases, extensions and flexions that make up dance with the eternal rhythmicity of life (the UR).

Schoop (1976) explained the significance of the UR experience in terms of dance therapy as follows:

> When I am intensely present in all my multifaceted totality, I feel that I am in balance. Thus, my approach to my work becomes an "attitude" rather than a "treatment." The application of any one treatment form would get in the way of my trying to understand the ununderstandable. If I face a patient with the freedom of all my capacities intact, I can more readily detect in him the parts that seem to be intact, as well as those that seem to be different.... I can feel assured that the patient contains all the same elements or possibilities that we all have; they merely differ in duration, intensity and arrangement. (p. 5)

62 Dance Movement Therapy

In summary, Schoop had two major concerns, both of which revolved around opposites. The first was helping individuals to experience, in a harmonious way, their conflicting emotions. The second, an outgrowth of the first, was helping individuals connect, first to their own immediate reality and then to the reality that went beyond the daily—an experience of the universality and uniformity of all living things, past, present and future. She believed that through the ability to contact the various sides and levels of one's own experiences one gained a deep understanding and connectedness with all living things.

Methodology

An overview of the Schoop approach reveals a format and rationale that is in some ways similar to that of the other pioneers. Schoop stressed the importance of teaching proper body use in order to build the individual's capacity for self-expression and exploration. Through movement, she believed that one's self-esteem could be improved via more efficient physical functioning. After building the body image through expanding the movement repertoire, developing increased body awareness and experimenting with postural attitudes, she gradually moved to thematic movement explorations, which she often initiated herself. When it was evident that the patients' tolerance of dynamic movement expression had increased and they had developed a sufficient movement vocabulary, Schoop, like many of the other dance therapy pioneers, moved to spontaneous movement expression in the form of improvisation. However, in contrast, Schoop stayed in this mode only long enough to bring out new personalized material. As this material surfaced, Schoop helped patients to organize their new experiences through movement "performances," that is, the planned reproduction and repetition of movement themes (Schoop & Mitchell, 1974). The process of formulating dance movement sequences served the function of slowing down the expressive process and in

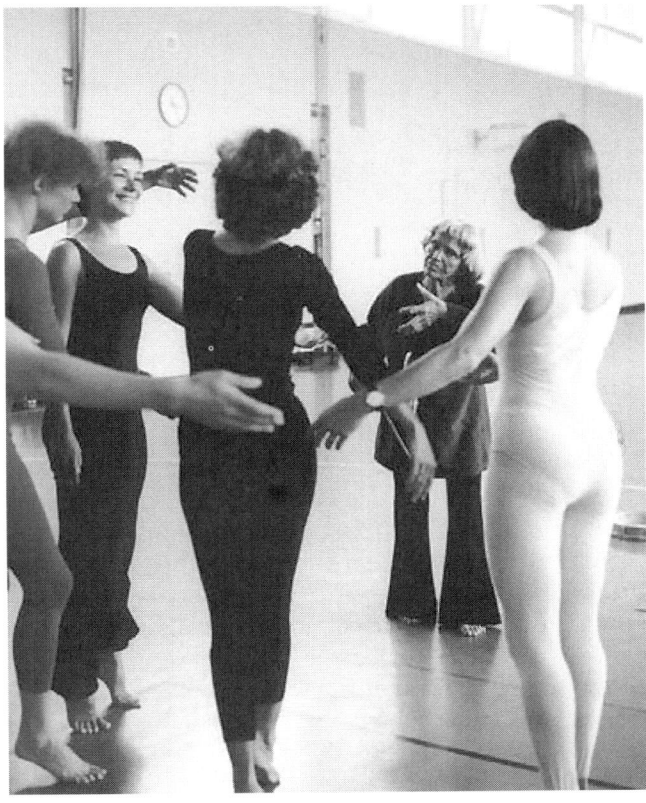

Schoop using her own movements to encourage interaction with her class (Photo courtesy Anthony Verebes)

this way allowed more time for the exploration of inner conflicts. Through choreographing conflicts, Schoop believed the individual could gain some control, insight and mastery over his or her problems.

Schoop combined four methods of developing the physical and emotional expressivities of her patients: 1) the educational approach; 2) rhythm and repetition; 3) the inner fantasy and 4) spontaneous movement improvisation and planned movement formulation.

Educational Approach

Schoop began by lifting the taboos against emotions. She believed that before patients could gain muscular control over the expression of their emotions, they first had to acknowledge their conflicts and then externalize them. She helped the patients achieve this through the use of humor and her own body. Schoop believed strongly in the healing aspects of humor, feeling that we all have much to laugh about, including the benefits of being able to laugh at ourselves. Because of her background in mime, humor was a vital part of Schoop and therefore naturally integrated into her work. The humor aspect of Schoop's work was usually only implied in her publications, but it is still common knowledge amongst those whom she taught (Mitchell, personal communication, 1987). Like a good comedienne, Schoop was able to abstract those universal aspects of personality and human conflict with which all individuals struggled and put them in a form that caused laughter and self-acceptance.

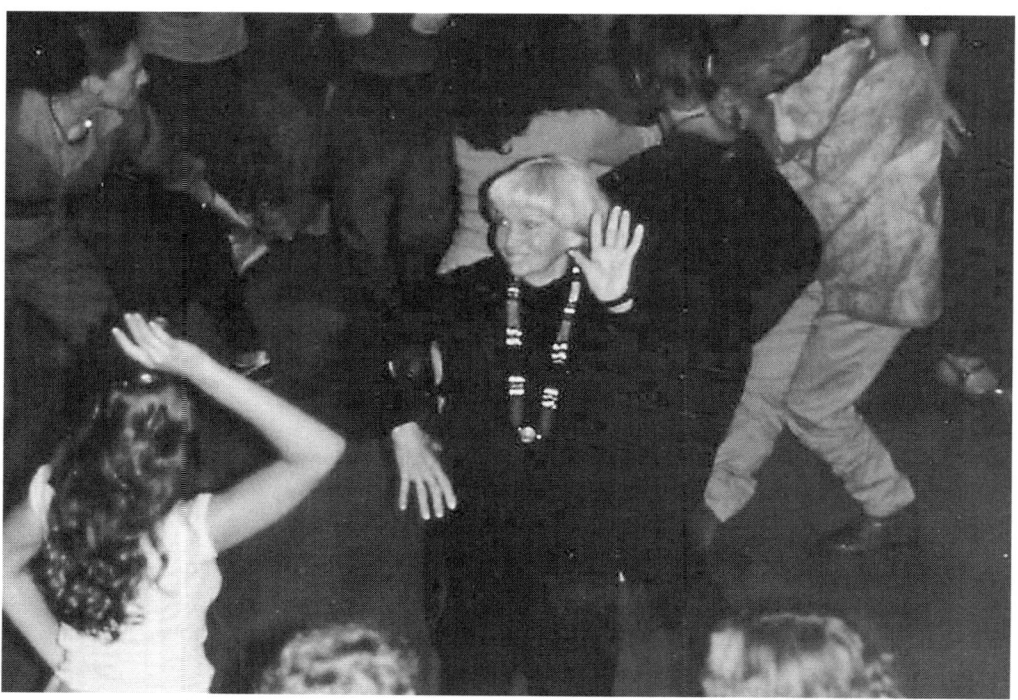

Trudi Schoop believed in spontaneous movement improvisation (Photo courtesy Anthony Verebes)

Schoop demonstrated this aspect of her approach—and attitude toward life—in *Won't You Join the Dance?* (1974). She described one of her initial sessions with hospitalized psychiatric patients. In this session, she eagerly decided to demonstrate a movement tantrum in the hope that this would release the patients' extreme inhibitions around feelings of anger. After acting out a complete, lengthy and exhausting tantrum, hoping that her withdrawn and solemn patients would be so moved that they would join her, she was instead greeted by blank stares and one slightly more aggressive patient who went up to her and asked, "Are you on Bennies?" (Schoop & Mitchell, 1974, p. 31). Schoop portrayed this colorful experience with humor and weathered the blow with minimal hurt. In spite of feeling a little foolish about this early plunge, she continued to develop her methodology by tailoring this original approach. Gradually she integrated her dramatic flair and her skills at characterization and emotional expression with her interactional skills and empathic nature. What emerged became the Schoop approach to dance therapy.

Schoop's skill at using herself actively, through drama and dance, to elicit the physical expression of feelings and ideas in patients has become one of the cornerstones of her work.

> She says the therapist should be like a very good actor. The patient will respond to the therapist if the therapist is really experiencing the feeling and projecting it fully, just as an audience responds to the feelings conveyed by a good actor. (Wallock, 1977, pp. 46-47)

In addition, by exhibiting various extremes of movement that served the purpose of exaggerating and reflecting patients' emotions, she helped them to laugh at and accept themselves in a new, less judgmental fashion. This style of intervention paved the way for the acceptance of conflicting emotions and in turn served to build an atmosphere of trust, which freed patients to explore their own internal cast of characters and conflicts.

After the taboos against emotions were lifted and the patients were more ready to accept themselves, Schoop proceeded by helping them learn about and experiment with their own body movement. The goal here was to increase the patients' body awareness, physical control and range of functional and expressive movements.

One method was the exploration of posture. To help the patients understand posture, she used alignment exercises integrated with the use of imitation, exaggeration and humor. For example, she had the patients imitate a posture and variations on common postures, which she deliberately exaggerated. She would also humorously imitate particular postures she saw in patients. This, the author believes, could be construed as ridicule and must be done with great delicacy and empathy.

> It certainly seems that when I demonstrate a patient's physical manifestation *humorously*, he is confronted by an affectionate and amusing image of himself. The stinging seriousness of his conflict appears to be lessened and for the time being at least, he doesn't have to defend himself against something when that "something" strikes him as funny. (Schoop & Mitchell, 1974, p. 76)

After this, she would exaggerate opposing postural styles in order to help clarify the differences and would encourage the patients to walk in various positions.

> We do the worst walks we can think of; we use every kind of ridiculous, overdone posture and gait, parading across the room pigeon-toed, splay-footed, knock kneed, bow-legged. We waddle, clomp and mince. We enthusiastically make different parts of our anatomies stick out, sag or flap. (Schoop & Mitchell, 1974, p. 86)

She further suggested that the patients imitated others, such as people at the hospital, friends, relatives, people on the street and so on. "… No one escapes our alignment inspection" (Schoop & Mitchell, 1974, p. 86).

Besides teaching about posture, Schoop helped the patients identify with their own bodies through the use of verbalization. She utilized words as a way to confirm and identify that a patient was in fact moving, by stating what part of the body was moving and how it was moving. For example, Eric swings his hand, Jane shakes her finger and Bill lifts his leg. After all body parts have been acknowledged in some action, she might play a waltz and then start a simple side to side swing, which would gradually increase in size until all body parts were united and committed to a single action (Schoop & Mitchell, 1974). Then she would encourage the patient to say, "This body that swings is mine, I am swinging" (Schoop & Mitchell, 1974, p. 102).

> To stress individual differences, I ask the patient to see and touch another person's body just as he learned to see and touch his own. As two partners face each other, I can give each one a different way of moving: round movements vs. angular, soft vs. staccato, slow vs. fast. Or they may show each other different expressions: silliness confronting sadness, boredom looking at happiness, anger watching friendliness. There is no end to the distinctions that can be made between the You and the Me as the patient struggles to develop a sense of identity. (Schoop & Mitchell, 1974, p. 102)

Another educational technique used by Schoop was the exploration of contrasting pulls in the personality. Her incorporation of contrasts into dance movement therapy techniques was one of her major contributions and is a style of working that is well-known and used by contemporary second and third generation dance therapists. The following describes one method Schoop used to explore opposing pulls in the personality:

> ... I purposely create split tensions in the bodies of my patients to make them conscious of what they are doing unconsciously. Energy-splitting can become quite a hilarious game, more difficult than you might think when it has to be done intentionally. In the course of a session, I may pick up split-body conditions that are being manifested by members of the group or I may rely on my own collection of "standard splits." We can move around with tight, contracted bodies or skip with "rag doll" arms and stiff "wooden" legs or run with one whole side rigid and the other side loose. (Schoop & Mitchell, 1974, p. 108)

After she encouraged a split-body exaggeration, like Evan, her goal then was to bring back unity and unison. Through the exaggeration of splitting the subsequent reunification could be made easier.

> As a beginning, I've found it best to work from the two extremes of tension. Almost anyone can grasp the idea of tightness or looseness and can make himself stiff or limp all over and then jump or run or dance about. When the patients are well acquainted with those two extreme possibilities, then they can be introduced to the degrees that lie between them. From the tightest, I can then ask for less ... less ... still less ... and finally, least. And from the loosest, more ... more ... still more ... and finally, most. The body becomes more flexible as the patient practices the tension scale and the patient can find that one degree in which his body feels most comfortable. He discovers his functional, basic level of energy. (Schoop & Mitchell, 1974, p. 109)

In the above passage, she described her "outside-in" approach. It combined the process of educating and sensitizing the body to one's active use of physical control. With this exercise, she was both supporting and teaching self-control through encouraging the mastery of physical extremes.

Schoop then guided the individual back to a more fully unified physical state.

> At last the whole body is ready to experience one degree of tension, sustain one level of energy throughout. To capture this oneness, I can adapt the entire body's tension to the tension in one of its parts. Starting with a clenched fist, for example, we lead the tension being felt by the hand into the whole arm. We move it across the chest and shoulders—involving the head en route—and down into the other arm. It is then spread downward through torso, legs and feet until the entire body feels like a fist. (Schoop & Mitchell, 1974, p. 109)

Rhythm and Repetition

Schoop's use of rhythm and repetition had many variations, but could be broken down into three basic approaches.

Using the first approach, externally prompted rhythmic action, Schoop generated the expression of a particular emotion by performing its universally associated action. The patients would then pick up on this through imitation. For example, to generate the expression of anger she had the patients repeat actions such as kicking or punching. In this way, she lifted the taboo from the emotion by giving the patients permission to express it physically.

Next, she transformed this direct release of emotion into dance form by adding the rhythmic component to the expression. This provided the patients with the tools to break the emotion down into its component muscular actions or specific muscular drives, thus facilitating externalization, control and mastery of expression.

This process leads to a neutralization of the often overwhelming emotion, which provides the patient with the necessary cathartic release but without the possible loss of self-esteem that might otherwise emerge in such emotional discharge. Now the patient has access to his or her emotions and has also acquired a new skill in movement. Schoop had now achieved her goal of unlocking the hidden side of the personality through nonthreatening means and cultivating this release through the positive reinforcement of the joy of self-expression and self-affirmation. The patient now had the movement tools necessary for communication and expression.

In the second approach, Schoop would take an educational role. She might request that the patients choose a feeling, whether they felt it or not and develop it fully into dramatic movement expression, which stressed rhythmic release. They were asked to work on it, repeat it and develop it until they were satisfied with the result. Like an artist, their task was to complete a finished product. If the emotion became personalized for them it was okay, but that was not the goal (Mitchell, personal communication, 1985). Instead, the goal was to build a flexible and strong expressive movement vocabulary. Schoop believed that this would generally prepare the individual for a more open, relaxed acceptance of life situations and emotions as they arose. In this way, the individual's need to block or deny circumstances that may have aroused charged and disturbing thoughts and feelings was reduced. This approach also built the individual's sense of control and mastery over emotional expression.

These exercises encouraged structured avenues of self-expression, which provided: 1) a sense of self-control, 2) trust of the body and therefore a deeper identification with one's physical self and 3) flexibility and strength in coping with life experiences.

It was a fundamental concept of Schoop's that we all have rhythmic ability, which at times seems inaccessible because it is repressed (Schoop & Mitchell, 1974). Her third method helped patients to release and explore their innate rhythmic motions.

For example, she might have asked the patients to act out various daily tasks such as combing their hair or getting dressed. In so doing, they were taught to become aware of their internal rhythm.

> For as long as necessary, the patients walk at their own speeds, clap their own rhythms, stamp in their own qualities and time patterns, without being dominated by music, drum or me. (Schoop & Mitchell, 1974, p. 119)

Thus, Schoop began by sensitizing the patients to the everyday rhythmic actions in their lives. They may not have previously been aware that these actions had any rhythmic value. After this was accomplished she proceeded to the next, subtler level of rhythmic awareness, the pulse. She asked the patients to take their pulses and sound out each beat.

> After a while, all pulses are located and the hall is filled with rhythmic sounds—some slower, some faster, some higher, some lower.... Soon the sounds even out, the fast ones slowing down and the slow ones speeding up, until all the voices are sounding in unison. At that point, the drum or the pianist can take over, continuing the rhythm created by the patients themselves. When the beat is firmly established, I can ask them to move their body parts to it. The fact that they are interpreting their own rhythms, not mine, makes them enjoy the performance much more. (Schoop & Mitchell, 1974, p. 119)

As in her other approaches to developing rhythmic awareness in patients, Schoop again would break down the rhythmic process into smaller parts. That is, she started with individuals beating out rhythms with beaters and body parts (arms, legs, etc.). Gradually, as a sense of security in rhythmic production was attained, the rhythmic action moved to the entire body, including the vocal chords, through the emission of sounds. In addition, she would subtly lead this into a group action by having the pianist pick up on the emerging rhythmic pulse. As a result, a strong group rhythmic activity developed, supported externally by the piano.

The merging of the group spirit was made possible as a result of the group's previous work on developing their own individual rhythmic awareness. Here one can see parallels between Chace and Schoop regarding their approach to the group. Both placed initial emphasis on registering and facilitating the expression of individual needs within the group and then gradually modified and organized these needs into united, empathic, rhythmic group action.

The process continued; Schoop explained:

> From rhythmical acceptance, we can move to rhythmical disagreement. I ask the patients to oppose my steady drum beat with their beaters: faster or slower or louder—whatever way they feel like beating, as long as it goes against mine. The room clatters and swishes and slaps, a ruckus of rhythmic revolution. Then they alternate, part of the time beating with me, part of the time against me, learning to say "I won't," as well as "I will." (Schoop & Mitchell, 1974, p. 120)

Once the group's attention was fixed to an external beat, Schoop moved again into a teaching role. Her goals were, as before, the building of a flexible and varied movement repertoire along with the encouragement of self-assertion and affirmation through movement.

The Inner Fantasy

Schoop was unique in her dedication to exploring, through dance movement, the fantasy life of patients diagnosed as psychotic. In order to bring the patient into the world as others saw it, Schoop believed in the importance of engaging the patient through understanding and temporarily joining the patient in his or her delusions, hallucinations and ideations.

> Don't artists move easily between two worlds as they realize a flight of fancy in a poem, a symphony, a sculpture, a dance? I would not want to try to stop the artist from seeing or hearing his fantastic images any more than I would want to prevent the imaginative play of a child. So I feel that rather than suppressing the fantasy of a psychotic individual, I would fly with him for a while then descend with him for a soft landing on this earth. In giving shapes to visions, he will create a world that fuses fantasy and reality. (Schoop & Mitchell, 1974, pp. 149-150)

Schoop was versatile in her methods of joining the patient in his or her world. She entered the individual's world by listening carefully, observing movement, asking questions and translating ideas and imagery into the reality of physical expression. Once the patient's ideas were transformed into their concomitant physical form through dance improvisation and enactment, they could be worked with in many ways. They could be molded, objectified, varied, discussed, reflected upon, controlled and even mastered, at least physically. Through this process, the patient may have had a greater feeling of control over the often-frightening symbolic content of feelings when they were expressed in concrete physical form.

The example which best illustrates Schoop's style of engaging a patient through making direct contact with his delusional system is in the case study of Luke[1] (Schoop & Mitchell, 1974). The following excerpts from this case demonstrate this and other aspects of Schoop's work.

The Case of Luke

Luke was a middle-aged black man who had a peculiar movement sequence by which he greeted Schoop and others.

> It consisted of three distinct, separate actions repeated one after the other, always in the same order. To begin, he would suddenly raise both arms in a sweeping arc, which ended with his hands forming precise, devil-like horns on his forehead. Maintaining this devilish or faun-like position, he would flatten his hands, palms turned down and, using them as if they were sharp cutting instruments, make slicing gestures along his neck. In the final movement he would drop his head on his chest and stroke his hair forward with soft, tender strokes. (Schoop & Mitchell, 1974, p. 164)

Initial contact:

> When Luke and I were seated opposite each other and he began his talismanic mannerism, I picked it up the second time around. Carefully and precisely I made the horns, bowed, sliced at my neck and brushed the top of my head. There was a pause. Luke's eyes were still downcast. He repeated the pattern and again I followed it. We did it a third time. Luke raised his head. His eyes looked straight into mine. And he smiled. I smiled back. (Schoop & Mitchell, 1974, p. 169)

Early movement explorations:

> ... Luke smiled when he came in this morning. We worked on runs, walks, skips and turns.... Later, I asked him if he would like to dance to the music Erica was playing. He listened to it for a while, then selected two scarves and fluttered them about for a while. It seemed to me that the softness of the scarves might be recalling tender feelings and that his body was reacting to them with staccato movements—like stuttering in motion. He was growing increasingly excited, so I asked him if he wanted to do his "favorite movements." He went through his pattern several times and I again accompanied him. I told him that he could feel free to do them any time he wanted to. (Schoop & Mitchell, 1974, p. 169)

---

[1] These excerpts are abstracted from a 31-page case study printed in Schoop and Mitchell's (1974) *Won't You Join the Dance?* In their book, they also include a reproduction of 14 of Luke's drawings.

In this example, Schoop, aware of the anxiety the scarves evoked (tender feelings), chose to encourage Luke to reinstate his defensive mannerisms and remind him that whenever his thoughts or feelings made him too uncomfortable he could return to these familiar gestures.

Body image and introduction of reality into Luke's delusional system:

> Luke was in a good mood and smiling a lot. First we touched our own body parts in time to a rhythm. When he touched his head or shoulder or knees, he doesn't give the picture of touching portions of himself; he looks as if he's touching strange objects. We worked with the beaters for a while, using them to touch each other's shoulders, elbows, knees. We stood up and did a few jumps and hops. Then I held out my hands to Luke and asked him to take them so we could dance together. He looked at them for quite a while, then looked away.... (Schoop & Mitchell, 1974, pp. 170-171)

Finally, with much hesitation, Schoop explained:

> ... he reached out and touched my fingers—not really holding my hands, but sort of petting them in short, light tappings. He still made faces and twisted his body and peeked at me, but these reactions were less extreme than they had been the first time. We did a few more exercises. When the time was up, Luke made his usual farewell horns. I told him that in Switzerland, people usually greeted each other or said goodbye with a handshake and I extended my hand. He took it, I gave his hand a firm clasp and released it. (Schoop & Mitchell, 1974, p. 171)

Development of trust, many sessions later—Luke explained the meaning behind his mannerisms:

> ... I still don't believe it! Luke came in very "normally." He said "Good morning" without the help of his horns. He removed his shoes and socks very naturally. He sat down opposite me and immediately went through his basic mannerism several times. Then he looked straight into my eyes and asked matter-of-factly:
> "Would you like to know what that means, Trudi?"
> "I would like that very much," I replied. "This," he said, demonstrating the bow and the horns with the index fingers extended, "is a salute to the white man. This," and he made that same first movement, this time using the pinky fingers as horns, "is the greeting of the Boy Scout or boy. This," the cutting gesture on the neck, "is wiping away the sweat, because I work so hard. And this," and he made the head stroking movement, "means that it's a hot day."
> "Thank you, Luke. Thank you very much." (Schoop & Mitchell, 1974, p. 178)

The following is a movement enactment of Luke's fantasies:

> ... "I went to school 'til I was five. I was a girl. Then I had a mom and dad. My dad brought me a beautiful suit when I was eighteen or twenty; it had long trousers. When I went to church on Sunday, I had a dress on. I was a girl. Now I am ... you know ... sort of a man or a boy."
> "Could you show me, Luke or act out for me, what you did and how you moved as a girl?"
> "I held my left arm with my right hand. And I walked like this!" And he walked about, flouncing up and down.
> "Luke, you are a man now. Show me how you walk today."
> And Luke walked a masculine walk better than at any time before! (Schoop & Mitchell, 1974, p. 183)

In this example, Schoop first went with the delusion and then in her final request employs reality testing of Luke's perception of his masculinity.

In the vignette that followed, Schoop invited Luke to act out his fantasies, thereby facilitating the expression and exploration of thoughts and feelings while simultaneously encouraging him in a direct symbolic interaction with her.

> ... I asked him if he would like to act out the ... scene with the wolf and the lamb.
> "Oh, yes. I want some water. I have to protect my family."
> I became the lamb and Luke the wolf. I scooped up a handful of water and offered it to him. He knelt down in front of me and drank it blissfully. When his thirst was quenched, we jumped and leapt and ran about like two wolves. His movements and gestures were marvelous to watch. Finally, we lay flat on the floor on our stomachs and lapped water from the "lake". Then we changed parts and repeated the same actions, he as the lamb and I as the wolf. After I had drunk from his hand, we hopped and skipped about like lambs and again drank together. At last, we stood up, became erect and walked together as "ourselves". And Luke's walk was amazingly different. His step was firm and secure. His body had straightened out. It was as if he had clearly grasped the posture difference between an animal and a human. (Schoop & Mitchell, 1974, pp. 185-186)

Here, Schoop emerged as the nurturing mother who, after several months of work with Luke, was able to engage this once severely defensive patient. Then, demonstrating her flexibility in taking different roles, Schoop encouraged Luke to reverse their respective wolf and lamb roles, in this way giving Luke a chance to experience metaphorically his own strength as a giving person. Finally and not surprisingly, when they stood up and returned to the reality of themselves, Luke's posture had changed. He was more "erect," "firm" and "secure" in his physical stance. These words, which Schoop used to describe Luke's physical state, seemed also to reflect his emerging positive identification with his masculinity. Through the depth of rapport and trust that Schoop established with Luke, accompanied by her continual reassurance that he was okay and that she liked him, Luke was gradually able to give up his defensive mannerisms and to accept his relationship with her.

Although these excerpts from the case of Luke illustrate several aspects of Schoop's methods, they primarily point out the creative and flexible interjection of herself into the patient's psychotic process. She is willing to enter into the fantasy, symbolism and gestures of her patients.

Finally, in discussing Schoop's use of fantasy, one must include her emphasis on the creative use of the group fantasy and support. Schoop generally preferred working with groups, whereby she actively integrated her belief in the power of the group process with her belief in the importance of expressing the individual's and the group's fantasies. One method Schoop employed was that of having members act as directors of their own imagination. This emerged through the participants' taking on various roles, that is, becoming the cast of characters in the enactment of a drama (Wallock, 1977).

The following excerpts from *Won't You Join the Dance?* (1974) provide excellent examples of Schoop's use of the patient's imagination within the group process. In the first example, each member became his or her own director and character and the space in the room became the stage or boundary for the emotional expression.

> ... the studio becomes a huge arena, surrounded by grandstands. I choose this particular space facility because there's simply no place to hide in it; within its vast circumference, a person is completely exposed on all sides. What's more, the idea of the arena is loaded with images from which the patients can draw: the politician, the bullfighter, the fire-and-brimstone preacher, the fashion model—any person who not only wants to be looked at, but *must* be looked at. One by one, the patients walk around the ring. Here comes the "King," proudly displaying the head that wears the crown. And here is a runner, bearing aloft a flaming torch for the world to see. And this is the "General", exhibiting the medals on his puffed-out chest. Every person thus imagines a reason for showing off some part of his body. (Schoop & Mitchell, 1974, p. 132)

This excerpt again demonstrates Schoop's reliance on mime and role-playing as a way to bring patients "out of hiding" and into parts of themselves previously repressed and/or fantastical.

The next case example demonstrates the way a group will frequently come together spontaneously to give emotional support and accommodation to a group member who is under extreme stress. This is the case of Alice.

> "They want to separate me from my friends on Venus," she sobbed. "They told me that's what they want to do! They said that's why they give me shock treatments!"
> "How would it be, Alice," I asked one day, "if you would tell all of us here in the group how your friends look and what they do that makes you love them so much?"
> "Well ...," she began hesitantly, "they're all so happy to see me when I come up to them. And sometimes Clandestine gives me a kiss." Nobody in the group had to be told what to do. Awkwardly but with affection, they shook Alice's hand. They patted her. They smiled. Their greetings must have pleased her, because she continued her description.
> "They lie on golden couches ... they drink out of golden goblets ... they fly all around on their golden wings. They have golden dragons—very friendly ones—to play with and ride on." And Alice began to teach her willing cast how these beautiful people moved and flew and drank and played. (Schoop & Mitchell, 1974, p. 147)

The last two illustrations could be referred to as group improvisations around specific themes, the first suggested by Schoop and the latter directed by the patient's own thoughts and feelings.

Improvisation and Planned Movement Formulation

The integration of movement improvisation with planned movement formulation was unique to the Schoop (1974) dance therapy approach. Schoop compared improvisation to "doodling" with the body, that is, "a process of nonverbal free association during which the individual permits his body to move spontaneously and unguardedly" (Schoop & Mitchell, 1974, p. 143). Schoop stressed the need to follow up the subjective experience that emerged during improvisation with the ego functions of self-observation, movement production and self-reflection. She accomplished this by helping the patient to reproduce significant aspects of his or her improvisational movement activities into planned and repeatable dance movement sequences. In this way, the individual was helped to organize (choreograph) and thus master physically the flood of unconscious stimuli, which emerged during periods of spontaneous improvisation.

> The time has come for the individual to present his subjective, free-floating feeling in an objective explicit form, with his body as the instrument for his composition. This production requires him to organize the forces of both his mind and his body.... As he develops a logical framework for his expression ... he is gaining the upper hand. (Schoop & Mitchell, 1974, p. 146)

This process served several functions. It helped in bringing previously repressed, unconscious id drives under the control of the observing ego. In this way, the individual worked toward gaining the ego's control over the id or if this ability of the ego had never developed, the ego may have acquired a degree of control previously out of reach. In the words of Schoop and Mitchell (1974):

> He is now able to experience that feeling without conflict and he can communicate it accurately and realistically. Other people can recognize it. They can react to it. And their response reinforces his own reality. (p. 146)

Finally, Schoop's thoughts on the strengths and limitations of the improvisational process in dance therapy, that is, when that process is not followed by structured movement formulation, are noteworthy:

> Once a person's feelings of conflict have been brought into the body, improvisation has served its main purpose. There's no point in going on and on with it, for no matter how many times the body "admits" to a feeling, it will continue to express it in the same manner, over and over. (Schoop & Mitchell, 1974, p. 146)

Schoop believed that creative work must be done with the energy and emotions released by the improvisation. If this energy was not used to help structure insight-oriented activities, the individual could become stunted in his or her growth and even become dependent on the cathartic experience, viewing it as an end in and of itself, void of internal integration, organization and meaning.

Summary

Schoop integrated educational and exploratory approaches during the therapeutic process. She intertwined her methods in a creative and flexible style. The sequence reflected here—movement education, rhythm and repetition, the inner fantasy, improvisation and planned movement formulation—appears to be more representative of her theoretical perspective than the actual sequence of her clinical work. As a result of Schoop's willingness to explore playful, expressive and creative interactions with her patients, she contributed many unique dance therapy techniques.

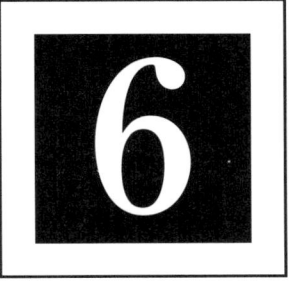

Alma Hawkins:
Humanistic Psychology, Imagery and Relaxation

Alma Hawkins (1905-1998) was chair of the Dance Department at the University of California, Los Angeles (U.C.L.A.) from 1953 to 1974. In 1963, she introduced dance therapy to U.C.L.A. and her work there evolved into a comprehensive dance therapy program. The program was eventually taken over by Irma Dosamantes-Beaudry.

Hawkins started her career in dance therapy in the early 1960s while working with Alfred Cannon, a psychiatrist at the Neuropsychiatric Institute at U.C.L.A. The two worked together with individuals and groups and with both adults and children. Hawkins worked at the Institute until 1977.

Hawkins studied dance extensively in the 1930s and 1940s with modern dance innovators such as Doris Humphrey and Hanya Holm (a Wigman disciple) at Bennington College in Vermont. Though she studied with professional dance artists, the primary emphasis of her work was in education.

Marcia Leventhal[1] stated that Hawkins "helped to put dance on the map in California" (personal communication, 1987) and continued:

> She has always been a totally committed and knowledgeable advocate of dance and because of her very respected position and the kind of stature and aura she carried at U.C.L.A., people with authority listened—taking dance into the mainstream and out of second-class citizenry. (Leventhal, personal communication, 1987)

In her advanced study, Hawkins was deeply influenced by the work of Harold Rugg, professor at Columbia University Teachers College in New York. Rugg was interested in the nature of creativity as it related to all the arts. He believed that movement played a fundamental role in the arts and was an integral part of the thought process (Hawkins, personal communication, 1985).

While teaching at U.C.L.A., Hawkins sought to increase her understanding of the nature of the creative process and the fully functioning person through the writings of and personal study with people such as Edmund Jacobson (relaxation), Robert Ornstein (modes of consciousness) and Eugene Gendlin (inner sensing). She worked with Valerie Hunt and they frequently discussed their common interest in movement. She also spent many hours discussing dance therapy with Mary Whitehouse, a long-time friend who taught dance therapy at U.C.L.A. for one year. Hawkins said:

> Mary Whitehouse and I shared many ideas. We did have much in common and I think a little of each of us rubbed off on the other. Our basic ideas were the same, but the approach sometimes differed. (personal communication, 1985)

Alma Hawkins' career has gone full circle—first working with dance, then developing a dance therapy program and now again teaching dance. She taught the fundamentals of choreography at Santa Monica College in Los Angeles. The course attracted artists, dance majors and leaders in dance therapy (Leventhal, 1984). Hawkins influenced several leading dance therapists, including Marcia Leventhal, Irma Dosamantes-Beaudry, Susan Lovell and Joanne Weisbrod.

---

[1]Leventhal, a protégé of Hawkins, was the first student intern who conducted sessions, directed research and assisted Hawkins from 1963 to 1965.

Theory

Leventhal, an associate professor and director of the Master's degree program in dance therapy at New York University, remembers her early training with Hawkins in the 1960s. She states:

> ... we always returned to the basic premise of Dr. Hawkins: that there is an inherent talent and creativity residing within each individual, waiting only to be guided and untapped. She has dedicated her life to the art of dance with the belief that there is no swifter, truer way for an individual to reach his/her fullest growth potential. (Leventhal, 1984, p. 7)

Hawkins felt that people search for a way to integrate mind and body, which have been separated in our culture for too long. The body self must be strong before we can see ourselves and relate in the larger sense: "We can't deal very well with the environment until there is a secure sense of self as an anchor" (Wallock, 1977, p. 96). Through the movement process, the individual can get in touch with his or her own feelings and thus be able to interact more meaningfully with the environment.

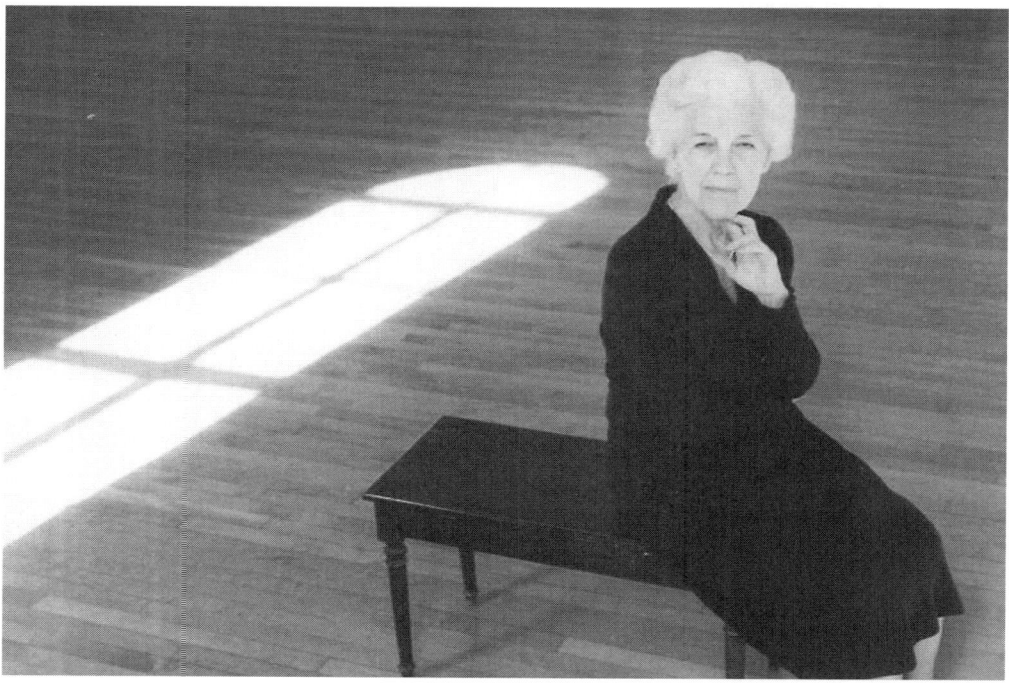

Alma Hawkins in her California studio, 1987 (Photo courtesy Mark Harmel)

Hawkins viewed the components of movement as energy, space and time. Like many of the other pioneers, she worked with "polarities", i.e., extremes and ranges of these three components, such as big/small, strong/weak, and with shades of polarities. This led to flexibility of range and patterning, which set an optimal mode for perception and experience. She stated:

> ... what I am trying to do is not *dancing*; rather we are stripping the experience down to the purest approach to movement.... The more I work, the more I see that movement and the body are related to perception. (Wallock, 1977, p. 90)

In this connection, Hawkins believed that relaxation was a highly significant factor affecting perception. She incorporated into her work the research of Edmund Jacobson concerning residual tension. Jacobson emphasized the need to identify and control tension in order to reduce anxiety, build body image and increase perception. A high degree of residual tension not only increases anxiety but also blocks perception. This results in a narrow, rigid pattern of response, which keeps one from his or her creative influences. According to Hawkins, "an optimal mode of handling information and functioning is being open to a wide range of sensory data ..." (Wallock, 1977, p. 90).

The person who has achieved a state of relaxation is better able to discover and release their creativity and natural energy flow, i.e., "authentic movement." Getting in touch with various levels of consciousness, he or she can then respond with more spontaneity and imagination. Energy flow and movement pattern thus become truly "authentic."

Authenticity in movement, according to Hawkins, implied that the externalized movement pattern was congruent with inner sensing (personal communication, 1985). Through relaxation, one opens the threshold to inner sensing (i.e., attentiveness to the inner self) and makes possible a new connection with previous experiences and memory traces. The movement that develops from this state can be filled with meaning and insight. Based on the work of Ornstein (1972), Hawkins saw this as involving the right hemisphere of the brain and made possible "an inner way of knowing, the intuitive, holistic sense rather than the linear, sequential way of experiencing and knowing" (Wallock, 1977, p. 81). From this evolved "body-self", i.e., the "ground structure for body image, body ego, [and] body boundary ..." (Wallock, 1977, p. 91).

Hawkins, in an interview with Susan Wallock (1977), described her own theoretical model as a "growth model" (p. 92) and specified humanistic psychology as one of her many influences. In an interview with Leventhal, Hawkins shared her thoughts on the relationship between dance as an art form and as a tool for healing. She stated:

> ... there is a basic movement process that can be directed toward therapeutic goals. It is this process that brings about the change. This basic movement process is in reality a creative process which can just as easily be directed toward an aesthetic goal and the achieving of an art object. It seems to me that in both art exploration and in dance movement therapy the basic process is the same. (Leventhal, 1984, p. 9)

Hawkins believed that as long as the creative process is based on "inner sensing, feeling and imagery, healing will occur" (Leventhal, 1984, p. 10). "Man seeks creative and aesthetic experiences because they enrich him ... help him become an integrated individual and help him feel in harmony with his world" (Hawkins, 1972).

Methodology

Hawkins saw her role as a dance therapist as a facilitator or guide rather than as a teacher or director. Her goal was to catalyze creative experiences that work toward putting individuals in touch with their thoughts and feelings, thus making it possible for them to more fully respond to internal and external stimuli. In the following quote, she described the development of her methodology.

> ... through the experience of trying not to use things related to dance technique ... I acquired a clearer understanding of the basic movement phenomenon. Eventually, I began facilitating movement events using the elements of movement: time, space, energy flow. I always allowed the experience to be directed or cued from what the patients were giving. Even though I knew enough not to teach dance or to do prescribed exercises, it took me a while to discover the true nature of basic movement. (Leventhal, 1984, p. 8)

Whether it was verbally or nonverbally, Hawkins supported whatever experience the individual was having in the session and suspended judgment. She may have facilitated the verbal discussion of movement experience by asking the individual questions such as, "Did you feel anything different happening today in the way that you were moving ...?" (Leventhal, 1984, p. 11). She did not believe in telling the individual what she saw in their movements or describing to them how they moved. Similarly, she did not interpret the client's movement response but supported their revelations as they occurred, believing that growth happens in time with the client setting the pace for his or her own insights. Hawkins' challenging role as the therapist was discovering the kind of experiences that best supported individuals in their journey toward self-realization.

Hawkins usually started a session with guided movement experiences that helped to focus attention and broaden experiencing. Then she turned to relaxation, which included attending to breathing. During the remainder of the session, individuals were involved in movement tasks that were motivated by imagery.

The images were always open-ended and allowed for self-directed response. Sessions frequently included experiences that allowed two individuals or a group to interact in response to an image and explore a movement idea together. Hawkins saw imagery as a developmental experience, ranging from concrete to abstract.

Imagery was an integral aspect of Hawkins' work. She described her use of it as follows:

> I began exploring the use of imagery in dance classes in the early 1960s. Then when I started working with dance therapy I experimented with a wider range of imagery—personal, concrete, abstract. And in recent work I have worked in greater depth, especially in the use of imagery as a means of facilitating "inner sensing" and the creative process. (personal communication, 1985)

Hawkins also worked with self-directed responses and "felt-level" experiences. The latter she described as experiences "derived from 'inner sensing,' which are different from pure emotion" (personal communication, 1985) in that they are purely bodily-felt experiences and perceptions put into movement. At the close of a session, the group comes together to share their experiences.

Summary

Hawkins' contributions as a therapist, artist and educator have influenced dance therapists, choreographers, dancers, actors and movement educators. Her major contribution has been in the area of integrating imagery and the elements of dance and creativity into a formal healing experience based on the tenets of humanistic psychology.

Discussion

Similarities and Differences Among the Major Pioneers

The contributions of six pioneering leaders during the 1940s and 1950s set a firm foundation for the practice of dance therapy today. By the early 1960s, the practice of dance therapy 1) had already serviced a broad spectrum of emotional disorders and 2) had utilized an equally broad range of practical interventions and facilitating techniques.

However, areas that were still underdeveloped were empirical research, experimental research and the establishment of a complete theoretical framework, which would serve to integrate the field's broad spectrum of theory and practice. Relying on established theoretical foundations of Freud, Jung, Adler, Reich and Sullivan, the integration of these more modern leaders was sparse and more often discovered, not through their own writings, but through verbal exchanges with the pioneers. The fact that the theory of dance therapy seems to have developed more slowly than its practice is perhaps in keeping with the nature of the dancer/therapist as essentially being an action-oriented individual, who aesthetically *feels* his or her way to the needs and realities of others, intuitively adapting to these needs, both verbally and nonverbally.

The similarities and differences among the original pioneering leaders in dance therapy can be explored by 1) the style of intervention (verbal versus nonverbal facilitation); 2) the degree of therapist control (directive versus nondirective approach) and 3) the predominant emphasis or focus of the therapist's attention (horizontal vs. vertical process [Siroka, personal communication, 1976] or, individual process vs. group process).

Style of Intervention

During the 1940s and 1950s, two distinct styles of dance therapy intervention existed. The first has been called the Therapeutic Movement Relationship and is characterized by the dance therapist's combined verbal and nonverbal participation in and facilitation of movement. The second is the empathic observer role, characterized by the primarily verbal facilitation of movement while the dance therapist quietly observes. While these styles of movement elicitation differ, the forms patients arrive at (mime, dramatic movement, improvisation and other styles of symbolic movement expression) frequently overlap. This overlap in movement form, but contrast in intervention or elicitation style, is demonstrated in the diversity of the major pioneers. Chace utilized the therapeutic movement interaction as a major vehicle by which she elicited these forms. Hawkins arrived at similar movement forms but did this through encouraging the patient's imagination and suggesting creative movement ideas. Patients of Whitehouse and Evan also came to these movement forms, although these dance therapists stressed free association through body movement, in addition to encouraging patients to enact images and dreams. Hence, while similar movement forms might evolve, the way in which these forms were catalyzed varied tremendously.

Degree of Therapist Control

The degree of therapist control ranges from the therapist allowing the patient to be self-directing to the therapist being in total control. All of the major pioneers were sometimes directive (teaching movement), structuring body awareness exercises, suggesting movement themes and/or choreographing.

Chace, through movement interaction, encouraged rhythmic expression. This expression, in conjunction with the therapeutic movement relationship, guided the individuals in their struggle for self-expression. Because Chace was always part of the patient's movement experience—guiding, narrating and reflecting—a large degree of therapist control was always present. On the other hand, Whitehouse and Evan sat to the side while their people improvised. They directed by helping individuals to formulate movement explorations, often around suggested or emergent themes. However, once the patient was involved in an improvisation, he or she was given independent time and space to explore conscious and unconscious thoughts and feelings. Reflection and discussion took place after the movement sequence came to its natural conclusion. Both Whitehouse and Evan spoke of the natural or inevitable ending of the patient's improvisation. The dance therapist allowed the improvisation to take its full course without interruption or direction.

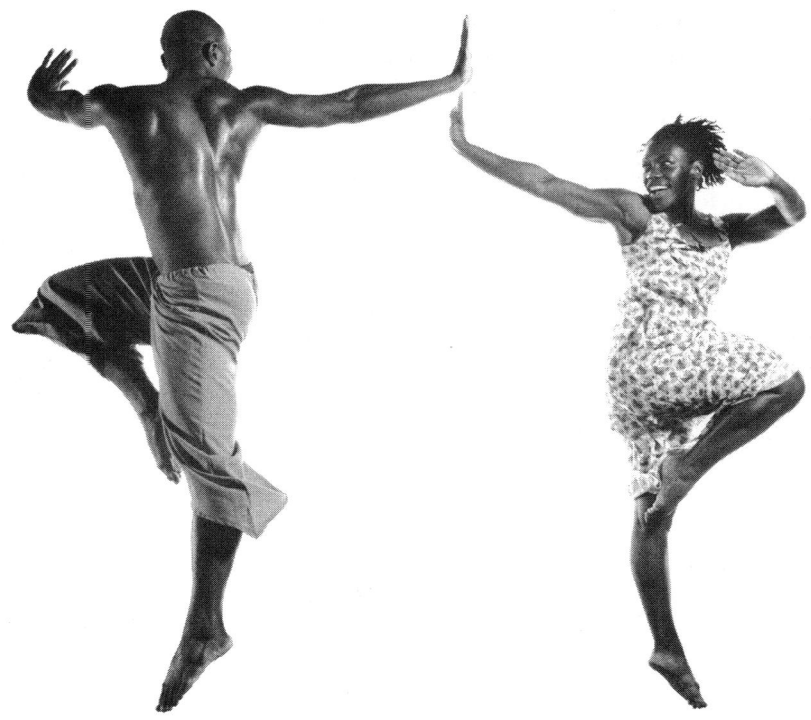

Dancers Gaetan Pettigrew and Christal Brown perform rhythmic expression (Photo courtesy Steve Clarke)

Schoop, like Chace, took a more directive role. Both Schoop and Chace worked with hospitalized psychotic patients and both tended to stay more in the moment, as opposed to delving into unconscious material. In addition, Schoop encouraged the choreographing of emotions to help patients cope in their day-to-day lives. Espenak, on the other hand, moved freely back and forth between directive and nondirective roles. She worked both in hospitalized settings and in private practice.

The pioneering leaders all took active control of dance therapy sessions, though in different degrees and through individual styles. All of the pioneers offered, either verbally or nonverbally, thematic and projective material for patients to explore. At no time were patients left to explore movement on their own without some kind of initial directive, ongoing guidance and narration, reassurance and/or reflection.

A pattern emerges amongst the pioneers. Those who worked with the more severely disturbed hospitalized patients tended to stay in the here and now, focusing more on conscious thoughts and feelings with a greater stress on patient/therapist interactions. Those who practiced privately with a healthier patient group delved more into the unconscious and early childhood material. In addition, they allowed for in-depth individual improvisation.

Major Focus of Therapist's Attention

The predominant emphasis or focus of the therapist's attention can be discussed in terms of the concept of "horizontal" versus "vertical" stress (Siroka, personal communication, 1976). "Horizontal" here refers to the process often seen in group psychotherapy whereby a specific or immediate theme of one individual is generalized or broadened so that it is applicable to one or more general needs of the group. In this way, what emerges is a continual process of mediating between the needs of the individual and the needs of the group. One example of the horizontal approach is Schoop's use of teaching patients many different movement styles. Through this educational approach, they can learn about themselves, others and about the overall possibilities of personality and behavior styles from which they can discover different aspects of themselves.

The vertical approach, on the other hand, delves more deeply into psychic conflicts and developmental needs of one individual, whether within a group or in a one-to-one format. The word "vertical" is used to indicate an individual emphasis, as is seen regularly in the work of Whitehouse, Evan, Espenak and at times in Schoop (most notably in her stress on the movement fantasy).

It is important to emphasize that the horizontal and vertical models can be used in either individual or group sessions. For example, though some dance therapists, like Evan, worked in both individual and group sessions, Evan tended to emphasize the individual, using the vertical process in both settings. Chace, though unique in her ability to reach deeply into the emotional life of her patients, worked primarily as a group dance therapist with a horizontal focus; that is, she moved with the emotional needs of as many group members as possible by mediating quickly and intuitively between these needs and modifying movement patterns to connect with the majority of group members. Chace fluctuated rapidly between group and individual needs, dipping into the individual process just long enough to establish contact and then reuniting the individual, through his or her movement, back into the group process. Chace also used the needs of the individual to deepen the group process, thus creating a reciprocal horizontal process.

Summary

While there are overlaps in the kinds of movements that are elicited, the method of elicitation distinguishes one dance therapist's style of intervention from another. In the area of control, all six major dance therapy pioneers exerted direction, but some emphasize verbal direction and others physical. Some dance therapists' major focus is on deep individual intra-psychic exploration, while others continually negotiate between individual and group needs, always bringing the emphasis back to the group's level of emotional expression.

SECTION C

Other Early Pioneers, Leaders and Contributors

 Dance Therapy Emerges in the Midwest

As noted earlier, the pioneers in dance therapy often studied with creative and modern dance instructors and then expanded this knowledge to develop the concepts of dance therapy, dance as a psychotherapeutic tool. Many of the early dance therapists in the Midwest were greatly influenced by Margaret H'Doubler, a "landmark dance educator" (Thomas, personal communication, 1986). Though not a dancer herself, H'Doubler fought for the inclusion of dance as an academic discipline in universities across the country. She began to teach dance at the University of Wisconsin in 1918 and retired in 1953. Published in 1940, her text, *Dance: A Creative Art Experience*, remains a classic.

Although H'Doubler did not practice or show an interest in dance as a form of therapy, her beliefs about movement led her students naturally into an exploration of dance therapy. She felt that the outer movement expression of inner feeling states and emotions acted as a means of keeping and restoring emotional balance. By the early 1950s there was a growing interest at the University of Wisconsin in dance and movement education as a process for dance therapy, on the part of H'Doubler's students, notably Rhoda Winter Russell and H'Doubler's colleagues Shirley Genther and Maja Schade. H'Doubler contributed to this trend, supporting student and faculty research in the area.

Utilizing humanistic educational philosophies of men like Dewey (Thomas, personal communication, 1987), H'Doubler taught "from the inside out," beginning with the person's sensation and perception of the movement, rather than "from the outside in," beginning with an external style and form. Her students were required to investigate music, rhythmic form, anatomy, physiology, physics, kinesiology, advanced biology and physical education theory, as part of their dance curriculum (Russell, personal communication, 1986).

H'Doubler's view of movement is reflected in the following statement by Russell:

> She aimed ... to develop kinesthetic awareness, perception and the ability to give adequate motor response; to discover and evaluate feeling states that accompany movement sensations; to experience the expressive power of movement; to gain the understanding that meaning and communication are due to the structure of the movement form. (Russell, 1970, p. 69)

Deborah Thomas, a leading dance therapist who did graduate work at the University of Wisconsin and became the director of Wisconsin's undergraduate dance therapy program, provides an example of H'Doubler in action. Thomas describes a class H'Doubler led in 1976, in celebration of the 50th anniversary of the Dance Major at the University of Wisconsin.

> ... she was asking the seated students to pay attention to the location and movement range of their shoulder blades (... with the aid of a skeleton). This felt very pleasurable and "new". Then she asked us to hold our arms extended straight forward from the shoulder while continuing exploratory movements of the shoulder blades. Later she added a lifted head with the gaze straight up. She then got the whole group walking more and more swiftly in this configuration across the whole length of the large gym, until they were running. It was an ecstatic flow of movement, built from inner exploration. It illustrated her technique of adding one element at a time for greater ease of perception (and coordination) and her practice of building from the student's own kinesthetic awareness rather than an external image. The resulting movement structure emerged "naturally" with a great sense of discovery and beauty. (Thomas, personal communication, 1986)

One can see from the quote above how H'Doubler's teachings could inspire her students to explore the use of dance as a form of therapy. In addition, Thomas says:

> At 80 she was a vivid, vitally interested person—she was interested in you! Her eyes and facial expression told you that you were special—and full of potential. She was looking for what would strike you—for signs of how you were going to interact with a particular idea. Her enthusiastic attitude was infectious and helped one overcome self critical hesitancies. (personal communication, 1987)

By the early 1950s, dance therapy was becoming a focus of attention and activity at the University of Wisconsin. Shirley Genther, a well-respected musician who was teaching music and rhythmic form and analysis, developed a special interest in psychodrama and the expressive therapies. She was one of the major forces behind the development of movement therapy at Mendota State Hospital, where several University of Wisconsin students did internships in dance therapy.

Genther, in collaboration with psychiatrists Thelma Hruza and later Edna Fitch, studied the use of creative dance with psychiatric patients. In preliminary sessions at the University of Wisconsin, they experimented with the combined use of dance movement and psychodramatic methods. Then, under the supervision of a staff psychiatrist at Mendota State Hospital, their methods were introduced to a group of severely disturbed patients. After doing relaxation exercises and simple body movements such as swings and discussing how the movements felt, the patients began to feel more comfortable with their bodies. As this comfort increased, "movement drama" was introduced to "reinforce and sometimes replace psychodrama" (Genther, 1954, in Rosen, 1956, p. 78). This concept of the movement drama reappears again in the late 1970s under the heading of "Psychodramatic Movement Therapy" (Levy, 1979).

Rhoda Winter Russell, a disciple of H'Doubler and a pioneer in dance therapy, was the first University of Wisconsin student to receive dance therapy training at Mendota State University Hospital (1951-54) and go on to develop and use those principles and techniques in psychiatric settings. Her studies in this area were supervised by Shirley Genther and her Master's thesis, "Motion and Emotion: The Choreography of Feelings" (University of Wisconsin, 1954), was supervised by H'Doubler.

H'Doubler's explorations of kinesthetic awareness and the connections between movement and human expression laid a foundation upon which Russell could work. Later, Russell traveled to Germany to study with Wigman. In her subsequent dance therapy practice and teaching, Russell integrated the pragmatic, unstylized approaches of H'Doubler, Wigman and later Alwin Nikolais to help clients "become fully themselves in movement" (Russell, personal communication, 1986). From this training and other influences, including Rational Emotive Therapy, Gestalt Therapy and Humanistic Psychology, she developed her own dance therapy methodology and initiated her own dance therapy training programs in New York City and Philadelphia. By 1956, she was in New York practicing as a movement therapist at Manhattan State Hospital and in private practice. It is interesting to note that among her trainees was Miriam Roskin Berger, a leader in the field and a former ADTA president. Berger's work reflects the influence of Russell as well as Marian Chace, with whom she also trained.

Maja Schade, a dancer, dance instructor and physical education teacher, was also at the University of Wisconsin during the early 1950s. Like Russell, Schade was influenced by the teachings of H'Doubler and also paid tribute to the ideas of Delsarte, Laban, Mensendieck and Kephart. At that time, she was becoming involved in the use of movement and relaxation as a healing tool. Her relaxation techniques, based on Jacobson's (1929) *Progressive Relaxation*, were described by Joanna Harris (1980), one of her former students, in terms of reassessing one's energy patterns and the use of imagery. Schade was also known for her work in physical correctives, particularly her use of structured therapeutic movement exercises.

It was also in the 1950s that Schade began teaching dance therapy in undergraduate courses at the University of Wisconsin. As part of their coursework, students were brought to psychiatric hospitals to work with patients (Kuppers, 1980). In addition, Schade helped to organize the first ADTA conference held at the University of Wisconsin in 1968.

Joanna Harris was a student of Schade, Genther and H'Doubler. Their influence, along with that of Mary Whitehouse, Merce Cunningham and developmental, Jungian and psychoanalytical psychologies, laid the foundation for Harris' work in dance therapy.

Although the University of Wisconsin was an important center for early dance therapy leaders in the 1950s, it was not the only source from which dance therapy in the Midwest took root. Other important leaders and contributors experimented independently during these formative years, notably, Alice Bovard-Taylor in Minnesota with psychiatric patients, Billie Logan in Minnesota with children with developmental disabilities and Norma Canner in Ohio (see Chapter 23) with psychiatric and cerebral palsy patients. In 1982, Jane Ganet Sigel spearheaded the first and only Master's degree program in Dance Therapy in the Midwest at Columbia College in Chicago. Sigel, originally a dancer and dance teacher in the Chicago area, heard of Marian Chace in the early 1960s and decided to leave Chicago temporarily to study with her in New York City. Sigel followed her instincts when she came to New York. She believed intuitively in the healing power of dance and had experienced this while teaching creative dance in the 1950s. Like so many of the pioneers, she witnessed and explored the therapeutic aspects of dance early on with her dance students.

Sigel brought the Chace technique back with her to Chicago in the early 1960s and began organizing with other individuals who were also paving new ground in this area—particularly Mildred Dickinson. About this early pioneering period, Sigel stated, "I felt alone. People were scattered around the Midwest, continuity ... was complicated by our distance from one another" (Sigel, personal communication, 1986).

In 1966, Sigel gave and received collegial support by becoming a charter member of the American Dance Therapy Association and later supporting the growth of this organization. In 1976, Sigel, along with Judith Fischer organized the first Midwestern Dance Therapy Conference. At the National Conference, which followed, 30 Midwest dance therapists organized themselves and initiated the first Midwest regional chapter.

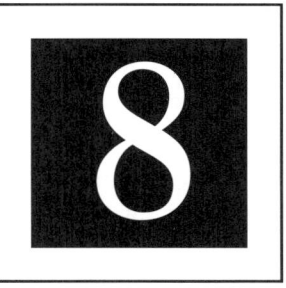

Pioneering Literary Contributions

This chapter discusses two pioneering literary contributions to dance therapy and outlines one of the first important studies analyzing the discipline.

First, Franziska Boas' (1941) article "Creative Dance" is reviewed in detail. Boas' article was the first comprehensive discussion of dance therapy techniques with children.

Also summarized here is Elizabeth Rosen's book, *Dance in Psychotherapy* (1957). Although now out of print, few books can compare to this detailed account of dance therapy with the hospitalized psychiatric population.

Finally, the 1956 study reviewed in this chapter analyzes the development of dance therapy at this early stage in its history. The study serves as a useful benchmark in reviewing the course of dance therapy through the years and how that course affects the state of the art today.

Part A. Franziska Boas: Seminal Concepts

Franziska Boas contributed two seminal articles to the literature of dance therapy in 1941. She later consolidated both articles into a comprehensive chapter for Lauretta Bender's (1952) book, *Child Psychiatric Techniques*. This consolidated article, entitled "Creative Dance," was reproduced in Costonis' 1978 book, *Therapy in Motion*.

The ideas Boas expressed in "Creative Dance" were clearly part of the whole climate of dance therapy theory and practice of which she was a part. In the 1940s, Boas was practicing dance as a therapeutic modality at Bellevue Hospital in New York. It was during this time that psychoanalytic thought, which was gaining widespread acceptance, merged with the concept of the "inner dance," which was prevalent in the first part of the century. Boas, who was influenced partially by this changing environment, integrated psychological concepts and therapeutic goals into her movement work at Bellevue.

It should be noted, however, that Boas was not primarily a dance therapist, but rather a teacher of creative modern dance. She was deeply influenced by her father, Franz Boas, the anthropologist. At the Sixth Annual Conference of the American Dance Therapy Association in 1971, Boas spoke about the relationship between dance-as-art and dance-as-therapy. The ideas she expressed reveal a definite drift to her original roots in dance, without the accompanying psychoanalytic terminology that was present in her articles. Clearly, Boas is first and foremost a dancer, teacher and researcher.

Boas attributed the development of her approach partially to her dance studies with Bird Larson and partially to her studies with Hanya Holm (Boas, personal communication, 1987). She was also greatly influenced by the work of Mary Wigman. Gradually, Boas evolved her own teaching styles in which she integrated technical movement skills with creative movement in a style she calls creative modern dance. She postulated that this creative and expressive approach to dance is inherently therapeutic.

> I make no separation between dance as an art and dance as a therapy. Every art has a therapeutic effect both on the artist and on the observer. It depends entirely on how you look at it; why you are dancing or painting or writing, etc.; why you are asking someone to take part in the activity. These things will determine whether the activity is for therapeutic purposes or not. Dance can be both therapy and art. (Boas, 1971, p. 26)

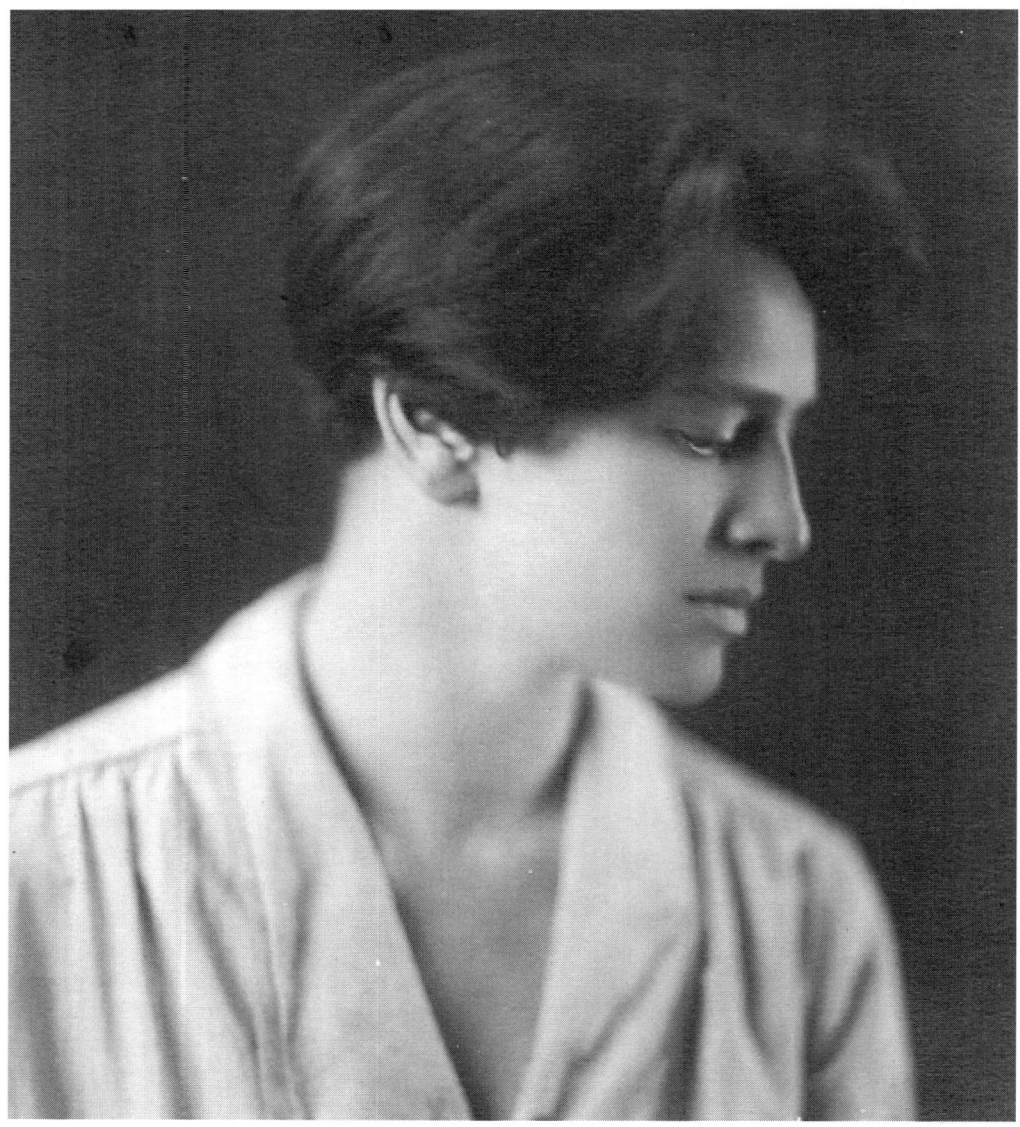

Franziska Boas as a young woman (Photo courtesy Gertrud Michelson)

The philosophy that Boas discussed looked at the function of dance in life and reflected her belief in dance as the expression of the human spirit.

> ... dance happens for its own sake. The movements become symbols of tensions, feeling and inner thoughts. To dance one must sense changes in weight, velocity, tensions and volume. One must be able to feel large and small space, dense and open space. One must be willing to allow the laws of motion to control the body and carry it where they will.... This requires the courage to "lose oneself" in the happenings which are going on within the body and mind. Mary Wigman has said, "One cannot dance without having encountered the spirit." (Boas, 1971, p. 22)

Dance, Boas asserted, has an innate power—a dynamic force that, if allowed, moves through the body and reveals the thoughts, feelings and the spirit of the dancer. This connection of dance to the spiritual aspects of people lifts certain aspects of dance therapy out of the realm of the sciences and reunites it, in part, with the arts. This concept is especially important to today's dance therapy. Many pioneering and contemporary leaders in the field are urging students to go back to dance in order to find the essence of dance therapy (results of 1985 survey; Evan, personal communication, 1980; White, personal communication 2003). There is deep concern expressed among these leaders that the newer generations of dance therapists are relying too heavily on the "vision" of other disciplines (e.g., psychoanalysis, bioenergetics, etc.), forgetting or perhaps never having truly understood and concretized for themselves, the inherent healing power of dance itself.

Creative Dance

In her article "Creative Dance" (1941), Boas' approach was articulated primarily within the context of her experiences at Bellevue Hospital working with children and in her studio work with dancers. At Bellevue, Boas incorporated into her creative dance techniques ideas and methods that grew mainly out of her association with Lauretta Bender and Paul Schilder.[1]

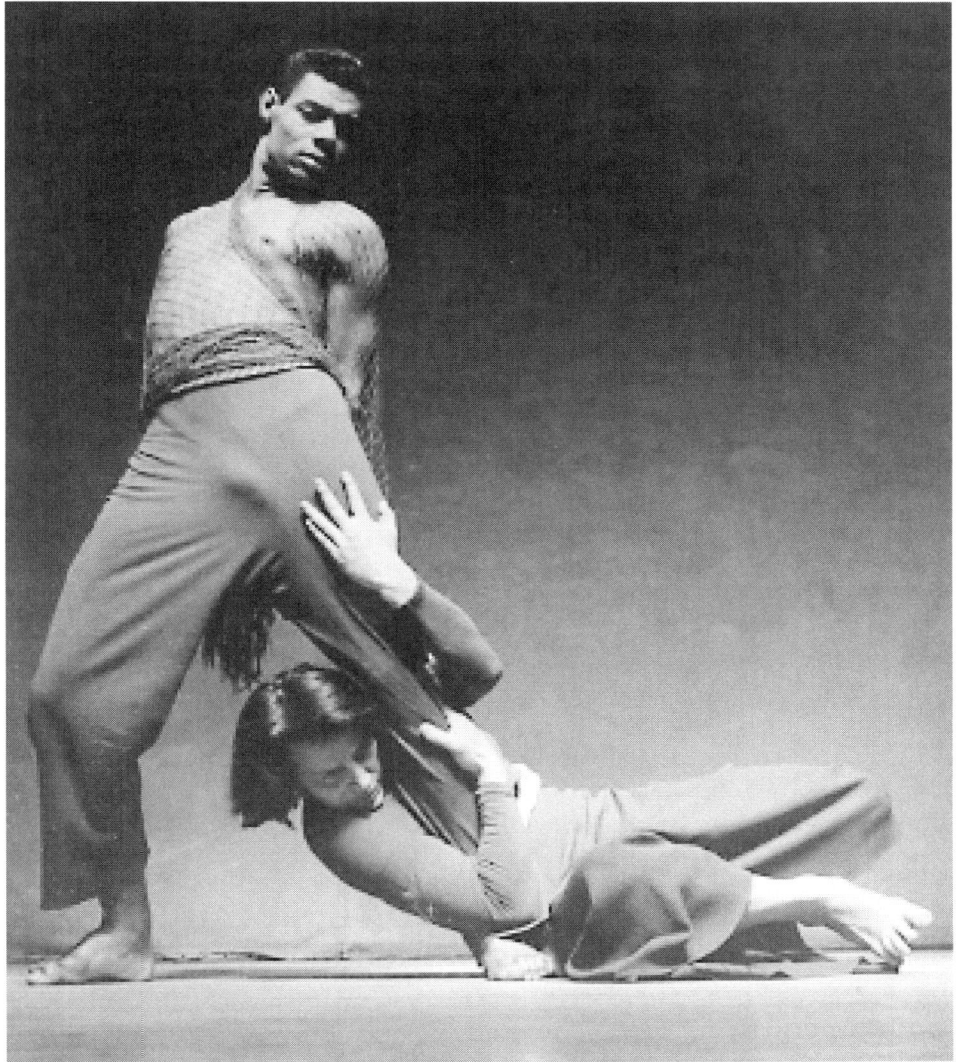

Claude Marchant and Franziska Boas in performance (Photo courtesy Gertrud Michelson)

---

[1] Lauretta Bender, a psychiatrist, is the author of *Child Psychiatric Techniques* (1952). Paul Schilder, a psychiatrist and psychoanalyst, is known for his classic work, *The Image and Appearance of the Human Body* (1950).

Boas was greatly influenced by Schilder's belief that the individual's movement behavior was the direct expression of his or her body image. She gave an example of a schizophrenic boy who wanted to try a backward somersault Each time he tried, he stopped short for fear he would die or lose himself. This exemplifies how an inadequate, fragmented or incomplete body schema (Schilder, 1950) can limit and define the parameters of self-expression available to the disturbed individual.

With Schilder's support, Boas stressed that just as the body image affects the movement repertoire, so deliberate changes in this repertoire can affect and develop the body image. This theory is basic to Boas' work. For this reason, she placed greatest emphasis on encouraging a variety of movement experiences. This meant, for example, subjecting individuals to new postures and extensive exploration of movement activities, which brought the body close to the floor (e.g., lying down, using all fours, etc.); having individuals work with eyes closed and using percussive sounds as a vehicle for encouraging movement responses. She postulated that the provision of new movement experiences external to an individual's usual preferences facilitated an awareness of self and an ability to explore dimensions of personality otherwise not available. For example, she used floor work to encourage the awareness and instinctual coordination of the animal or primitive being within us.

> Everything which disturbs or changes the relation of the individual to the vertical plane (gravitation) affects the motor mechanism of the entire body. The whole system of postures is fundamentally different when an individual is lying on the ground or when he is standing. Even when he is standing upright the muscle tone is very different according to whether the head is turned forward or to the side. The whole distribution of tone changes with every change of position of the head. (Boas, 1978, p. 115)

Boas believed that human beings, as part of a civilized culture, continually struggle with unsatisfied primitive and chaotic impulses. She emphasized the importance of allowing children to experiment freely and indulge in chaotic and formless expression before attempting to shape, form and structure their creative movement experience. She believed that it is the satiation of these early primitive impulses toward freedom that enables children to eventually develop their own integrated movement styles. That is, the sublimated expression through movement and dance of thoughts, feelings and fantasies evolves in a spontaneous and natural way, rather than in a rigid or stylized fashion.

> This type of investigation and learning should be allowed to continue to the point of saturation, then the disorganized movements and chaotic themes begin to form themselves into rhythmic repetitions and recognizable fantasies. In other words, the primitive animal-like impulses may furnish material for sublimation into an art expression. (Boas, 1978, p. 118)

The role of the "teacher-therapist" is to be sensitive to the student's readiness to move beyond this early stage, to a stage that Boas called "subconscious sublimation" (1978, p. 118). Subconscious sublimation is a more organized and symbolic level of motility. Boas pointed out that not all children would be able to make this transition. When sublimation is blocked, two behavior patterns may occur. The first is the individual's retaining a chaotic infantile style of movement; the second is the adaptation of movements for escape in defense against natural primitive desires.

Boas believed that the greatest obstacle to psychophysical integration is the fear of experiencing the self in a new and different light. This is often expressed as a fear of falling, loss of control or loss of a body part.

> The feeling of his own physical strength and the ability to control and direct it is a stage the dancer reaches after having freed himself from anxiety and fear over the dynamic violence of primitive motility and its associated emotions. For the dancer, anxiety and fear of dynamic movement spring from insecurity in the concept of his own body image and from the resistance to consecutive changes in himself. Exploration of the dynamic power of movement brings to the fore instincts of self-preservation, destructive and constructive drives and through their mastery brings about an understanding of these elements. (Boas, 1978, p. 130)

The major part of Boas' work was dedicated to helping children and adults experience, through dance movement, these "unconventional" aspects of personality. In order to free muscular rigidities, she devised many techniques that allowed individuals to explore diverse movement styles and still remain in control. She provided movement ideas, themes and situations, which gave individuals permission to relax the usual controls of the ego and superego and encouraged the controlled use of physical regression for the purpose of self-discovery.

Projective Technique

During the 1940s, Boas and Bender were synergizing their efforts in the study of projective technique at Bellevue Hospital with Margaret Naumberg in art therapy and Adolf Wollman in puppetry. Other pioneers of this technique were Sidney Levy (a strong proponent of dance therapy and mentor of the author), who specialized in the study of symbolism in animal drawing, Karen Machover, who specialized in figure drawing as a projective technique and Henry Murray, who developed the Thematic Apperception Test. The seminal thinking in projective techniques that evolved at this time enriched Boas' already developed style. The use of animal projections, role-playing and storytelling were an integral part of Boas' dance movement work.

Boas believed in and actively utilized dance as a form of expression of affective and cognitive processes. She stressed that dance is more than the physical or mechanical action of muscles and joints, but is also the expression of the individual's subjective concept of his or her body. In her work, she combined the active use of movement in the form not only of dance, but also of drama and role-playing, with the verbalization of fantasies. The use of dramatic play as a tool for the projection of one's thoughts and feelings onto external objects and ideas is demonstrated in the following excerpt from Boas' work.

> ... Several children began to ride on the teacher's back. Carrol ... played at being a buffalo and butted the children and the teacher. Then he tried to make a double animal by putting his arms around the waist of a crawling boy and crawling behind him.
>
> Benjamin was a chicken attacking children. The chicken was killed by a child; it came alive and was killed again. Finally it was really "dead" and should be buried. The children "dug" a grave and "covered" him up. They all wanted to step on the "grave" and then left him. Carrol did not take part until Benjamin was buried. Then he crouched next to him, closed his eyes and performed a kind of sorcerer's dance. He had a slight vibration in his body and passed his hands back and forth over Benjamin's head and body. When the children came back he pushed them away. (Boas, 1978, pp. 126-127)

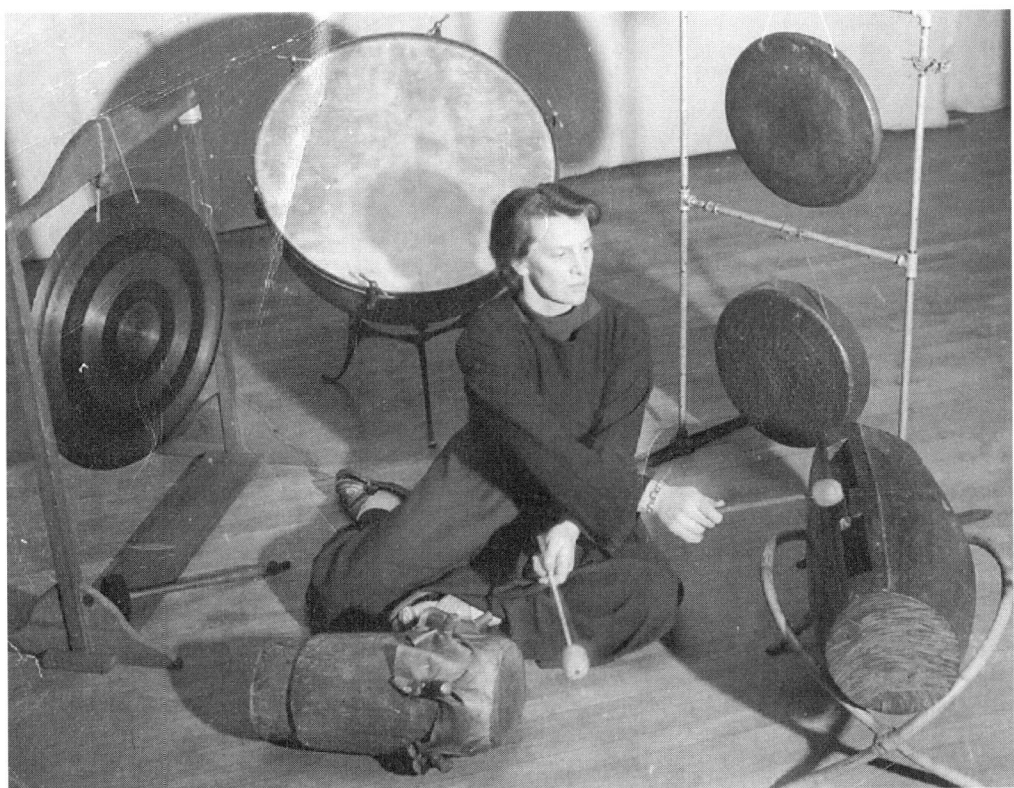

Boas was known for her innovative use of percussion instruments (Photo courtesy Gertrud Michelson)

Boas encouraged the development of an animal activity by positioning children supine on the floor and asking them to explore different movement activities from this position.

> From these exercises the usual development is into animal fantasies with their characteristic movements of crawling on all fours, propelling the body across the floor without the use of hands or feet, rolling over one another, jumping like frogs. Certain children prefer to retain their human character. This leads to dramatic dance games of shooting animals or of animals attacking humans or horse and rider games. (Boas, 1978, p. 128)

Boas indicated how the development of one child climbing on another could often lead to other kinds of movement activities and fantasies, such as

> ... diving into water and swimming, animals jumping from trees onto and over objects and each other.... These are soon combined with more complicated rhythms such as cartwheels and somersaults remembered from the work on the floor. (1978, p. 129)

One can see in Boas' work her tendency toward dramatic movements, role-playing and the active use of the child's imagination. She combined play activities and story telling with a concentration on the growth of movement skills and simultaneously integrated the movement fantasies that these play activities provoked. Her stress was twofold: improved motility, integrated with the acknowledgement, acceptance and development of the concomitant psychic fantasies.

Boas' use of dramatic play demonstrates the emphasis she placed on pure expression. She did not speak in terms of analysis and interpretation. In fact, she was deeply concerned that premature analysis or interpretation could stifle the creative and expressive process (1978).

Use of Music and Sound

The use of music and sound was an essential aspect of Boas' work with children. Like Evan, she used musical instruments extensively.

> Recognizable rhythmic and dynamic [movement] patterns grow out of tension in the individual and tensions in the group.... Most of these patterns demand externalization in sound. Some require a rhythmic drumbeat, others a mellow gong tone or a sharp cymbal crash. A musical accompaniment...[has] to be created... Sounds fill space with substance. (1978, p. 121)

Boas explained that the use of percussion in the background could act as an auditory guide to provoke certain actions and reactions as well as to reinforce emerging patterns of mobility. Like Chace, she used repetition as a way to impel the development and expression of new and dynamic movement patterns. She speculated that the sensory impression of the percussive beat might have a deep psychological influence. Furthermore, rhythmic sound tends to invite even the most resistant children into participation and often acts as a safety guard for feelings. That is, feelings are expressed within auditory guidelines or sound boundaries. This helps put a lid on expressions of, for example, hostility, which otherwise may surface out of control. The repetition of sound adds a sense of play or unreality, thus creating an atmosphere in which it is safe to express oneself.

Boas emphasized that by playing percussive instruments the therapist could help direct the flow of the emotional expression through the use of crescendo, accelerando, retardando and diminuendo.

> The sounds emerging from percussion instruments in themselves have specific qualities which relate to space, time and tension. The drum bounces its listeners in space and creates a desire for rhythmic action. The cymbal softly played cuts space and spreads out in all directions horizontally. The gong fills space and suspends the hearer in it. Sharp sounds produce strong tension and penetrate space. Soft sounds produce weak tension and fill space. Regularly reproduced sounds produce repetition of movement and activate space. Crescendos produce increase in tension and fill space with activity. Descrescendos decrease tension and quiet the space. Accelerandos increase speed of movement and activate space. Retardandos decrease speed of movement and empty space of action. (1978, p. 121)

In summary, Boas used music and sound as structure to expedite several major aspects of the therapeutic process. These include: focusing encouraged by rhythmic repetition; control and guidance of self-expression; broadened use of movement and release of vocal expression with dance action.

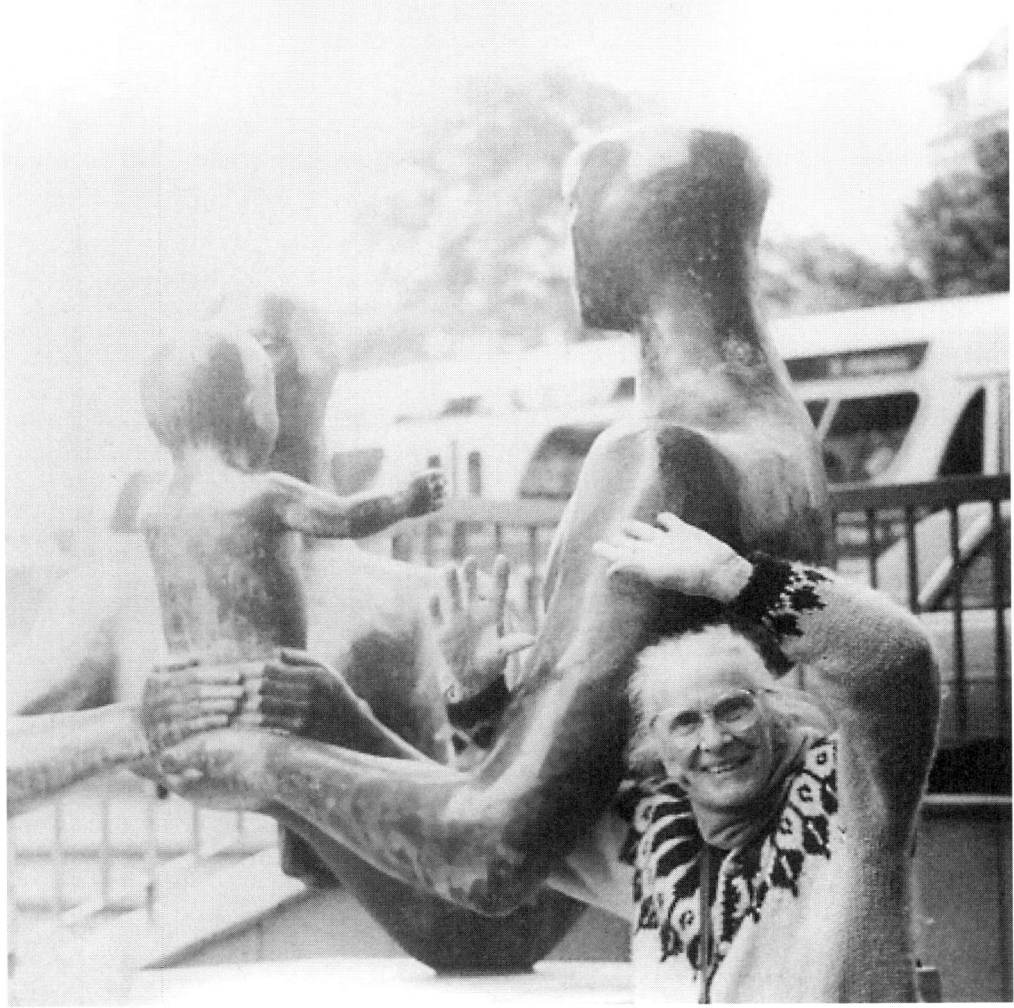

Franziska Boas, 1986 (Photo courtesy Gertrud Michelson)

Movement Improvisation or Psychomotor Free Association

A technique that Boas used in her private studio work as a dance teacher and is used widely today is that of psychomotor free association during dance, a technique similar to Whitehouse's active imagination. Like Whitehouse, Boas often initiated this by having students work with closed eyes, while moving spontaneously to sustained gong tones or in silence. Most students began with self-conscious and/or frustrated movements, such as adjusting hair and clothes or collapsing, stamping feet and so on, but were then encouraged to go beyond these reactions. Boas urged them to enact the movement as soon as the thought or impulse appeared, thereby establishing a free and constant flow of information from mind to body.

During this process, Boas stated,

> ... gradually more and more movement is experienced and larger gestures are made. The body begins to respond to the various shifts of weight and begins to travel through different space levels following the laws of inertia, impulse and momentum. Emotional reactions become manifest and changes in tension begin to create a dynamic and rhythmic flow of movement. During these activities the instructor is constantly encouraging by words and sounds the externalization of gestures and movements which begin to make their appearance. Eventually only the percussion sounds are continued and the body moves by itself. (1978, p. 132)

She continued:

> There is a logic in the development of one movement into another both in the body and in the use of space. To the trained observer any interjection of an arbitrary movement can immediately be discerned. This is a sign of a break in concentration and usually takes the form of some habit movement pattern which the pupil considers "safe," that is, either it covers up the externalization of a "forbidden" fantasy or sensation or it prevents exploration into the unknown. (1978, pp. 133)

This style of work grew directly out of the modern dance movement championed by Mary Wigman during the early part of this century. Boas, in her 1971 ADTA presentation, referred to Wigman and to Wigman's disciple Hanya Holm (Sorell, 1969) concerning their delineation between "active" and "passive" movement. Boas stated:

> Active movement is consciously self-directed, while passivity allows movement to happen. Anyone who has experienced passive movement will know that there is a heightened consciousness of tensions, space relations, emotions, which is arrived at through a period of stillness. Passivity can lead to extreme activity, precisely because of this sensitivity to all stimuli both internal and external. (1971, pp. 22-23)

It is this "passive" approach that Boas was referring to in the eyes closed approach to improvisation. It is very similar to the approach used by Whitehouse and the Whitehousian distinction between the "I move" (active) and the "I am moved" (passive) experience. Both Whitehouse and Boas were deeply influenced by Wigman's ideas about improvisation. What differentiated Whitehouse's work, in part, was her reliance on Jungian analytic concepts to define what she observed in the movement process. This approach to improvisation or psychomotor free association used by both Boas and Whitehouse in their studio work continues to be used today by many Whitehouse disciples and others who work primarily with the often high-functioning adult population. Elements of this form of improvisation can also be seen in the work of Hawkins, Espenak and Evan.

Summary

Boas pioneered in the integration of dance and movement into a psychotherapeutic modality in two settings. The first was as part of a research team, which included the work of Lauretta Bender and Paul Schilder at Bellevue Hospital in New York. The second was within her studio working with dancers. Boas integrated three major ideas prevalent at that time: 1) the building of body image through movement explorations, 2) the use of projective techniques in psychotherapy and 3) the use of free association.

Boas, influenced by the changing view of dance and psychology so prominent in the 1930s and 1940s, helped to usher in a new form of expressive and creative dance that integrated both the aims of the art of dance and the science of mental health.

Part B. Elizabeth Rosen: Trial and Error

Elizabeth Rosen wrote the first book on dance therapy, *Dance in Psychotherapy* originally as her Ed.D. and published by Columbia University Teachers College in 1957. This manuscript stands out as the first comprehensive study of dance therapy within the hospital milieu. Because Rosen stopped practicing soon after her study was completed and because the book was taken out of print, her contribution has not always received the recognition it deserves. Much of the following discussion of Rosen's work is based on this pioneering publication.

Rosen directed the dance therapy programs at Hillside Hospital and Manhattan State Hospital and taught a course in dance therapy at Brooklyn State Hospital in 1959. Her students included two prominent dance therapists, Phillis Lipton and Claire Schmais. Rosen developed her own style of intervention through a process of trial and error. She drew a correlation between the patients' emotional needs and the roles they assume in a dance therapy group situation.

In her book, Rosen discussed five major aspects of dance therapy: 1) the broad objectives of dance therapy, 2) educational and creative styles of movement facilitation, 3) the therapist's role, 4) patient reactions to dance therapy and 5) dance therapy in a hospital setting.

Rosen outlined three broad objectives of dance therapy: physical, social and psychological, with specific aims depending on the individual needs of the patients. For example, the physical objective for lethargic patients was to condition their bodies through simple techniques such as bending and stretching as a way to get them accustomed to physical activity. For manic patients who needed to avoid stimulating activity, the stress was on structured techniques, which demanded disciplined body control along with relaxation techniques.

The social objectives varied, depending on the patients' capacities for social interaction. The objective for the severely withdrawn was to arouse some responsiveness through kinesthetic reaction to rhythm and movement. For patients who had problems with aggression, the objective was to teach social control by channeling their aggression into dance movement responses. In the case of the more socially mature patients, cooperative group activities and group improvisations were emphasized.

The overall psychological objective was to help the patients use dance to express and satisfy individual needs. The withdrawn and more timid patients were given continuous support and reassurance. Feelings of unity with and acceptance by the group were fostered by the use of simple, rhythmic group movements performed in circle formation with the patients holding hands. Folk dances and ballroom dancing provided a satisfying social experience for self-conscious patients who would feel threatened by more unconventional forms of dance, while the dramatic dance offered a socially acceptable way for the more aggressive patients to express hostility. Patients with exhibitionist tendencies were given opportunities to lead the group and improvisations and pantomimes were stressed.

Rosen viewed the therapist's major role as twofold: first, to provide individual support and second, as a group catalyst. Because of this dual role, she brought in an assistant leader to co-lead the groups.

In her discussion of the hospital atmosphere, Rosen covered a broad spectrum of concerns that pertained specifically to dance therapy in the hospital setting. In particular, she noted several problems that she faced in regard to the hospital milieu and to the formation of a group. The physical environment was very distracting, with a constant stream of people walking in and out; there was no confidentiality because the doctors and nurses could see the patients. The broad age span within the group created special problems in that the older patients had different physical needs and abilities from the younger ones. There was a constant shift in patient load, with discharges, new admittances and transfers. Also, shock therapy and psychotherapy were often scheduled at times that overlapped with the dance sessions. These factors, she believed, reduced the effectiveness of the group as a cohesive, integrating force.

Hillside Hospital: The Open Ward

Rosen's social objective of creating a sense of belonging to a group was realized most fully on the open ward. The dance sessions were elective for the open ward group and each came with a desire to dance. These patients required much less support from the leaders and were able to use a variety of group structures without loss of group identification. In addition to the circle formation, patients were able to work in small groups, in lines or scattered throughout the room. The clique of "regulars" that came to the dance sessions became a tight-knit group, very close to each other and deeply committed to the dance therapy sessions.

Many of Rosen's patients were motivated to join the group by a desire to learn how to use their bodies effectively. They wanted to acquire better body control and coordination and to expand their range of movement. Here, they were expressing solid ego-oriented needs for control, mastery, effectiveness and so on. They recognized that learning the basic skills of dance would help them reach these goals.

Accordingly, at least one third of each session was devoted to technical exercises. The patients were trained in all the fundamentals of body technique and rhythm, which were presented in a highly structured form moving from the simple to the more complex. With frequent repetition of these basic tools, the patients gradually developed a repertoire of movement techniques and simple folk dances, which provided them with a feeling of accomplishment.

The most challenging approach for these patients was the use of dramatic ideas and themes. Concepts that were not too threatening or personal, such as "storm," "searching," or "sorrow," were used to stimulate creative expression in movement. Rosen noted that certain words and ideas are deeply rooted in cultural traditions and evoke stereotyped reactions that tend to cover up real emotional responses. Like Boas and Evan, Rosen believed that by applying the "free association technique" to movement, the motor responses to certain words and ideas could be used as a projective method. For Rosen's patients, learning how to project the feeling and quality of certain concepts opened up new avenues of communication through movement. It also helped them to appreciate dance as an art form rather than merely as the perfection of technique and body control, which, as mentioned earlier, was the initial motivation that prompted most of them to join the dance sessions.

In regard to the overall results of the improvisational work of the open ward group, Rosen stated:

> While the majority of patients did develop a sense of ease and confidence in movement which enabled them to participate freely in the creative work of the group, individually they exhibited frustration and conflict about doing anything alone. Improvisations were willingly attempted when everyone "did them together" and when no special point was made about "showing it" to the others. (1956, p. 122)

Nevertheless, once the group had established cohesion, the creative movement experience became more personally meaningful to the patients and they began to recognize that these activities were therapeutic. Some found their identity through dance. For example, one patient, who was diagnosed as catatonic schizophrenic with initially a poor prognosis, began to realize her potential as a dancer through this program. On discharge from the hospital, she aggressively pursued a successful career as a dancer. Another patient became attached to the dance therapy process, feeling he was getting more from it than from his psychotherapy. He said:

> From the beginning I felt (or hoped) that this dance form had potential importance for me. Something made me seem to yearn for this type of expression. Buried feelings pushed for the opportunity to be freed and perhaps more accurately, I pushed the feelings, trying to find some way of expressing them through the use of my body.
>
> Modern Dance helps me experience feelings which I have seldom been able to express or release. For example, when you make a conscious effort to express joy through movement, this feeling is released to some extent and you learn what it feels like. And familiarity with a feeling will probably decrease resistance to expressing this feeling in other situations. Anxiety about expressing feeling is reduced. (Rosen, 1956, p. 129)

Manhattan State Hospital

As was the case at Hillside Hospital, the purpose of the dance therapy program at Manhattan State Hospital was research and observation. Rosen directed the project with the cooperation of hospital staff members.

The dance sessions were held twice weekly for 15 weeks, with each session lasting approximately one hour. The group originally consisted of 12 female patients between the ages of 20 and 40 who were selected on psychiatric referral. Of these, two dropped out and the study covers the remaining ten. All of these patients were diagnosed as psychotic-catatonic or paranoid. All were considered chronic and had undergone either electric shock or insulin therapy during the previous two years. Their general characteristics were physical deterioration, slovenliness, sluggishness, docility and acquiescence.

The dance sessions took place in the recreation hall, a large open room and an attendant brought in the patients. In the initial session, the patients entering the hall showed no response to the lively music that was being played or to the leaders who were moving about freely, nor did they react to the physical spaciousness of the large room after being confined in the narrow halls of the wards. Rather, they passively followed the attendant to one part of the hall where they sat down and waited quietly until the session formally began. Only then did they come out on the floor to dance. They followed this same routine in all the subsequent sessions.

During the first few sessions, the patients were introduced to very basic types of movements, including running, skipping and waltzing with rhythmic accompaniment and relaxing and stretching techniques. All of these exercises were very simple, presented in highly structured and repetitive form. The goal of the leaders during this introductory period was to assess the abilities of the patients, to offer them support and reassurance and to help them get used to the medium of movement. Throughout this time, the patients responded automatically, without interest or personal involvement. The activity seemed to have no meaning for them and they performed without conscious awareness.

Rosen, suspecting that the techniques being used were too structured and simple, decided to adopt a new approach that might challenge the patients to express their feelings in words and movement. She introduced two methods. The first was a direct question technique presenting an idea or theme. Questions such as "How does one show anger?" were asked to stimulate the patients to express themselves verbally and in movement. This method was successful in arousing some individual responsiveness.

The second method, the interpretation of music, evoked a much less-intellectualized kind of movement and feeling than the direct question method. The patients responded best to familiar music, such as lullabies, military songs, hymns, folk songs and jazz recordings. The rhythm and quality of the music and its cultural and personal associations seemed to arouse and awaken the patients' "flashes of recognition, penetrating deeply into long-forgotten memories.... Patients who had previously appeared totally out of contact could thus be drawn into a reality response" (p. 161).

Musical selections from other cultures were also used. The patients did not respond well to the strange rhythms of Far Eastern music, but African tribal music and the drum rhythms of Haiti were extremely successful. It was discovered that movement responses were generally freer and less-stereotyped when the music was more primitive, as was the case with the African and Haitian music. The patients abandoned themselves to the power of the rhythm and their movement interpretations were uninhibited, almost instinctive. Sometimes, the patients responded as a group, spontaneously creating a dance with unity; other times they responded individually.

The change in approach from simple movement techniques to creative expression through the interpretation of music and the dramatization of ideas aroused responsiveness from the patients. While the response during the early sessions was detached and mechanical, the dance took on extra meaning when the patients were encouraged to "do it their own way." Verbalizations increased noticeably and the patients began to react with greater awareness to the leaders, establishing various kinds of relationships with them. Rosen does not describe exactly how this came about, that is, whether she moved with the patients, directed them or just put on music and waited.

This greater responsiveness to the encouragement of creative expression versus the use of simple movement techniques is very interesting in light of the common assumption that the more disturbed the population the greater the need for structure. This assumption had been supported at Hillside Hospital where the less disturbed open ward patients responded well to improvisational work while the more disturbed patients needed structure. Yet, at Manhattan State, where the patients were severely disturbed, the opposite was true.

The patients at Manhattan State Hospital were able to achieve *some* degree of group participation through the physical act of dancing together and there were occasional moments of group unity. While major interactional changes did not occur, the patients' "... kinesthetic response to movement and rhythm ... proved to be the most effective means of initiating social participation...." (p. 181). In addition, on the individual psychological level,

> ... the dance did offer certain patients a usable medium for self-expression and a means of releasing ideas and feelings previously unexpressed. It provided a whole new area for acting out conflict and fantasy. (Rosen, 1956, pp. 182-183)

Summary

Rosen categorized her findings regarding patient reactions to dance therapy into the following patterns:

1. *Withdrawn.* The patients who reacted according to this pattern were generally submissive, obedient and detached. Their responsiveness to movement was basically an empathic one and they were highly dependent on the support of the leader. They responded best to techniques involving simple and natural movements of the body performed in a circle formation with a strong rhythmic accompaniment.

2. *Self-conscious.* These patients were generally apathetic, keeping careful control over their emotions and were extremely conscious of being watched or observed. They participated in exercise techniques and in social dancing but were embarrassed by more creative or primitive movements and avoided all free, expressive improvisations.

3. *Aggressive.* These patients were hostile, suspicious and very defensive. They used dance to express their aggressive feelings, often manifested in strong, thrusting movements and frequently argued with the

leader and criticized the other participants. Finding the structure of the circle or group dance too restrictive, they responded best when performing dramatic improvisations or pantomime.

4. *Exhibitionist.* These patients used the dance to satisfy their need for approval and recognition. When they were being watched and admired by others they participated with great enthusiasm. Otherwise, they either quickly lost interest or became disruptive.

5. *Intellectual.* These patients were generally intelligent but unable to express real feelings. They were attracted to dance as a means of releasing emotion and participated enthusiastically in dramatic improvisations, verbalizations about the dance and interpretations of music.

6. *Voyeuristic.* These patients did not participate in the dance but were very involved as spectators and felt a strong identification with the group. They often responded with small body movements or rhythmic swaying.

Rosen's *Dance As Psychotherapy* was an important contribution to the discipline of dance therapy. It provides an in-depth, detailed and systematic discussion of the initiation and development of two early dance therapy programs. Although not published until 1957, Rosen's study began long before dance therapy was a recognized profession in 1952. Rosen's scholarly approach elicited support from both the psychiatric and psychological professions. This enabled her to work closely with other hospital staff and as a result her study became a collaborative effort in which each contributor benefited from the expertise of the others.

Central to Rosen's work as a dance therapist was her willingness to experiment. When she found, for example, that patients were not responding to simple prescribed movements, she abandoned her initial concept of teaching movement and moved to improvisation. Rosen actively pursued a trial and error process of treatment, with few—if any—preconceived ideas about how things "should" evolve. This flexibility was the cornerstone of her success with the most regressed patient groups. She is unique in her use of improvisation and free association with hospitalized patients in addition to structured dance experience.

Part C. Dance Therapy Study

In 1957, the Dance Therapy Study Committee of the American Alliance conducted a study for Health, Physical Education, Recreation and Dance (AAHPERD), National Section on Dance. Its purpose was to assess the state of the art and practice of dance therapy and to explore the future of the field. This study was done in two parts, one in the United States and one in England.

For the study conducted in the United States, 56 questionnaires were sent to people in the dance and recreational fields. Additional questionnaires were sent to interested psychiatrists or administrators. The questionnaire inquired about their backgrounds, their definition of dance therapy, their methods and their views on opportunities within the field.

Twenty-five dance therapists and eight administrators (including four psychiatrists in administrative positions) responded. Twenty of the dance therapists who responded worked in mental hospitals, clinics or agencies. Five of them worked with patients who were blind, hearing impaired, developmentally disabled or had orthopedic or neurological disabilities. From their responses a workable definition of dance therapy was reached:

> Dance therapy is the use of dance as a carefully guided tool to produce desirable physiological, emotional and/or behavioral changes in emotionally or physically handicapped persons. (Hood, 1959, p. 18)

These changes were found to be in the areas of "alleviation or correction of physical difficulties, release of tension, development of awareness, acceptance of self and others, effective social interaction" (Hood, 1959, p. 18).

In regard to the training of these early leaders, the questionnaires revealed that most had degrees in physical education, recreation or music therapy. In dance training, some had very little and others had extensive backgrounds; only one had none. Seventeen had studied modern dance and one-third had experience in several dance forms including modern, tap, ballet, jazz, folk, square and ballroom. Nineteen studied psychology and about two-thirds had on-the-job training. Eight studied with Marian Chace directly and three studied with Rudolf Laban.

Dance therapy was found to be one of the newer and less known treatment modalities. It was considered "experimental, improvisational, [and] uncharted ..." (Hood, 1959, p. 18). However, responses from the questionnaires revealed that the use of dance as therapy was received enthusiastically in the setting where it had been tried. Dance as therapy was reported as being used for: 1) the experience of feelings (e.g., sexuality, hostility, depression); 2) physical benefits; 3) interaction and 4) as a bridge to verbal interaction with others, hence, as preparation for psychotherapy.

The committee that conducted the study suggested that dance educators should become familiar with dance therapy techniques and research. They stated: "Dance therapy has grown out of the educational approach to dance; in turn, research in dance therapy may contribute to dance education" (Hood, 1959, p. 72).

The companion study conducted in England revealed that the use of movement as therapy was more firmly established and was recognized by more psychiatrists in England than in the United States during the mid-1950s (Wooten, 1959). While American dance therapists at that time came from a wide variety of backgrounds and experimented with various techniques, the vast majority of English dance therapists (including all of those who responded to the questionnaire) based their work on Laban's *Art of Movement* (Wooten, 1959).

Five dance therapists, one psychotherapist, one psychiatrist and one lay analyst responded to the questionnaires sent out in England. Of the five dance therapists, one worked very closely with a psychiatrist, three worked independently of psychiatrists, but all had some patients who were also under psychiatric care. Many psychiatrists in England at this time viewed dance therapy as an alternative to psychoanalysis and sometimes referred patients to a dance therapist. However, most of the people who came to dance therapists did so because they were under stress but did not want to consult a psychiatrist.

All the dance therapists who responded to the questionnaire used movement as the only therapy for some patients. Five uses of movement therapy were identified:

1. Movement as communication, that is, as a means for making initial contact and establishing rapport with the patient;
2. Group movement for social adjustment;
3. Movement as creative expression for the individual, that is, as a means of bringing the unconscious to consciousness and thereby helping the individual get in touch with his/her inner state;
4. Movement as expressive of the individual, that is, the dance therapist could learn about the individual's personality and capabilities by notating and analyzing his motion rhythms using Laban's framework and
5. Movement as an impressive agent, that is, movement has specific meanings in terms of the individual's personality.

Wooten explains:

> The impression made on the individual by his use of effort and space is specific and predictable, each aspect of his personality being linked with a definite aspect of movement. For example, man's sensory self is linked with his use of weight, his intuitive self with time, his thinking mind is linked with his use of space, his feeling or emotional self with flow. (Wooten, 1959, p. 76)

As is clear from numbers 4 and 5 above, English dance therapists in the mid-1950s were greatly influenced by Laban's teachings. However, this "new development" was not, at that time, "widely recognized or understood," but showed "great promise" as "a valuable means for reintegrating the disturbed personality" (Wooten, 1959, p. 76). In the United States, it was not until the mid-1960s that Laban Movement Analysis became important to the work of dance therapists.

The Dance Therapy Study, conducted by AAHPERD's National Section on Dance, was an important benchmark in the history of dance therapy. Done in two parts, one in the U.S. and one in England, its purpose was to assess the state of dance therapy practice and to explore the future of the field. The results reflected some important trends that helped to define the profession in terms of its roots in dance psychotherapy, its goals, its acceptance as a discipline, the therapists who were practicing and the clients they served.

Discussion

Outline Depicting the State of the Art by 1960

The following outline depicts the state of the practice of dance therapy in the early 1960s. The outline was derived from an analysis of the clinical contributions of the major pioneers discussed in Chapters 1-8. The items designated by Roman numerals represent overall categories of intervention. Listed beneath these major headings is a breakdown of the various methods used alternately by the pioneers. Interestingly, the outline indicates that by the early 1960s, dance therapy had already achieved a very broad and complete base of practice. What the following decades would bring to the art of dance therapy was not so much new techniques, but a more in-depth, well-defined understanding of why the practice of dance therapy works, that is, theoretical foundations. While dance therapy techniques are being refined and expanded for specific patient-client groups, it is clear that the practical foundations were well developed and extremely diversified quite early in the history of the discipline.

DANCE THERAPY OUTLINE DEPICTING THE STATE OF THE ART BY THE EARLY 1960s

I. Warm-up and Body Awareness Techniques Included:

   A. Articulation of body parts (e.g., rotations and swings),
   B. Rhythmic movements, explorations and games,
   C. Repetitive movements,
   D. Education in the rudiments of movement,
   E. Introduction to basic dance steps (e.g., folk. social etc.),
   F. Use of props (hoops, scarves~ percussion instruments~ etc.),
   G. Relaxation and breathing techniques,
   H. Exploring tension fluctuation and extremes,
   I. Exploring contrasting movement themes (extremes and gradations)
   J. Body awareness techniques,
   K. Postural explorations,
   L. Projective techniques and
   M. The use of music as a facilitator of movement and as a background support.

II. **Expressive Dance Movement Activities Included:**

   A. Psychomotor free-association through:
      1. Improvisation,
      2. Active imagination,
      3. Dream interpretation,
      4. Fantasy explorations,
      5. Reenactments of childhood memories,
      6. Projective techniques,
      7. Spontaneous dance movement interpretation of music and
   B. The exploration of ambivalence and emotional conflict through:
      1. Role-playing,
      2. The exploration of contrasting movement themes—spontaneous and choreographed and
      3. Choreographed explorations of emotions.

III. **Dance Forms Used by the Pioneers at Various Times Included:**

   A. Rhythmic action and repetition,
   B. Exaggeration of expression,
   C. Improvisation,
   D. Choreographed or planned (rehearsed) movement,
   E. Dramatization,
   F. Folk,
   G. Modern and creative,
   H. Ballet,
   I. Social,
   J. Ethnic and
   K. The exploration of movement dynamics—variations in space, weight and time (e.g., sustained movements vs. fragmented movements, direct movements vs. indirect movements, light movements vs. heavy movements).

IV. **The Therapeutic Interaction with the Dance Therapist Included the Therapist:**

   A. Mirroring and reflecting patients' feelings back to them through a dance movement interaction,
   B. Reacting and responding through movement to patients' needs and nonverbal communications,
   C. Engaging in playful movement dialogues as in the creation of games, fantasies and dramatic movement interactions,
   D. Verbally narrating and reflecting the conscious and unconscious thoughts and feelings of patients during the dance movement process,
   E. Empathizing, observing and listening and
   F. Teaching body movement and guiding the patient through the personal unconscious to the collective unconscious.

V. The Early Dance Therapists Used Verbalization for the:

A. Elicitation of thoughts and feelings,
B. Facilitation of insight,
C. Exclamation of thoughts and feelings while moving,
D. Reflection and narration of the psychomotor process,
E. Identification of the body in stillness and in action—naming body parts and what they are doing,
F. Facilitation of movement and
G. Interpretation and integration.

VI. Group Dance Therapy Techniques Included:

A. Shifting of leadership roles within the group;
B. Changing group constellations:
   1. Dyads and triads,
   2. Small clusters,
   3. Large group,
   4. Individual action within the group,
   5. Circle—clasped and unclasped hands and
   6. Various line formations,
C. Promoting the rhythmic group relationship,
D. Promoting supportive empathic group interaction (verbally and nonverbally),
E. Supporting the satisfaction of various role needs through controlled acting-out and
F. Role-playing.

VII. Music and Rhythm Were Designed To:

A. Help organize patients' thoughts and feelings into expressive action,
B. Support and encourage self-expression,
C. Facilitate improvisation,
D. Reflect patients' moods and needs,
E. Facilitate rhythmical action and expression,
F. Motivate and activate,
G. Create emotional responses and
H. Help modulate emotions and activity levels.

UNIT II

Subsequent Development of Dance Movement Therapy

The dance therapists discussed in Unit I made significant contributions to dance therapy in the 1940s and 1950s, at a time when it was not yet a recognized or organized profession. Their contributions paved the way for a period of rapid growth that began in the late 1960s and was inspired, to a large degree, by the development of the American Dance Therapy Association in 1966. The association was organized to "establish standards of professional competence, to encourage training and education to fulfill these standards and to effectively communicate to those in allied fields and to the general public the aims and achievements of dance therapy" (ADTA, 1966).

In the years that followed, with the ADTA's successful achievement of these goals, the profession made the transition from infancy to early adulthood. Many innovative leaders emerged in the late 1960s and 1970s with unique contributions to the field through their positions in the ADTA, as teachers and creators of educational programs and through publications. These leaders laid the professional foundation, which enables today's dance therapists to practice privately and in recognized educational institutions as well as mental health, medical and psychiatric facilities.

In addition to contributing to the professionalization and institutionalization of the field, leading dance therapists during this period also contributed to the expansion of dance therapy theory and practice. The evolution of the work of the major pioneers of the 1940s and 1950s is clearly reflected in the work of the succeeding generations of dance therapists, who were trained either directly by one or more of the pioneers or by their disciples and who have expanded upon the approaches of their mentors in a variety of ways.

Some, for example, have carried on the work of the pioneers, broadening and clarifying specific theories and techniques or adapting them for use with particular populations. Others have integrated into the approaches of their mentors ideas and methods from other related fields. Still others have developed approaches that incorporate aspects of the work of two or more pioneers and in recent years there has been a merging of east coast and west coast influences. These trends can be seen as an extension of the tradition set by the original pioneers themselves, many of whom developed their approaches through a merging of influences from, for example, their experiences as modern dancers and/or creative dance teachers and from pre-existing theoretical frameworks.

Because of the rapid growth of the field during this period and the proliferation of dance therapists who have made contributions, the focus of Unit II shifts away from individual dance therapists and revolves instead around key developments in dance therapy theory and practice. Section A examines the impact of Laban Movement Analysis, introduced in the United States by Irmgard Bartenieff. Section B focuses on other areas of theoretical and practical expansion, specifically, the integration of psychoanalytic thought by dance therapists on the east coast, the expansion of the Whitehousian approach by dance therapists on the west cost and the incorporation of other action-oriented psychotherapies.

SECTION A

Laban Movement Analysis and Dance Therapy in the United States

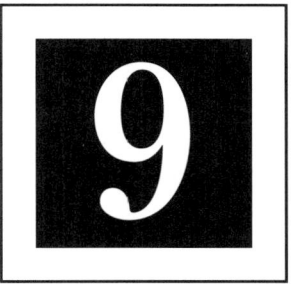

The Theoretical Contributions of Laban and Lamb

Rudolf Laban's theories, which originated in the early 1900s, were integrated by English dance therapists into the therapeutic use of dance and movement in the 1950s. Warren Lamb was a protégé of Laban who expanded on Laban's original concepts. It was not until the mid-1960s, however, that the theories of Laban and Lamb became popular among dance therapists in the United States. At that time, when dance therapy was still a fledgling profession, Laban's teaching provided a method of movement analysis and a system of notation that placed dance therapists on their own professional ground, giving them a language for describing patients' movements and eliminating the need to rely on less accurate jargon borrowed from other disciplines.

Various terms are commonly used in referring to Laban's work. The term "effort/shape" refers to Laban's effort system and to Lamb's shape system. Some dance therapists, who do not use Lamb's shape system, simply use the term effort, while those who use Laban's complete theoretical framework refer to "Laban Movement Analysis," "Labanalysis," or "LMA."

Laban viewed body movement in a complicated and multifaceted way. He saw its potential use as an expressive medium of both conscious and unconscious thoughts, feelings and conflicts and also a vehicle through which societies pass on traditions, coping behaviors and religious rituals.

> Man moves in order to satisfy needs. He aims by his movement at something of value to him. It is easy to perceive the aim of a person's movement if it is directed to some tangible object. Yet there also exist intangible values that inspire movement. (Laban, revised Uliman, 1971, p. 1)

Laban continually impressed on his readers the variety of ways in which we express ourselves and our particular styles of coping through what he terms our movement configurations. For example, some individuals meet a problem energetically with quick, direct actions, while others circle an issue in a sustained manner for several days before coming to a conclusion.

Laban also stressed the individual's capacity, as compared with that of animals, to change his or her style of communication and adaptation through both conscious and unconscious mechanisms. Comparing animal movements to human movements and correlating his thoughts concerning the complexity of the human movement potential with one possible cause of human conflict, Laban said:

> It appears that the effort (exertion) characteristics of man are much more varied and variable than those of animals. One meets people with cat-like, ferret-like, horse-like movements, but one never sees a horse, a ferret, a cat exhibiting human-like movements. The animal world is rich in effort manifestations, but each animal genus is restricted to a relatively small range of typical qualities. Animals are perfect in the efficient use of the restricted effort habits they possess, man is less efficient in the use of the more numerous effort shadings potentially possible to him. It is not surprising that more numerous and vehement conflicts should arise in human beings possessing the capacity for such manifold and often contradictory combinations of effort qualities. (Laban, revised Ullman, 1971, p. 11)

Laban's keen observational skills and his attention to form and content grew out of his theater and performing background and his interest in architecture. His investigation of movement began in Central Europe, where he experimented with three different forms of movement: traditional forms in fencing and ballet; modern forms, which led to the development of the early modern dance style of Central Europe and formalized work movements (Dell, 1970). Out of this experience Laban developed a system of movement description called Kinetography Laban or Labanotation, describing what body parts move, when and where.

Later, when Laban was asked to conduct efficiency studies for British industry during World War II, he investigated the qualitative aspects of movement, that is, how a person moves. This resulted in his development of a system of movement description that attempted to describe all the possible ways we move in terms of the concept of exertion (effort). Later, growing out of Laban's work, Lamb's (1965) concept of "shape" was introduced as a correlate of "effort" (Dell, 1970), resulting in "effort/shape."

Basically, effort/shape is "a method of describing changes in movement quality in terms of the kinds of exertions [effort] and the kinds of body adaptations in space [shape]" (Dell, 1970, p. 7). These two distinct though interconnected concepts are widely used by dance therapists today.

Effort

Effort describes movement dynamics in terms of four motion factors: space, weight, time and flow. Each movement factor has two opposing possibilities called "elements": the individual's use of space can be either "direct" (the shortest distance between two points) or "indirect" (circuitous); the use of weight can be "strong" (using greater exertion) or "light" (using less exertion); the use of time can be "quick" (sudden) or "slow" (sustained) and finally, flow can be either "bound" or "free" (representing the ease or restraint of the movement).

It is impossible to isolate one movement factor or element. Each movement factor is dependent on certain other factors. What varies is the intensity and combination of movement elements, which dominate at a given moment. Thus, in observing the movement of a patient, the therapist tries to discover which movement factors or elements are present as part of the larger movement configuration and context.

In using effort, movement characteristics are often discussed in relation to personality attributes. The movements seem to come alive and have more meaning when discussed in this way. However, this can be misleading and convey emotional overtones not actually inherent in the individual's movement behavior. Also, one must be cautioned against possible judgmental aspects of the effort terminology when used in

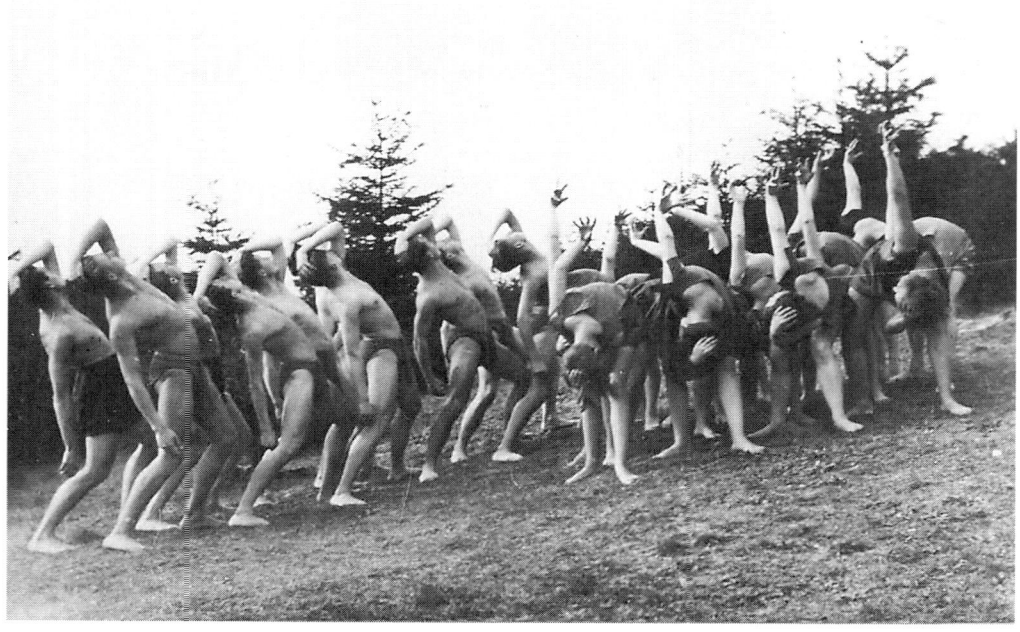

Rudolf Laban's Movement Choir (early 1900's)—exploring large group movement (Photo courtesy The Laban-Bartenieff Institute of Movement Studies, New York)

this way. For example, an indirect use of space does not necessarily mean an inability to cope with space or life directly, but rather a preference for a certain style of coping. Similarly, concerning the strong versus light use of weight, an individual who uses mostly movements of "strength" does not necessarily have a stronger or more assertive personality than an individual who uses "lightness."

To guard against making simplistic interpretations of personality structure, therapists need an understanding of movement from a psychological, anthropological and sociological perspective. Moreover, the therapist must not lose sight of the whole movement process and get lost in the parts.

Shape

Warren Lamb (1965) introduced the concept of shaping. Whenever an individual makes a change in his or her use of effort elements, a corresponding shape change occurs. Shape describes the "where" of movement, that is, where the body forms itself in space. There are three kinds of shape changes that are observed in Laban Movement Analysis:

1) shape flow, 2) directional movement and 3) shaping movement.

For shape flow, the observer looks at changes between body parts moving towards or away from each other. For directional movement, the observer looks at the paths of movement in space, which are either arc-like or spoke-like. These one- or two-dimensional movements tend to be characteristic of functional activity. For shaping, the observer looks for adapting or molding movements such as holding an infant. These are usually two- or three-dimensional movements.

The primary leader responsible for the timely introduction of Laban and Lamb's concepts in the United States was Irmgard Bartenieff. Bartenieff was a pioneering leader in dance therapy and a protégé of Laban. In Chapter 10, the relevance of LMA and effort/shape will be explored through a discussion of Bartenieff's contribution.

The concept of shape flow was derived from the work Forrestine Paulay was doing with Judith Kestenberg. The concept of directional movement was developed from the work that Paulay and Bartenieff were doing in the choreometrics project—a cross-cultural study of movement style—with Alan Lomax at Columbia University.

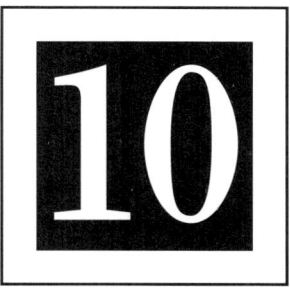

Irmgard Bartenieff Brings LMA to America

Irmgard Bartenieff (1900-1981) played an important role in the history and development of Laban Movement Analysis (LMA) and its application to dance therapy and physical therapy. She pioneered the integration of LMA with her career as a physical therapist. Out of these two disciplines, Bartenieff created her own approach to body movement education known today as the Bartenieff Fundamentals (Bartenieff & Lewis, 1980). This approach to body movement is re-educational in that it develops movement efficiency and expressiveness by emphasizing the spatial aspects of movement and incorporating them into efficient motor organization.

Born in 1900 and raised in Germany, Bartenieff was part of the early European modern dance movement of the 1920s. In 1925, she began her studies of Rudolf Laban's work in movement analysis. In the 1930s, Bartenieff had her own dance company, which toured Germany. She was impressed with Mary Wigman's work, but did not want to be influenced solely by Wigman's technique (personal communication, 1980). As Adolph Hitler rose to power in Nazi Germany, Bartenieff, like Espenak and Polk, fled to the United States, bringing along her knowledge of LMA. She began teaching at several key places, including Bennington College, Columbia Teachers College, the Brooklyn Museum, the New School for Social Research and the Hanya Holm Dance Studio in New York (personal communication, 1980).

Bartenieff received her degree in physical therapy from New York University in 1943 and later worked with polio victims at the Willard Parker Hospital in New York. It was there that she began experimenting with movement techniques, an experience that later contributed to her development of the Bartenieff Fundamentals and of a philosophy based on the use of movement to promote mental health. In the 1950s, she continued to work with children with disabilities at Blythedale Hospital in Valhalla, New York and resumed her studies with Laban in England during the summers.

In her physical therapy work at Willard Parker and Blythedale Hospitals in New York, Bartenieff was particularly respected for her ingenuity in reaching children depressed by severe physical limitations, devising special games adapted to their needs and abilities. She emphasized the mobilization of movement forms, which integrated emotional and motivational needs with physical needs (Bartenieff and Lewis, 1980). She was greatly influenced by her teacher, George Deaver, whose motto was: "activate and motivate" the patient (Bartenieff and Lewis, 1980, p. 1). Having personally experienced the hardships of escaping from Germany and supporting her family in the United States, she was well aware of the role of motivation in personal growth and in the ability to change and adapt. This concentration on activation and motivation later became her most natural means of working with both patients and students.

In the early 1960s, Bartenieff became associated with Israel Zwerling, professor of Social Psychiatry at Albert Einstein Medical College Hospital and director of the Day Hospital at Jacobi in the Bronx, New York.[1] At the Day Hospital, Bartenieff was involved primarily in research projects, observing and notating nonverbal communication and interaction in family and group therapy sessions. She also began to explore the use of movement as an expressive medium for psychiatric patients. On one occasion, Zwerling happened to observe her intervention with one severely disturbed catatonic patient and was deeply moved by her ability

---

[1] Noted movement researcher Martha Davis (Bartenieff & Davis, 1965) was first introduced to Bartenieff and LMA at the Day Hospital. Davis assisted Bertenieff in her work and later at Bronx State Hospital, and has become a leading proponent of this form of movement analysis.

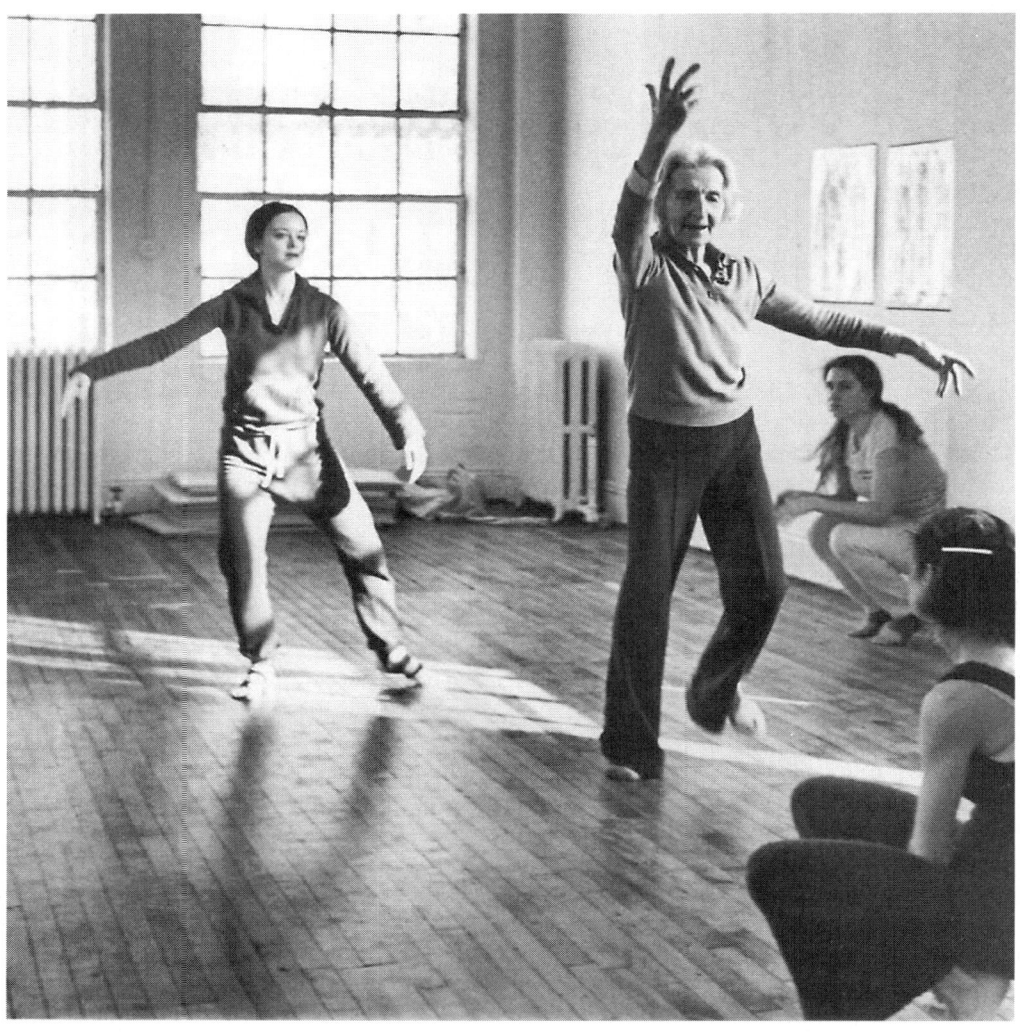
Bartenieff asserted that a successful dance therapist activates the patient's "independent participation in his own recovery" (Photo courtesy The Laban-Bartenieff Institute of Movement Studies, New York)

to draw this and other individuals out through movement (Davis, personal communication, 1980).[2]

In the mid-1960s, Bartenieff went with Zwerling to Bronx State Hospital and continued her work in dance therapy research. Whereas at the Day Hospital she worked with outpatients, at Bronx State she adapted LMA as therapy for inpatients with severe developmental disabilities.

It was at Bronx State Hospital that Bartenieff's work became formally integrated with the discipline of dance therapy.[3] Her contributions to the field were timely and crucial. She offered a system of movement observation, analysis and notation that could be used to guide, direct and describe dance therapy sessions. This was at a time when dance therapists were in need of a language that could communicate their clinical

---

[2]Zwerling was extremely supportive of Bartenieff's work, respecting her both for her interaction skills with patients and for her talents in movement analysis and research. He was a major proponent of the creative arts therapies, emphasizing body movement for research purposes, for diagnosis of family interactions, and most importantly as a form of primary therapy. (Zwerling, 1979)

[3]Elissa White and Claire Schmais soon joined Bartenieff and her assistant, Martha Davis. Their collaboration led to the development of the Dance Therapy/LMA program at Bronx State Hospital, which became a major training ground for dance therapists. (See *Chapter 11*)

experience. Laban's and Lamb's contributions, applied practically and expanded by Bartenieff, represented a partial solution to this problem.

Bartenieff maintained an active interest in movement research throughout her career. From the 1940s through the mid-1970s, she was a prominent faculty member at the Dance Notation Bureau (DNB) in New York City. Together with Davis and Paulay, she pioneered a training program at the DNB. It was there that many dance therapists were first introduced to Laban's work. In the late 1970s, Bartenieff and several colleagues left the Dance Notation Bureau to open their own training institute designed to specialize in LMA education. Bartenieff was a founding member and the first president of this new institute, the Laban Institute of Movement Studies in New York City.[4]

At the age of 80, Irmgard Bartenieff made her final contribution to the field of human body movement: her book entitled *Body Movement: Coping with the Environment*, coauthored with Dori Lewis and published in 1980.

Theory and Practice

Bartenieff's work stressed perceiving movement as a complex interrelated whole.

> What is critical to the comprehension of these perceptions is that they be understood as a whole—without fragmentation. Change in any aspect [of movement] changes the whole configuration. (Bartenieff & Lewis, 1980, p. x)

This perspective of body movement as a continually fluctuating process influenced Bartenieff's thinking in every area of movement analysis and intervention. Her conviction was that:

> ...behavior must be understood in relation to neurophysiology and total organic functioning. The effort-shape theory of movement is based on an organic model of behavior. The major hypothesis [is] that neural processes, adaptation and expression are integrated in movement. Every movement in any part of the body is at once adaptive and expressive; it functions as a coping mechanism while at the same time it reflects something about the individual. (Bartenieff & Davis, 1965, p. 51)

Bartenieff believed that each individual's movement style was an amalgam of his or her congenital activity type, psychological influences and the cultural milieu (Bartenieff & Lewis, 1980). Respecting the individual's unique physical expression of these influences, she worked creatively to help her patients make better use of what was already present in their movement repertoires.

Focus on Potential Movement Expression

In clinical work with patients, Bartenieff always looked at the total movement configuration with a major focus on the potential movement expression. The idea that potential movement was inherent in one's physical actions and movement preferences derived from Laban's concept of "a diminished effort." If an effort was diminished, it remained present, but in small quantity. Hence, there existed the beginning or partial utilization of certain effort and shape factors that were only partially activated. Bartenieff did not attempt to explain, in formal psychological terms, why a specific movement factor might appear only in its diminished state or why a certain quality of movement would not actually fully materialize. Instead, this was simply accepted and incorporated into the total configuration.

Bartenieff cautioned the therapist against pointing out to a patient what movements they were lacking or requesting that the patient consciously work at producing a particular movement. Rather, she believed the therapist should study the total movement configuration available to the patient and then nonverbally engage him or her in movement activities, which, in accordance with the individual's specific movement preferences, would eventually draw out the diminished movement factor or element.

In the following statement, Bartenieff described the circuitous process of reaching an individual who, for one reason or another, was not employing directness within his or her movement repertoire:

---

[4]After her death in 1981, the institute's name was changed to the Laban/Bartenieff Institute of Movement Studies.

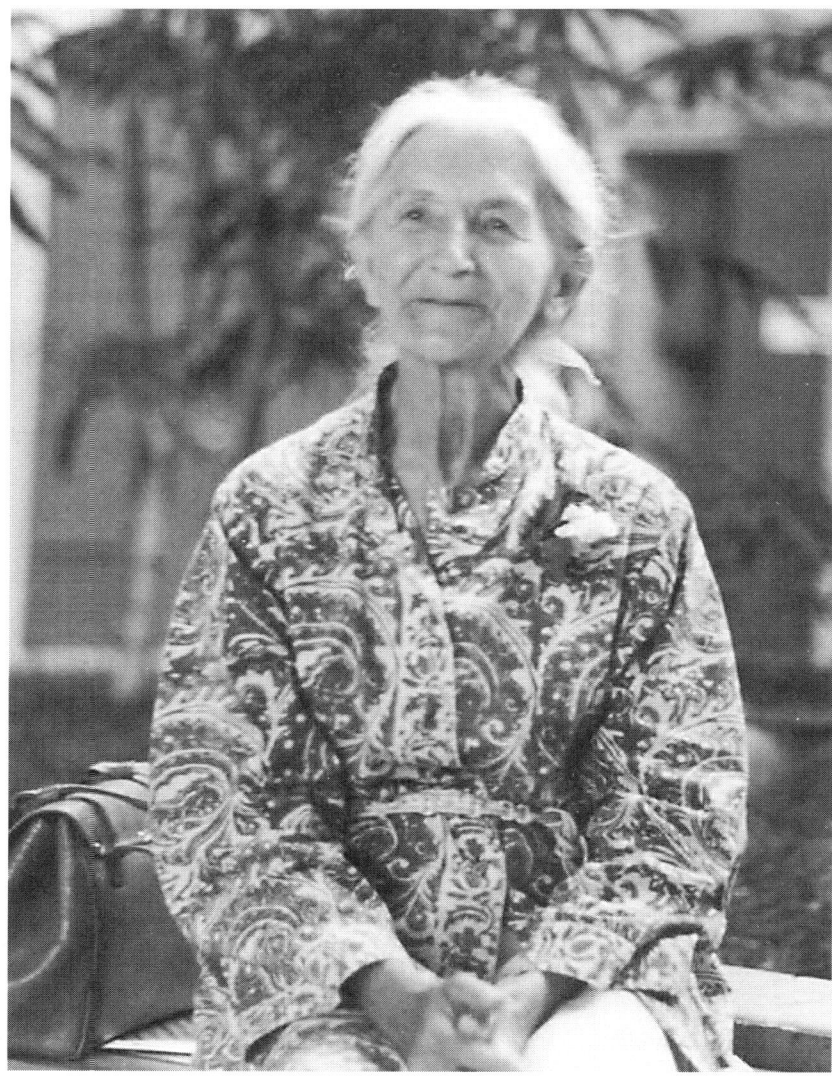
Irmgard Bartenieff (Photo courtesy The Laban-Bartenieff Institute of Movement Studies, New York)

> ... the Directness deficiency ... should be treated in the context of the patient's whole organization of Effort combinations and the accompanying spatial shape actions. The therapist may first start to explore all combinations of the patient's repertoire, such as Flow with Weight (Strength or Lightness), Flow with Time (Sudden or Sustained) and soon, from there, the therapist may gain access to the use of Directness in combination [with other movement factors]. (Bartenieff & Lewis, 1980, p. 148)

This was perhaps the essence of the Bartenieff philosophy and the resulting methodology, that is, finding the correct activities that supported the development of specific muscle systems, which, in turn, affected certain emotional attitudes.

Another approach Bartenieff used, mostly among patients with mental retardation, to help an individual develop a specific effort element—in this case "directness" (a space factor)—was playing physically active games. Since active games often require clear spatial intent on the part of the players, such activity would support the expression of this effort factor in a non-threatening and often pleasurable way.

Bartenieff viewed dance therapy within a humanistic framework. Instead of focusing on the limitations or pathology of the personality as viewed through the body structure and movement behavior, Bartenieff looked at the total movement profile, with a major focus on the potential movement expression.

Motivation and the Use of Space

In helping hospitalized individuals to explore their movement potential, Bartenieff stressed the need to activate and mobilize the "movement impulse" (the motivational factor behind movement).

> My task, defined for me by this climate of stasis and regression [i.e., the hospital milieu], was to find ways of keeping alive the movement impulse. This problem has continued to remain central to all my work with the emotionally disturbed and dealing with it is the key to dance therapy. (Bartenieff & Lewis, 1980, p. 9)

She found that movements that emphasized the creation of spatial designs (i.e., circular, angular, spoke-like, etc.) elicited important emotional responses and attitudes in patients. Particular spatial pathways activated during dance explorations inspired the somatic externalization of specific thoughts and feelings. Through the incorporation of spatial designs, Bartenieff could further develop the patient's expressive movement vocabulary. However, she stressed that in order to successfully introduce spatial concepts, the dance therapist must be comfortable with and aware of the patient's intentions. Only if the therapist is attuned to the patient can he or she facilitate the patient's psychophysical connection to space via dance. If the dance therapist is successful he or she can activate the patient's "independent participation in his own recovery" (Bartenieff & Lewis, 1980, p. 3).

The Bartenieff Fundamentals

Out of her early experience working with both individuals with physical disabilities and individuals with mental illnesses, Bartenieff later developed six specific body movement exercises, which are described in her book *Body Movement: Coping with the Environment* (1980). These basic exercises, called the "Bartenieff Fundamentals," provided the individual with "a means of becoming aware of some primary experiences of the self and being led from that to a clearer feeling of oneself in relation to others" (Bartenieff & Lewis, 1980, p. 146). They were specifically designed to help the individual integrate body feeling with emotional feeling and expression. "The functional and expressive contents of movement are two sides of the same coin" (Bartenieff & Lewis, 1980, p. 145).

The Bartenieff Fundamentals were also designed to enable individuals to unify their perceptions of three simultaneous activities: breathing, muscular fluctuation and feeling. She purposely limited her verbal instructions, omitting statements such as "this is how you breathe." Instead, she encouraged her patients to develop a personal sensitivity to their body processes by having them do movement sequences that supported the integration of the physical and emotional experiences of the self. The Fundamentals attempted to replace intellectualized movement endeavors, which Bartenieff felt only further fragmented the mind and body, a state often already overemphasized in the disturbed individual (Bartenieff & Lewis, 1980).

The Fundamentals grew out of Bartenieff's early-held belief that contacting the motivational aspect of the individual's movement is the key to integrating physical expression with emotional expression, that is, unifying mind and body. In emphasizing the strength, potential and uniqueness within the personality, Bartenieff supported the individual's self-acceptance. This, in turn, encouraged a more total actualization of the individual's movement potential, along with a more flexible and complete expression of self.

Focus on Community/Society

While the motivational aspect of movement focused mainly on the individual's relationship to self, Bartenieff also emphasized the individual's relationship to others and to society. She recognized the need not only for the integration of mind and body but also for establishing a healthy balance between internal and external demands on the personality.

Because the reality of life is that we do not live in isolation, Bartenieff emphasized movement as a tool that could bridge the gap between internal and external, thereby integrating the subjective and the objective aspects of the individual's life.

> By projecting feelings into space through the body, the movements themselves are immediately communicative ... The experience of building one's own organic structures in space can subtly build confidence in one's self. To do this with others helps to develop a sense of supportiveness from the community and

an ability to make adaptations for the interdependence of that support. (Bartenieff & Lewis, 1980, pp. 144-145)

Her stress on bringing the subjective out into communicable form, adapting and shaping it so that it could be relayed, demonstrated her belief in the importance of the community and communal aspects of dance.

According to Bartenieff, the therapist's role was one of helping patients to find a satisfying mode of behavior that would enable them to live peacefully with themselves and with society. This could be viewed as developing ego controls. She stated:

> When the focus of the therapist is only on the subjective, isolated, body level without any relation to space or ... structure, there is a great danger of getting the patient stuck in single aspects of his/her problem and increasing the fragmentation of his/her movement activity. (Bartenieff & Lewis, 1980, p. 144)

> What is most important for patient and therapist is to keep both intellect and feeling accessible and functional without fragmentation. The dance therapy discipline should not be permitted to deteriorate into amorphously indulgent self-expressiveness. Nor should it become so structured by mechanical measurements that the parts become greater than the whole. (Bartenieff & Lewis, 1980, p. 151)

Summary

Bartenieff's emphasis on the perception of body movement as a complex, integrated whole permeated every aspect of her teaching and her work and was one of her major contributions to dance therapy. Her greatest contribution, however, aside from bringing Laban's theories to the United States, was perhaps her ability to communicate to others her dynamic understanding of the structure and function of movement.

Zeitgeist at Bronx State Hospital

In the mid-1960s, around the time Bartenieff began working at Bronx State Hospital, she and her disciple Martha Davis wrote an article entitled "Effort/Shape Analysis of Movement: The Unity of Expression and Function" (1965). This article presented the following three assumptions regarding the use of LMA:

1. Is a replicable technique for describing, measuring and classifying human movement;
2. Describes patterns of movement that are consistent for an individual and distinguish him from others and
3. Delineates a behavioral dimension related to neurophysiological and psychological processes (Costonis, 1978, p. 90).

In accordance with these beliefs, Bartenieff used LMA as an observational, diagnostic and assessment tool in her work at Bronx State. Her work became formally integrated into the discipline of dance therapy in the late 1960s when the dance therapy staff at Bronx State was expanded and training programs were instituted. These developments were due largely to the pioneering efforts of Elissa Queyquep White and Claire Schmais, in collaboration with Bartenieff and Davis.

Certified movement analyst White began working part-time at Bronx State in 1967 as a family therapy research assistant to Israel Zwerling, the hospital director. Zwerling's research did not involve LMA, but White, coincidentally, was simultaneously training in LMA with Bartenieff, using the family therapy session at Bronx State as the subject of study. Later that year, White was employed there working half time in research and half time in dance therapy. Soon afterward, Claire Schmais, who was teaching part-time at Hunter College, also joined the staff.

Schmais and White had met each other in the mid-1960s at a meeting of dance therapists interested in forming an association and had become "friends and comrades" while working together, along with others, to form the ADTA (White & Schmais, personal communication, 1986). Both Schmais and White had previously taken courses with Bartenieff at the Dance Notation Bureau. They also had both taken a well-known dance therapy course with Marian Chace at the Turtle Bay Music School, Schmais in 1961 and White in 1963. In addition, Schmais had interned with Chace at St. Elizabeth's Hospital in Washington, DC, for one year. Their joining the staff at Bronx State resulted in the historical and timely coming together of two previously distinct movement disciplines: the Marian Chace technique of dance therapy carried on by Elissa White and Claire Schmais and the contributions of Laban and Lamb carried on by Irmgard Bartenieff and Martha Davis.

Soon after arriving at Bronx State, Schmais and White discovered that the progressive and innovative atmosphere at the hospital presented opportunities for expanding the use of dance therapy there.

> Dr. Zwerling literally opened the locked doors at the hospital and created a climate that was receptive to new ways of working with patients. Because our primary interest was in dance therapy we became intrigued with the possibility of setting up a dance therapy program at Bronx State Hospital. (White & Schmais, personal communication, 1986)

After consulting with the nursing supervisors and with the chiefs of services, Schmais and White began giving dance therapy orientation sessions for nurses and their staffs. The purpose was to "help them understand the role of dance therapy in the overall treatment plans of their patients, how they might best participate when they joined in the sessions with us and how we could contribute to their understanding of movement behavior" (White & Schmais, personal communication, 1986). These orientation sessions eventually became a part of the regular training for new attendants and student nurses.

As the demand for dance therapy sessions increased, White and Schmais set up a six-week therapy training program for mental health workers and other staff interested in using this modality. The program focused on elementary dance therapy techniques in an effort to increase the trainees' awareness of their own movements and the movements of their patients in sessions and on the ward. After completing the training, most of the participants began conducting dance therapy sessions on their wards. Though all of them liked to dance, none had the in-depth dance training and dance teaching experience on which to base their dance therapy training. Unfortunately, it was not possible at that time to provide the ongoing support, dance training and supervision they needed.

> Though the outcome was disappointing, as it did not increase the use of dance therapy throughout the hospital, these trainees were always tremendously helpful as assistants in sessions. Their training in observation helped them talk about their perceptions of the patients' movement behavior, be it in a dance therapy session or on the ward. (White & Schmais, personal communication, 1986)

In the meantime, the dance therapy staff at Bronx State was increasing. White became the director of the first dance therapy unit at the hospital and by the late 1960s had facilitated the hiring of three full-time and five part-time dance therapists. This was a major triumph in that dance therapy was—and at times still is—fighting for professional recognition. As the dance therapy staff increased and because Zwerling's philosophy was that all staff should have continuous education, White began classes with first-year psychiatric residents, introducing them to dance therapy and movement observation. These classes evolved into ongoing sessions with the residents at the hospital and became an integral part of their psychiatric training.

In 1969, in response to continued requests for dance therapy training, White and Schmais began giving one-week, intensive introductory dance therapy workshops. Because of the burgeoning interest in dance therapy, people came from all over the country to attend these workshops. Those who desired further training were able to volunteer at the hospital. As a result of their experiences conducting these workshops, Schmais and White began to "formulate a philosophy of dance therapy training which involves the importance of understanding and knowing individual style, developing movement observation skills and knowledge of how movement interaction affects the group in dance therapy" (White & Schmais, personal communication, 1986).

They felt that given this philosophy and the enthusiastic response to training, Schmais (at Hunter College) should apply to the National Institute of Mental Health for a curriculum development grant. In response to this request, the Experimental and Special Training Branch of NIMH's Division of Manpower and Training Program contacted Schmais. She was requested to design a prototypical dance therapy-training program on the Master's level. In 1970, Schmais, White and Davis wrote the grant proposal for Hunter College.

In planning the program, they utilized their own combined experiences in dance therapy practice, training and movement research to develop an intensive, full-time, 30-credit program consisting of coursework continuously integrated with field experience. At that time, all field experience was planned for Bronx State Hospital.

In developing the program, Schmais and White examined the needs of the profession. Educational standards were necessary to protect the public from incompetent practitioners. To protect students from inadequate education and training, employment criteria was established for occupations including civil service on the local, state and federal levels.

In accordance with the philosophy of dance therapy training on which the program was based, movement observation, which included effort/shape, became a part of the required curriculum.

LMA as a Dance Therapy Tool

Schmais and White developed ways of using LMA as a tool for self-observation, providing a means for dance therapists to analyze their own movement patterns and identify their movement prejudices and preferences. This is equivalent to the need for a psychotherapist to know his or her own emotional repertoire, preferences and needs, so as not to unconsciously influence clients or overemphasize certain aspects of their needs while possibly ignoring others. This concept, frequently referred to as countertransference, becomes particularly relevant in connection with the "therapeutic movement relationship," an essential part of the Chace approach.

In this relationship, the intimacy and immediacy of the movement interaction style of the dance therapist is especially important and difficult to monitor. Since the essence of the therapeutic movement relationship is the dance therapist's ability to react and interact spontaneously with the patient through the medium of dance; it is essential that the therapist have practice in many movement possibilities. In this connection, the study of LMA can help therapists learn about their own movement preferences and prejudices and expand their own movement repertoire. It can also aid in understanding the meanings and impact behind the subtlest of communications that take place between patient and therapist.

Often a dance therapist's movement training includes choreography and performing experience, as well as a broad spectrum of movement styles. Many dance therapists, through their intense dance training, have already struggled through certain problems regarding movement preferences, strengths and weaknesses; hence, a certain degree of self-awareness and body-awareness has been developed. According to White (personal communication, 1987), "if the dance therapist receives a solid dance movement training at the age appropriate time, 'movement thinking' is internalized."[5]

However, for some dance therapists with extensive dance backgrounds, LMA can serve as an accessible and efficient cognitive tool for organizing what is already known and integrated on a body level. In other words, the Laban system of movement analysis can help the dancer/dance therapist make the transition from an internalized kinesthetic sense to an intricate cognitive understanding of movement behavior. Having access to this body of knowledge allows the dance therapist to record and process minute fluctuations in movement repertoires. In this respect, LMA is a valuable tool for planning treatment goals and augmenting diagnostic impressions of patients.

The contributions of Schmais and White in developing Laban Movement Analysis as a training tool marked a major attempt to make dance therapy into a professional, unique, complete and documental method of psychotherapy. What differentiated this method of psychotherapy from other methods was its idiom—body movement. In short, the medium was movement in the form of dance action and the system for observing and recording interaction, process and change was Laban Movement Analysis.

The LMA/Dance Therapy Bronx State tradition continued under the direction of Miriam Roskin Berger, a former student of Bartenieff, Chace and the Midwest pioneer, Rhoda Winter Russell. Berger was part of the Zeitgeist at Bronx State, arriving there in the late 1960s. She created its unique Creative Arts Therapies Department, which she headed from 1970 to 1990 and where hundreds of dance therapy students from all the academic programs trained. A former dancer with the Jean Erdman Theatre of Dance, Berger wrote one of the earliest academic studies of dance therapy in 1956. She has developed her concept of dance therapy from a synthesis of her studies in psychology, LMA and the aesthetic, creative elements of dance. Dance, she states, "is an art which uniquely combines feeling and form through bodily experience" (Berger, personal communication, 1992.) In addition to her work in the United States, Berger has been a major leader in the development of dance therapy training programs around the world (see *Chapter 26*).

---

[5]This may help us to understand how the six pioneering dance therapists developed their work in dance therapy without the additional resource of LMA. For example, Marian Chace, Blanche Evan, and Liljan Espenak were all thoroughly trained in the dynamics of dance in addition to the kinesiological aspects of body movement.

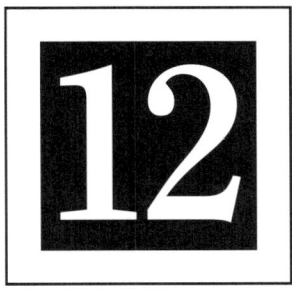

Marion North: Personality Assessment and Treatment

Marion North, a protégé of Laban and one of the leading dance therapists in England, has made several important contributions to the practice of dance therapy. Her work typifies the clinical use by English dance therapists of Laban's terminology as a tool to diagnose, assess and plan treatment programs for patients. As mentioned previously, this reliance on Laban's movement framework as a guide for dance therapists is an integral part of dance therapy in England. This is in contrast to dance therapy in the United States, where other theoretical frameworks such as psychoanalytic, ego-psychological, humanistic and Gestalt Therapy are often utilized in addition to Laban's concepts.

Theory and Practice

North views dance therapy primarily as an adjunctive therapy. She sees as ideal the integration of several forms of therapy, stressing the importance of combining movement work with other types of psychological intervention, whether it is in other creative arts (art and music therapy) or in the form of psychiatric or psychological treatment.

A major theme that underlies much of North's work is the interrelationship between movement, behavior and personality adjustment. She views Laban Movement Analysis as a complex and comprehensive theory of movement that can be used to assess personality in regard to its strength, potential and limitations, as well as to formulate body movement treatment goals.

North stresses that the strength of movement therapy is in its ability to meet the individual at his or her own level of development and that each individual's modes of expression and adaptation are unique. Hence, she attempts to guide individuals by using their movement repertoire as the building blocks for further development, integration and modification.

> I see the special value of movement as a therapy, in that it can assist the psychological and physical growth of a child according to the stage of development which he has reached, it can help the gradual unfolding process of differentiation and self-realization, according to his own capacity. The aim is not toward any "ideal" or "average" person and therefore there is no "norm." (North, 1972, p. 229)

Implied in the above statement is the concept of the infinite variety and complexity of movement possibilities, which is basic to the Laban, Bartenieff and North philosophies. Both North and Bartenieff stress that each individual's movement patterns must be seen in their total complexity without preconceived ideas of good or bad movement styles. North emphasizes the importance of noting the individual's movement "needs" (1972), but at the same time she reminds us that movement aspects in reality cannot be dissected and worked on in isolation.

> It is essential to aim for a whole and coordinated movement pattern, rather than to pinpoint a deficiency or disbalance and work on that; indeed, this may well cause a rebound into a deeper state of distress. (1972, p. 41)

Like Bartenieff, North tries not to lose sight of the person as a whole. All movement aspects, she believes, "are interrelated and therefore as one aspect changes, the whole balance is different and a new situation arises" (1972, p. 159).

North's stress on the whole person, as well as her recognition of the complexity and uniqueness of each individual's movement style, demonstrate her sensitivity to the individual's particular struggle on both an intrapersonal and interpersonal level. In her assessments she looks at individuals and observes their interactions in both the expressive and adaptive aspects of their movement repertoire (1972). However, she continually reminds us that the assessments she makes and the movement suggestions that they produce are not to be fed back to the patient like a prescription.

> Every human being reacts in his own way to the challenges of life and is in a state of continual change ... Movement therapy is an artistic medium and, as all therapy, needs an experienced and sensitive therapist, able to guide when necessary and able to leave alone when necessary. Although there are basic principles which should be understood, no set system of rules is given which should be followed. (1972, p. 229)

In contrast to Bartenieff, who emphasized pure movement knowledge, North makes the jump from a movement base to personality concepts. In order to verify her belief in the psychological value of LMA as an assessment tool, she attempted to correlate movement characteristics of children with personality traits. She conducted a study, described in her book *Personality Assessment Through Movement* (1972), in which she observed the movement of 12 children over a period of two school terms. Through her movement observations, she deduced certain personality characteristics using effort/shape and behavioral concepts. She then compared her movement analysis of these children with a report on the behavior and personality of the same children compiled by their schoolteacher and derived in part from the results of the Children's Apperception Test, an I.Q. test and a questionnaire depicting certain personality and behavioral characteristics. She discovered a particularly high correlation between her own assessments and the teacher's reports.

Through her study, North demonstrates the value of Laban Movement Analysis not only as an objective, nonjudgmental system to scientifically describe movement behavior, but also as a way to correlate various movement tendencies described in LMA terminology with personality characteristics, including the strength, potential and limitations of the personality. She concludes that through her study "a fair case has been made out for the accuracy of [personality] assessment through movement" (North, 1972, p. 229).

There is little scientific evidence for the correlations that North makes beyond this initial study. Some dance therapists have expressed concern about over-interpreting movement and thus introducing an element of judgment into movement analysis. We can only speculate, as North did, that certain movement patterns are indicative of certain personality traits, much as we accept without scientific proof the existence of an id, ego and superego because clinical experience indicates their presence. In light of this, North's study represents a preliminary attempt to depict personality traits and coping styles through the concreteness of movement behavior and is thus an important step toward developing a psychology of movement. As will be shown later, Kestenberg also conducted a study attempting to concretize accepted psychoanalytic theory through the minute notation of complex movement characteristics.

As has been shown, North's stress is on personality assessment and body movement treatment goals. She does not go into depth in the area of dance therapy practice or outline any single approach or methodology. However, some of the particular methods she uses and their relation to her philosophy of movement are illustrated in the following case study. In this study, North relates, through a movement vocabulary, a treatment plan for a 34-year-old female patient who was seen by North for three years, from 1960 to 1963.

This patient, who will be referred to as J., was suffering greatly with intense feelings of deadness, negativity, remoteness and unreality, compounded by intense fears to the point of phobias. She felt stuck inside herself and wanted desperately to get out.

In her movement description of this patient, North notes that she looked fairly healthy with no severe restrictions or physical deformities. There was mobility in the center of her body but a lack of integration or connection between the movements of the upper and lower body parts. There was pronounced tension in her shoulder girdle and top of the spine, but there was mobility in her joints. J.'s hips were narrowly held, with a lack of the necessary tension that usually helps in keeping balance, especially when moving away from symmetrical alignment. She kept her hands in a closed position, though not bound.

In the movement sessions, North's first goal was to establish the patient's trust in the therapist. North believes that therapy "is a cooperative effort, guided by the patient or the therapist at different times" (1972, p. 109).

In beginning with this patient, North felt it important to suggest movement sequences simple enough to master but hard enough to provide a challenge. She used a highly directive approach, suggesting a movement sequence, which confronted or engaged the conflict J. experienced over her tendency to go "inside herself" rather than "getting out."

> A strict pattern was therefore chosen, one which gave room both for some immediate achievement and some obvious failure ... [The pattern chosen was] gathering in—a grasping, closing movement, contrasted with a scattering, opening movement. This was taken in the hands, the upper part of the body and finally with the whole body, including a shift in weight. (North, 1972, p. 109)

In this case, she chose a movement sequence that alternated between a gathering/grasping action and a scattering action. She carefully broke down these opposing actions by encouraging only the use of the hands at first and then gradually moving to the whole body. In this way, she attempted to help the patient build movement links between opposing tendencies in the personality. This is illustrated in North's response to J.'s comment that she "ought to try very hard to be 'out' ... [referring to her movement choices] and not enjoy the inward movement" (1972, p. 109). North explained:

> ... this was not the object of the movement [exercise]—... all of us are "inside" at some time and ... it is a normal and, indeed, desirable attribute, but what we wanted her to find was her way or route between the natural inward and outward experience. The route between, i.e., the movement itself, as distinct from a static state, was at this time most important. This understanding helped the patient not to concentrate exclusively on the opposite side to the one she was experiencing: this would have been unhelpful and probably cause an even stronger rebound into her own inward escape. (1972, pp. 109-110)

It should be pointed out that in this particular case, the client stated her problem by discussing her opposing drives and thus gave North permission to begin the exploration of these opposites.

One has the sense in North's work that she closely monitors the movement experiences that the client is having. She discusses the experience with the patient as if it were a joint task of shaping and forming the thoughts, feelings and experiences of each movement sequence the patient is practicing.

> Each session demands acute observation of the subtle differences and developments and quick adjustment to the constantly changing situation: a mixture of encouragement at the right time and place, comments on aspects unachieved and illustrating new implications and tasks. (North, 1972, p. 109)

The philosophy that comes through over and over again in North's work is one of going with a patient's patterns of movement from the point where they begin and then gradually adding, altering, modifying and extending movement sequences. In other words, instead of rejecting the original movement patterns, she tries to use those patterns to build new sequences.

A second and unique aspect of North's work is her stress on building and practicing movement sequences. Patients are encouraged to practice what they experience and are taught in the sessions. North believes that altering the patient's movement sequencing behavior can directly affect his or her habitual patterns of response. "To perform the movement, wholeheartedly, concentration is required and the close relationship between the movement and the inner feelings and attitudes works in a very direct way on the personality" (North, 1972, p. 110).

In addition to her work with movement sequences, North also works with patients in a fashion that attempts to combine held positions with transition movements. She first has the patient practice certain positions, which the patient is instructed to hold in space. After the position is mastered, the pathways or transitional sequences that lead from one to the next are experienced and practiced. In deciding on these positions and transitions, North employs the movement language and definitions of Rudolf Laban. The sequences that North instructed J. to follow were:

1. A rising, lifting movement to high;
2. An advancing, extending movement forward;
3. A closing, covering movement backward and down and
4. An opening movement spreading sideways. (1972, p. 110)

North describes a moment of great satisfaction and achievement for J. As she did the first transition, a rising, lifting movement to high, she experienced the movement traveling through the center of her body, thus connecting, for the first time, the upper and lower parts of her body. She also commented on a new sensation of experiencing the ground beneath her feet.

At first glance, it might appear as though North's work emphasizes prescribed movement programs as a way to influence personality change. However, not all of her work is done with as much structuring, as was the case with J. North did encourage J. to create her own movement sequences, but J. was not ready. The directive intervention style that North used with J. is being stressed here, in that it is one clear way in which she has integrated Laban's work into a psychomotor therapy.

An analysis of North's writing and examination of other case studies reveals that her use of effort/shape to plan treatment programs serves as a guideline that should not be followed rigidly. She stresses the need to take into account not only the unique movement patterns of patients, but also their personal needs and life circumstances. This more flexible philosophy is also demonstrated in her emphasis on the patient/therapist interaction and relationship.

The Laban Centre

North's work was reunited with Bartenieff's during the formation of The Laban Centre at the University of London's Goldsmiths College. In 1984, The Laban Centre at the College and Hahnemann University in the United States established a formal relationship. Under the direction of Dianne Dulicai, the Hahnemann graduate program in dance therapy was replicated at Goldsmiths College. Over a four-year period, the program was adapted to meet the British standards for accreditation. This allowed the Centre to offer a Master's program in Dance Movement Therapy. The introduction of the American curriculum by Dulicai necessitated a rejoining between two of Laban's protégés, Marion North and Irmgard Bartenieff, whose professional directions diverged when Bartenieff left England.

Application of Laban's work in the United Kingdom has gone in several directions, including education and business, while Bartenieff in the United States applied Laban's work to psychotherapy. Dulicai, who was a protégé of both North and Bartenieff, was instrumental in bringing their work together in the new program. In addition, numerous Laban students such as Walli Meir, Simone Michelle, Warren Lamb and Valerie Dunlap in the United Kingdom and Jody Zacharias, Kedzie Penfield and Martha Davis from The Laban Institute of Movement Studies in the United States facilitated the development of the program.

Dulicai believes that all aspects of Laban's teachings can be integrated into dance therapy education. At Hahnemann, Laban's concepts were tailored to the entire curriculum. Dulicai states, "my gratitude to the contributions of Laban and personally to Irmgard Bartenieff, Marion North and Martha Davis is honored in these academic programs..." (Dulicai, personal communication, 1992).

Judith Kestenberg: Movement Profile

The organization of concepts borrowed from the work of Rudolf Laban and Warren Lamb into a theory of development and the application of this theory to dance therapy was advanced by the work of Dr. Judith Kestenberg, psychiatrist and psychoanalyst. Although her work included training dance therapists in her theories and methods, Kestenberg did not have a background in dance and did not call herself a dance therapist, but rather a "movement retrainer." Her work, however, represents a distinct orientation to dance therapy practice and movement analysis.

Kestenberg's work grew out of her long-term collaboration with the Sands Point Movement Study Group sponsored by Child Development Research (CDR).[1] Based in part on the theoretical formulations of Laban and Lamb, Kestenberg expanded on LMA, adding subsystems of movement patterns to effort/shape patterns and correlating all movement characteristics with psychological phenomena, creating a developmentally and psychologically coherent profile. More specifically, the Kestenberg system views minute variations of movement patterns, rhythms and preferences with regard to their relevance to psychosexual stages of development, affects, defenses, adaptive functioning and self and object representations. These can be correlated with the developmental assessment work of Anna Freud (1965). Kestenberg's theoretical formulations also incorporate the work of Hartmann, Winnicott, Mahler and others.

Kestenberg's integration of LMA concepts with psychoanalytic theory culminated in the formulation of a diagnostic movement profile that measures psychomotor development. This profile, known today as the Kestenberg Movement Profile (KMP), is a complex series of graphs that chart several aspects of a child's movement repertoire using primarily the effort/shape movement descriptive vocabulary. These movement characteristics are then correlated within the psychoanalytic developmental framework.[2]

The Use of Kestenberg's Work in Dance Therapy

The clinical implications of Kestenberg's work—that is, the concretizing of psychoanalytic thought through the study of body movement patterns—serve as a theoretical foundation supportive of and immediately applicable to the practice of dance therapy. Several of today's dance therapists who have been trained extensively in Kestenberg's work have made contributions in this direction.

Martha Soodak, who was formerly on the board of Child Development Research and is also in the Academy of Registered Dance Therapists, has used this approach in her practice since 1973. Soodak, a dancer, began using dance in 1951 for therapeutic ends with children. She met Kestenberg at the Dance Notation Bureau in 1969 and this resulted in an association that centered on the therapeutic aspects of expressive movement and movement training. Soodak has worked as a dance therapist in collaboration with Dr. Esther Robbins in New York.

Concerning her use of the KMP, Soodak states:

---

[1] Other members of the Sands Point Movement Study Group at that time were Dr. Jay Barlowe, Arnhilt Buelte, Dr. Hershey Marcus and Dr. Esther Robbins. Martha Soodak joined in 1969.
[2] A complete and definitive description of the work of Kestenberg and the Sands Point Team can be found in *The Role of Movement Patterns in Development 2*. (Kestenberg & Sossin, 1979)

Although a person well trained in movement has in mind a rather complete concept of the range of human capacity, it is very useful to have a structure which describes, defines and analyzes this, taking it from the realm of intuition into that of objectivity. The profile ... serves as a framework for orientation. It provides terminology for defining and interpreting movement events which arise during the therapy and at the same time, it places them into a developmental context. So, the therapist can see what the patient's strengths and weaknesses are, what [strengths] need to be shored up, what can be safely worked with and what should be deftly sidestepped....

During the course of my work, I have ... observed fixed characteristics of holding or moving which I term 'body defenses.' The use of the profile terminology promotes accurate description of such defenses....

In working to correct these distortions, I keep in mind that while defenses may be counterproductive, they serve ... to keep a person functional. Thus ... I do not immediately seek to remove patterns, but rather to build in the [patients'] capacity to support alternative ways of doing things. Only when it is clear that the patient has the capacity to support movement without the undesirable habits do I address it directly.... (personal communication, 1986)

Another dance therapist trained in Kestenberg's work is Penny Lewis (formerly known as Bernstein), author, educator and founder of the Dance Therapy Master's Program at Antioch New England Graduate

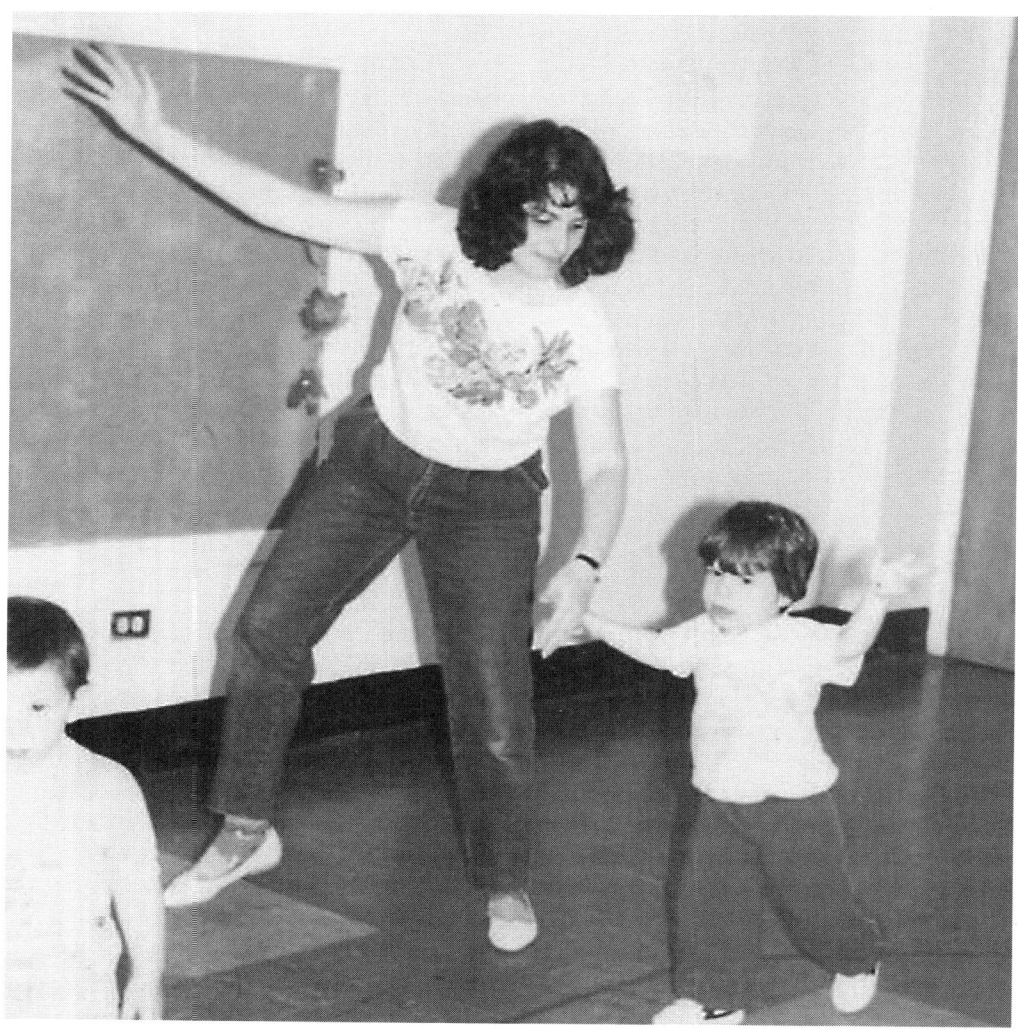

Susan Loman, preventive work with children (Photo courtesy Center for Parents and Children, Long Island)

School and the Dance Therapy Master's Specialty at Goddard College. Lewis has been a leader in her adaptation of the Kestenberg System to the clinical and research needs of the dance therapist. In her article "Recapitulation of Ontogeny: A Theoretical Approach to Dance Movement Therapy," Lewis (Bernstein, 1973) discusses the importance of establishing a theoretical framework for the practice of dance therapy. She cites aspects of Kestenberg's movement framework and discusses it using concepts of functional and adaptive behavior versus dysfunctional, maladaptive behavior. She believes that through the observation of one's movement patterns, adaptive versus maladaptive behavior can be diagnosed, as can the developmental level of the patient and hence, his or her movement needs. She gives examples of adaptive/functional movement patterns for each of Kestenberg's developmental categories and juxtaposes this with its maladaptive/dysfunctional counterpart.

Susan Loman, the director of the Dance Movement Therapy program at Antioch New England Graduate School and former student of Lewis, went on to receive extensive training with Kestenberg in the late 1970s. Loman used the profile as an assessment and intervention tool in her prevention work with infants, children, parents and families at the Center for Parents and Children in Long Island from 1979 to 1987, co-directed by Judith Kestenberg and Arnhilt Buelte. She has also been teaching Kestenberg's system in the United States and abroad.

One application of the profile that Loman finds helpful in preventive work is "attunement," a concept that is comparable to kinesthetic empathy. The infant or young child feels comforted by those whose movement patterns "attune" to his and thwarted by those whose movement patterns "clash." In each phase of a child's development, different rhythms become prominent and necessary for the child's successful mastery of developmental tasks. When parenting figures are unable to adapt their personal movement preferences to synchronize and/or harmonize (both forms of kinesthetic empathy) with the child's, the child may become hampered in his or her psychodynamic growth.

In her work at the center, Loman trained interns to detect, with the help of the KMP, "clashing" movement patterns between child and adult and to recognize maladaptive movement styles in the child as a result of these clashes. Once the above is analyzed, the dance therapist is able to "attune" to the child's and adult's movement patterns and in this way begin the process of promoting healthy functioning and making up for early deficits and frustrations. Parents are also helped to move more synchronously and comfortably with their children, that is, to attune to their children.

In this respect, Loman compares aspects of the work to Winnicott's (1957) "holding environment." This concept, which is so often referred to as "starting where the patient is," pervades the dance therapy literature. After "attunement" is established between therapist and patient, the dance therapist can begin to facilitate the development of new adaptive and expressive movement patterns to eventually replace destructive, maladaptive and repressive behaviors. Various games, tasks, movement interactions, images, props, tactile stimulation and other dance therapy techniques are specifically designed to stimulate new forms of interaction, coping and self-expression. All of these interventions are based on the findings of the profile.

At the Center, dance therapists work either with the child or adult alone or with the parent and child together. During sessions, dance therapists try to "foster greater empathy between parent and child through their movement interactions, to remove obstacles to developmental progression and to strengthen the child's resources" (Loman, 1981, p. 2). The interventions used at the center span the entire range of dance therapy methodology discussed thus far. What primarily differentiates the Kestenberg approach is its emphasis on prevention and the use of the profile as a guide to treatment.

In her 1981 presentation for the ADTA, Loman noted that dance therapists could incorporate the principles from the profile without necessarily constructing a complete profile, a process that is extremely time-consuming. In this regard, Loman stated, "a dance therapist with knowledge of [and training in] the profile can still apply its principles to her work with clients even if a complete profile is not constructed" (1981, p. 5).

Since 1989, Antioch New England Graduate School has sponsored KMP conferences on topics including research and works in progress and applications to a variety of clinical populations. Two books stimulated by conference presentations have been published by the graduate school: *The Kestenberg Movement Profile: Its Past, Present Applications and Future Directions*, edited by Penny Lewis and Susan Loman and *The Body Mind Connection in Human Movement Analysis*, edited by Susan Loman with Rose Brandt.

Discussion

LMA: Varying Views

While the practical applications of Laban Movement Analysis vary greatly among dance therapists, there are, generally speaking, two major views concerning its use in the field.

One school of thought is represented by the views of Elissa White, whose work was discussed earlier. In review, White emphasizes LMA as a tool that can be used by dance therapists in the following ways: to record patients' movement dynamics; to provide a format for developing treatment plans; to analyze patient/therapist interaction; to develop the dance therapist's ability to observe his or her self; and for research.

Virginia Reed, another leader in the integration of Laban's work with dance therapy, was a close friend and colleague of Bartenieff. For Reed, Laban's work is a psychotherapeutic philosophy and a dance therapy methodology in and of itself. Reed emphasized LMA as an integration of a philosophical, anthropological, psychological and physiological view of life. She believes that inherent within this system is a therapeutic philosophy that sees life as a continually developing, growing and changing process. Several other dance therapists certified in LMA, including Monica Meehan McNamara, Cece Ritter Flax and Bonnie Robbins, have worked to further explore this holistic concept of Laban's work (see also Reed, Chapter 25).

Diana Levy (personal communication, 1987), the first dean of the certification program in LMA at the Laban Bartenieff Institute, sums up this school of thought in the following statement: "My experience teaching LMA for many years has led me to believe that personal integration of those concepts which are most fundamental to the LMA framework is a therapeutic process."

SECTION B

Further Expansion of Dance Therapy Theory and Practice

The Evolution of East Coast Influences

As Laban's theories were influencing dance therapy during the late 1960s and 1970s, some dance therapists were also beginning to incorporate psychoanalytic concepts into their work. This chapter discusses the contributions of two East Coast leaders, Elaine Siegel and Zoë Avstreih. Their work provides a general overview of the psychoanalytic concepts that Siegel and other dance therapists began espousing in the late 1960s that have become an important part of the dance therapy literature.

Part A. Elaine Siegel: Psychoanalytic Approach with a Touch of Chace

Author of the book *The Mirror of Our Selves: A Study in Dance Movement Therapy* (1984), Siegel completed a dance therapy-training program with Espenak in 1964. Her dance background includes training in classical ballet and in Haitian and African dance. To broaden and clarify her understanding of personality with special concern for how the psyche and soma interact, Siegel turned to the study of psychoanalytic thought.

Siegel has integrated her psychoanalytic knowledge with her understanding of body movement and psychotherapeutic treatment. In her article "Psychoanalytic Thought and Methodology in Dance Movement Therapy" (1974), Siegel points out one essential difference between the psychoanalytic model of therapy and dance therapy. This difference centers on the issue of verbalization versus somatization. She states:

> The psychoanalyst ... is firmly convinced that "somatization" ideally should be [kept at] a minimum and confined to "trial action" within the psychic structure so that the ego can then decide what action to take in the real world. (1974, p. 29)

In contrast, the dance therapist is frequently encouraging the physical expression of emotion on various levels.

Having pointed out this seemingly broad rift between psychoanalytic treatment and dance movement treatment, Siegel then points to the similarities:

> First and foremost, both therapies are essentially developmental in nature, expecting the client to grow out of an inefficient, fixated or infantile mode of existing into a nearly normal one. (1974, p. 30)

Siegel also refers to the significance of the transference relationship as instrumental in the growth of the client in the dance movement therapy situation. Like many of the original pioneers, she refers to the parallel between improvisation in dance therapy and verbal free association in psychoanalytic treatment, noting that both methods of exploration work to release unconscious thoughts, feelings and associations.

> Depending on the state of treatment, the dance movement therapist may then lend herself as a catalyst to a cathartic reaction or interpret via dance movement and verbalization, much like an analyst who hears, reconstructs and interprets the patient's past from verbal remembering and the observation of affect states. (1974, p. 30)

Siegel emphasizes that different populations require different kinds of movement intervention. In addition, what the dance therapist can do with a patient who is seen privately several times a week cannot be done in weekly sessions in a hospital setting. Whereas Siegel sees movement therapy as a form of treatment which can, through the positive transference relationship, help an individual regress to the fixation point and hence work through previously unresolved conflicts, she does not see this as feasible or advisable in the usual hospital setting or for all patients. For example, Siegel cites the child with autism who never advanced beyond the very early stages of development and who is still attached or merged with the mother:

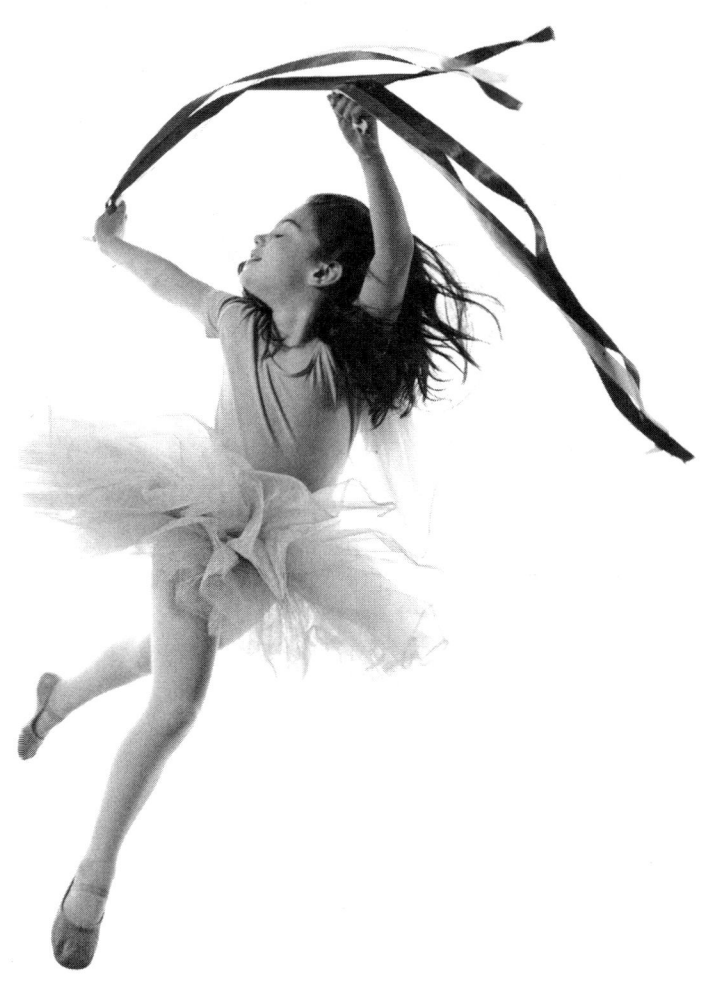

Model Zoë performs ballet as personal expression (Photo courtesy Steve Clarke)

"He needs another chance to live through the body-image building stages of the mother-child dyad" (Siegel, 1974, p. 30). In such a case, the patient is already in a state of regression and the focus of the dance therapist must be on building in the awareness of self and others. This can include holding, touching, breathing together and so on, activities not usually appropriate for the neurotic client. Similarly, while Siegel sees the therapeutic movement relationship as one way of fulfilling early childhood needs, she also works as an empathic observer with clients who can benefit from more independent work and free association.

Siegel encourages the dance therapist's respect for the uniqueness of individual psychomotor expression. She believes that the individual's personality cannot be separated from the cultural influences that helped to shape and form it. Thus, an individual's movement is reflective of both inner impulses and outside influences, as the latter give external form and shape to the former. As a result, external forms such as ballet, modern dance or flamenco dance can become authentic expressions of the self if the individual in earlier years cathected to these particular styles through visual and/or bodily experiences and attached unconscious significance to them.

In this respect, Siegel's view of body movement is contrary to Whitehouse's view that "authentic movement" comes directly from the unconscious with no structuring from cultural influences, and seems to coincide more with the belief that "all movement is authentic" (Kalish-Weiss, personal communication, 1980). Siegel believes that the concept of "authentic movement" places expectations on the patient to express him or herself in a specific way. For Siegel, no single methodology or movement form is appropriate for all individuals. Each individual is the result of a complex interrelationship of early experiences and memories. The therapist must be able to perceive, respect and appreciate this complexity in order to find the appropriate and meaningful style of intervention.

One can see how Siegel's earlier experiences with both the extreme intellectual control of ballet and the pure emotional discharge of primitive dance have led to her belief in the need to find a constructive and meaningful balance and integration of conscious and unconscious influences. Siegel does not attend only to the unconscious aspects of the personality, but is equally concerned with preserving and developing the ego functions of the individual. In this respect, she is aligned with the thinking of the ego-psychologists, who stress the integration of the unconscious with the conscious aspects of development. Whereas Siegel sees Haitian and primitive dance as expressions of the unconscious, she sees ballet as potentially the expression of the patient's ego-ideal, that is, when used correctly, but warns that it also has the potential of being the expression of the punitive superego, if introduced anatomically and psychologically incorrectly (Siegel, personal communication, 1980).

Siegel believes in Hartmann's concept of working in the conflict-free ego sphere (Siegel, 1974, 1980) and building the individual's adaptive resources. The defenses of the individual as manifested in bodily actions will dissolve, Siegel contends, when enough ego strength has been encouraged and successful therapist/patient contact has been made. However, she cautions that this should not be pushed or encouraged prematurely (Siegel, personal communication, 1980).

Siegel notes that a close examination of Chace's writing reveals continual references to the concept of meeting the individual on his or her level of development and readiness for interaction and communication (Siegel, personal communication, 1980). Siegel believes that Chace, in picking up on the patient's movements, is accentuating the ego by making contact with the patient within the conflict-free ego sphere, hence broadening and expanding the healthy and adaptive aspects of the patient's total functioning. She contrasts this with other mental health disciplines whose emphasis is on illness and on constant interpretation of pathology.

In her work, Siegel differentiates between catharsis and abreaction. She sees catharsis as a part of therapy, but not its goal. "Catharsis, with its emphasis on the temporary absence of ego and conscious thought, can be either too frightening or addictive" (Siegel, 1979, p. 90); whereas the psychoanalytic concept of abreaction Siegel views as a potentially more gradual process of letting go. Abreaction supports the active presence of the observing ego, hence allowing previously repressed thoughts and feelings to gradually emerge and become integrated into the existing ego structure. Abreaction integrates a degree of catharsis with insight and reflection while catharsis is primarily an emotional release.

Along similar lines, Siegel stresses seeing the patient as a whole, implying the integration of the unconscious with the conscious. She emphasizes the importance of verbalization as integration of the nonverbal expression, again placing stress on the whole person with utilization of all his or her strengths and abilities. In conjunction with the need for verbalization and interpretation, Siegel notes that movement can at times be a defense against one's thoughts and feelings. The dance therapist must therefore be on the alert for when to encourage and when to discourage the patient's use of movement.

Finally, though dedicated to dance, Siegel prefers the word "movement" in describing her work, since the term "'movement therapy' includes all forms of moving one might employ with any kind of patient during a given session" (1979, p. 92). This can include holding a patient, breathing with an autistic child and other early steps that she believes build the ego strengths of the patient and hence prepare him or her for more dance-like activities. In short, the word "movement" covers a broad spectrum of styles and levels of body movement participation and intervention.

In summary, many aspects of Siegel's methodology overlap with that of other dance therapists discussed so far. Her work synthesizes, modifies and refines many of the original contributions of the pioneers. An overview of her methodology reveals the use of exaggeration of movement styles for the purpose of reality testing, exploring the unconscious meanings of actions and intensifying bodily felt experiences and emotions. She also uses mirroring and the movement interactional dialogue as well as the patient's self-touch and touch of the therapist to help in developing a sense of boundaries in moments of more severe regression. Siegel believes in discussing and interpreting movement events and behavior. Stress on interpretation is determined by the particular needs of the patient. She works with and without music and moves on a continuum, from the use of balletic exercises to help patients construct images and movement themes, to pure improvisation or sitting with and rocking a child with schizophrenia. In essence, it appears that for Siegel the client's needs are first and foremost. Though she views these needs in formal psychoanalytic terminology, her interaction with patients can best be characterized as flexible and reflective of the moment.

Part B. Zoë Avstreih: Psychoanalytic Perspective Integrating Chace and Whitehouse

Zoë Avstreih, former Coordinator of the Graduate Dance Therapy Program at Pratt Institute, is a psychoanalyst and dance therapist. Like Siegel, she has been deeply influenced by her psychoanalytic training, specifically in the area of object relations theory and self-psychology. Avstreih began her dance therapy studies at Hunter College, where she studied the Chace technique with Schmais and White. She received further training from Siegel and Evan. Avstreih is currently the director of the dance therapy program at the Naropa Institute.

In "The Emerging Self: Psychoanalytic Concepts of Self Development and Their Implications for Dance Therapy" (1979), a paper presented at the 1979 Annual American Dance Therapy Association Conference, Avstreih presented clinical studies in which she analyzed the psychodynamic needs of five patients and described the therapeutic movement intervention styles she used to meet each patient within his or her developmental level. Avstreih's approach centers on the developmental process, using Mahler's concept of separation/individuation as a base. She emphasizes the importance of the transition from contact perception to distance perception and finally to spatial organization. She states: "The need for contact perception versus distance perception and the ability to sense oneself and others as continuous in space reflects the degree of separation achieved" (1979, p. 7). In this connection, it is particularly important for the dance therapist to determine the most appropriate distance for establishing contact with the patient. Depending on the patient's level of development, too much closeness might be perceived as engulfing, while too much distance could be perceived as abandoning.

Avstreih incorporates into her theoretical framework Winnicott's (1958) concepts of the "Holding Environment," the "Primary Illusion" and the "Good-Enough Mother." The "Holding Environment" defines the child's inner and outer worlds. Through the mother's "empathic, non-intrusive holding" (Avstreih, 1979, p. 3) or lack of it, the child develops either a sense of self-worth or of emptiness. If the mother is empathically attuned to her child's needs, the child will come to believe that he is creating what he needs. This is what Winnicott calls the "Primary Illusion," that is, the illusion of self-sufficiency. This provides a sense of security and is important in the child's later development of the ability to love and care for others.

The "Good-Enough Mother," through her nurturing, reflects to the child his feelings about himself. "If she is not able to reflect accurately the child's affective states," Avstreih says, "he will not be able to develop a reliable sense of self" (1979, p. 5). Thus, if the sense of self has been blocked by a "non-responsive, non-empathetic" maternal figure, the dance therapist can fulfill this role by providing a reflective image. Through her own unique and direct use of self, the dance therapist can help to reconstruct any missing aspects of the child's early developmental experiences and hence, to reintegrate the body image of the child.

The dance therapist works within what Winnicott (1958) has called the "transitional space." Belonging neither to external reality nor to the individual's internal reality, the transitional space "... is the space of therapy. It is here we help to build the bridge which connects and separates the inner with the outer and the self with the object" (Avstreih, 1979, p. 22). It is in the transitional space "... the psyche of the therapist and patient can play, i.e., join in the spontaneous affective exchanges which were so lacking in the early maternal environments" (Avestreih, 1979, p. 7).

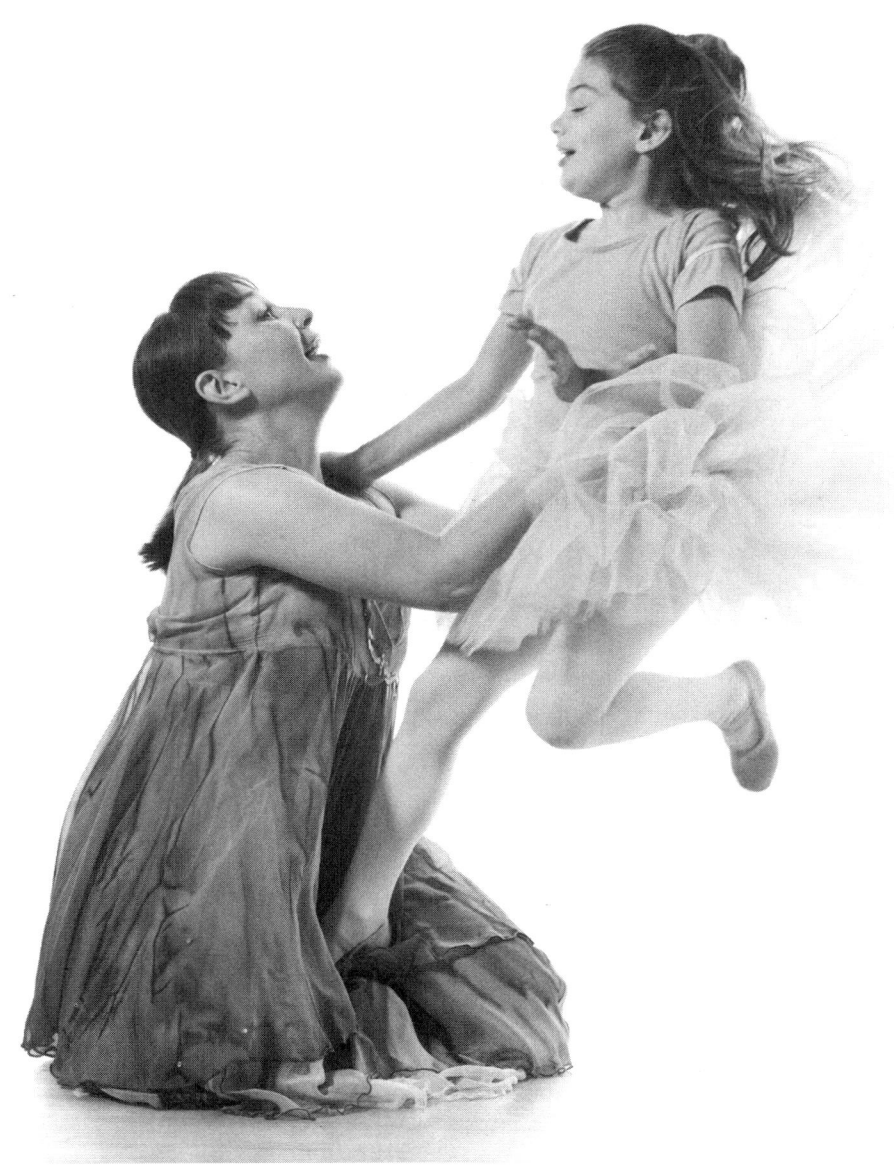

Models Kelly Swindell and daughter Zoë (Photo courtesy Steve Clarke)

This can be illustrated by Avstreih's work with an adult patient named Marcia. Marcia did not feel comfortable with her body and displayed

> ... a general giving-in-to-gravity ... and a tendency towards quick, self-related, gestural movement.... [She] was hypercathected to her body which led to a great deal of somatization and she felt an overwhelming sense of emptiness and isolation. (1979, p. 9)

Her movements, which were stiff and forced, were intellectually motivated rather than from feeling or experience. Finding the dance studio uncomfortable for its lack of outside stimuli, she kept asking for more structure and exercises. Believing that Marcia "lacked the primary educative experience which exists in the mother/child dyad" (1979, p. 10), Avstreih decided to move with her. Avstreih used her own body as "a mirror to serve as a bridge enabling ... [Marcia] to rediscover her body parts and gain a sense of mastery over them" (1979, p. 10). Avstreih then structured a play-like situation in which they alternated initiating and joining in movements. As the child begins to develop a stable body image through "reflective interaction with the mother" (Avstreih, 1979, p. 10), the adult (in this case, Marcia) who had been deprived of this "feeding" develops a sense of self through interaction with the therapist.

For several years, Avstreih has also been exploring reflective interactions through the work of Whitehouse and Chace. She believes that there is a correspondence between the therapeutic stance of the psychotherapist working from a self-psychology framework with that of the "witness" as described originally by Whitehouse and elaborated on by Adler and Chodorow (see *Chapter 15*).

She notes that Chace emphasized the role of the dance therapist as the nonjudgmental observer ("witness") and, in addition, emphasized the benefits of the dyadic union and interaction between patient and therapist. Avstreih, however, differentiates the empathic responses utilized in the Chace technique from the pure nondirective experiencing role of the "witness/mover" relationship. She believes that the Chacian dance therapist, though initially witnessing the "mover" (patient), utilizes the therapeutic movement interaction to help the mover be organized and expressive.

In response to this use of the therapeutic relationship, Avstreih states "as soon as there is an intervention or interpretation of any kind (guidance is a form of interpretation) the role of the 'witness' is altered and the witness stance is no longer in its pure form" (personal communication, 1987).

The witness does not direct the mover as he or she engages in dialogue with the Self, the Jungian concept of the "Divine-Within," the archetype of wholeness that resides in the unconscious. The witness maintains total respect for the integrity of this inner journey, allowing the deep knowledge of the unconscious to become manifest in movement and image. Writing, drawing and speaking may follow movement, facilitating the process of making the unconscious conscious. The "witness," like the mover, is taught to attend to his or her own subjective and unconscious process and the insights obtained on both sides are, when indicated, shared (Adler, 1985; Avstreih, personal communication, 1987). This differentiation brings Avstreih to an important question: is the "witness/mover" relationship really therapy? Just asking this question is, in and of itself, a contribution.

In conclusion, Avstreih's practical extension of the works of Winnicott, Mahler, Spitz, Kohut, Kestenberg and others has further clarified the contributions of dance therapists such as Chace and Siegel and has rounded out the overall picture of dance therapy as a form of in-depth psychotherapeutic treatment.

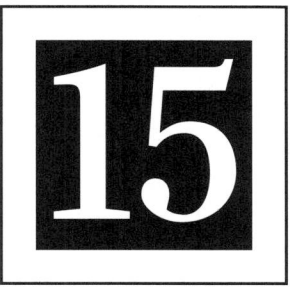

The Evolution of West Coast Influences

While many dance therapists, particularly on the East Coast, welcomed the introduction of effort/shape and psychoanalytic concepts and incorporated these in varying degrees into their work, others perceived this trend as contrary to the early and major tenets of the field. These dance therapists continued to emphasize a more experiential approach, which avoids labeling or diagnosing. This trend was particularly evident among dance therapists on the West Coast, especially those who were influenced directly or indirectly by Mary Whitehouse and who generally work with a fairly healthy nonhospitalized population.

This chapter reviews the literary contributions of dance therapists who, in carrying on the teachings of Whitehouse, have broadened and/or clarified aspects of the Whitehousian approach. Some have focused on the Jungian aspects of Whitehouse's work and others on "authentic movement" and/or movement experiencing. It should be pointed out that the discussion focuses on the expansion of Whitehouse's teachings. The influence of the other major West Coast pioneers, including Hawkins and Schoop, can also be discerned in some of the writings reviewed below.

Expansion of the Whitehousian Approach: Non-Jungian Aspects

Three dance therapists who have written about their use of non-Jungian aspects of Whitehouse's teachings are Irma Dosamantes-Beaudry, Diane Fletcher and Janet Adler. Their work is representative of an approach that generally stresses inner attending to the body and to body-level experiences and bringing these internal experiences forward into movement. This is in contrast to the Chacian approach, which is more interactional.

Part A. Irma Dosamantes-Beaudry: Experiential Movement Psychotherapy

Dosamantes-Beaudry (formerly Dosamantes-Alperson), a clinical psychologist as well as dance therapist and former director of UCLA's masters program in Dance Movement Therapy, contributed numerous articles espousing techniques and theories of what she calls "experiential movement psychotherapy." This refers to a form of therapy that integrates movement, imagery and verbalization and incorporates several aspects of the Whitehousian approach.

She prefers the title "movement psychotherapy" to "movement therapy" because she feels the latter can be mistaken for the body therapies that do not incorporate the emotions.

Dosamantes-Beaudry was strongly influenced by her dance therapy training with Alma Hawkins and by Whitehouse disciples Joan Chodorow and Janet Adler. Her influences were Nikolais in dance and Gendlin, Perls, Freud, Sullivan, Rogers and others in psychology. Although she is a clinical psychologist, she does not believe in applying medical labels to the individuals she treats and basically feels that the difference between the way the dance therapist functions in a psychiatric hospital setting versus in private work is based more on the different demands of the setting itself than on the diagnosis of the individuals seeking treatment.

Dosamantes-Beaudry views movement as an excellent device to facilitate the integration of the intuitive-preverbal level of human functioning with the rational-verbal level. Referring to Gendlin (1971), she states:

Personality change is promoted when a person is able to make contact with a bodily felt level of experiencing ... and is able to verbalize or make explicit at least some portion of it. (1974a, p. 211)

Referring to Wallen (1970), Dosamantes-Beaudry lists three ways that individuals commonly avoid the "bodily-felt level of experiencing": 1) poor perceptual contact with one's body and its environment (i.e., being unaware of what various body parts are doing at any given time); 2) blocking the open expression of an urgent need and 3) repressing an unacceptable reaction, such as anger. "When we distance ourselves from our experiential body process," she states, "we literally cut ourselves off from the kinesthetic and sensory input on which we rely to know our various feeling reactions toward ourselves and the world" (1974a, 211). Effective therapy, therefore, must place the patient at the center of his or her own experience.

Dosamantes-Beaudry delineates two styles of movement or two experiential modes: the receptive mode,

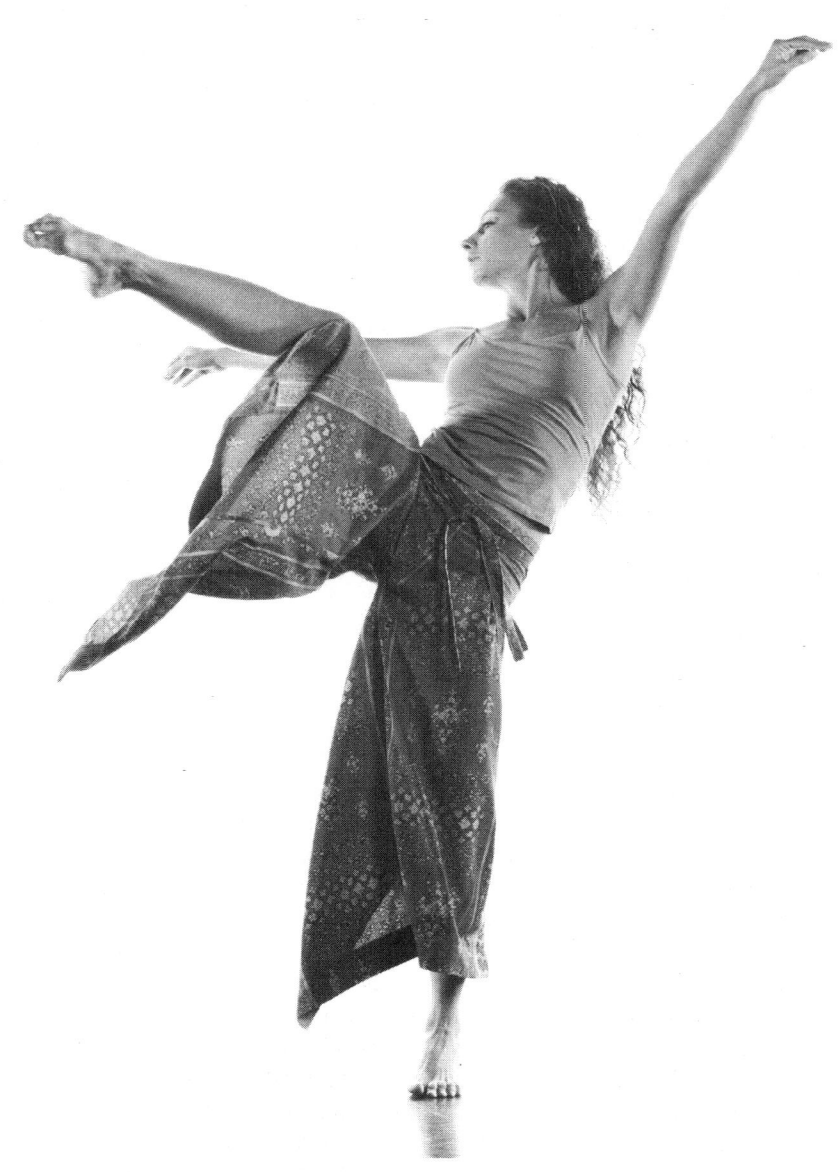

Dancer Rebekah Kennedy expresses freedom of movement (Photo courtesy Steve Clarke)

where attention focuses inward on internal events; and the action mode, where attention focuses on external events. In the receptive mode, the client focuses on internal stimuli, allowing sensations, feelings, images and thoughts to emerge and flow naturally. Movements in this mode are subtle and often difficult to detect. They are referred to as "shadow movements" or "internal-intrapsychic movements" (Dosamantes-Alperson, 1979b, p. 21). Examples include changes in body tension and breath flow. Having the client lie down with eyes closed can facilitate such movements. This reduces external stimuli and enables images, memories and associations to emerge.

The receptive mode is illustrated by the case of Sharon, a 32-year-old woman who complained of breathing problems and tension in the neck and chest areas. Dosamantes-Beaudry suggested that she lie down, eyes closed and focus on the tightness in her chest. Soon Sharon formed an associative image of a block of ice, which began to melt as she concentrated on it. A physical release was observed in her body. "Her chest muscles became relaxed, her breath flowed more smoothly and tears streamed from her eyes in an automatic way" (Dosamantes-Alperson, 1979b, p. 23). As Sharon permitted herself to relax, she could breathe more deeply and was able to cry and to verbalize her emotional reaction to the experience.

Images that occur during the receptive mode are referred to as "hypnogogic images." They are "preconscious, preverbal visual symbols characterized by changing thematic content, motion, vividness, affect and relative autonomy" (Dosamantes-Alperson, 1979b, p. 25). They allow the client to actually relive situations from the past, merging them with the present. This can lead to new insights into unresolved conflicts.

> ... the movement psychotherapist can assist the transformation of the physical form to the visual symbol by first helping clients discriminate the physical or bodily qualities they experience and then encouraging them to allow an image to develop which shares similar attributes to the physically experienced one. (Dosamantes-Alperson, 1979b, p. 24)

Then, after the imagery phase, the therapist facilitates physical identification with the image and externalization of the image through movement.

> The value of moving *an image* rather than simply focusing on an image without movement, is that clients can take the visual experience into their bodies, allowing a physical identification to be made between their internal sensations and the imagined situation. They can empathize physically with all aspects of the image and thereby gain an awareness of the attitude they hold toward each revealed experiential element. (Dosamantes-Alperson, 1979b, p. 26)

While in the receptive mode the individual's attention is focused inwardly, in the action mode attention is focused outwardly. "When clients move in the action mode, they reveal how they approach and deal with the external world of objects and people" (1979b, p. 27).

In this mode, the patient moves with eyes open, moving deliberately and exploring the surrounding space. Movements are "overt and readily detectable." Terms used in this mode are "movement style" or "movement range," and the process is categorized as "external-interactional movement" (Dosamantes-Alperson, 1979b, p. 27).

Many clients, especially those without experience in dance or other physical training, will need to become "desensitized" or "disinhibited" before they can move without feeling self-conscious. The therapist can facilitate this by creating a relaxed and conducive atmosphere, which "offers clients the opportunity to discover physical and movement aspects of themselves while providing an opportunity to exercise a safe degree of self-direction" (Dosamantes-Alperson, 1979b, p. 27).

The client begins to express his or her personality as he or she moves with more confidence and spontaneity in this mode. There is increased self-awareness as the client learns which types of movement are comfortable and which are uncomfortable and as he or she becomes aware of differences and similarities between his or her movement and that of other group members.

The following case study illustrates the external-interactional mode of movement. Dosamantes-Beaudry describes a session that took place on Halloween Eve, in an all women's group. One of the members came dressed as a witch. Because of her dramatic appearance it seemed to Dosamantes-Beaudry that "this woman needed to be acknowledged by the group for that part of herself represented by the witch character" (1979b, p. 29).

The client was encouraged to become the center of the group and to express the witch's character through movement. She used expansive, undulating movements, sometimes seductive, sometimes aggressive. She was encouraged by the therapist to move with and relate to each group member individually. This role gave the woman a sense of power and control. The group members, in turn, responded to her:

> Some allowed themselves to be bewitched, letting themselves be overpowered and yielding to her. Others rejected her attempts to overpower them by asserting their own strength against hers. (Dosamantes-Alperson, 1979b, pp. 29-30)

The discussion that followed the movement session brought out the feelings the issue of power aroused in each member of the group.

In comparing the receptive mode with the action mode, Dosamantes-Beaudry says:

> ... internal-intrapsychic movement provides a bridge between less conscious and more conscious levels of experiencing and acting. Through external-interactional movement which takes place in the action mode, clients can ascertain how they cope with the external world and the sort of impact they have on the world. (1979b. p. 30)

It appears that movement in the receptive mode is less willed and less overt than movement in the action mode and relates to the Whitehouse concept of "I am moved" as well as Hawkins' stress on attending and relaxation. Contrarily, the action mode involves more willed and overt movement and more interactional movement. This more closely connects to what Whitehouse called "I move."

In early sessions, Dosamantes-Beaudry has her clients work within each of the two modes in order to help them explore their range of movement and increase their awareness of and sensitivity to their own bodies.

As sessions progress, greater use is made of the person's "imaginative responses" (Dosamantes-Alperson, 1974a, p. 212). As the client's movements grow in range, sessions become less dependent upon the external structure imposed by the therapist and become more self-directed. The therapist then becomes more of an observer than a guide, interceding "only when the client encounters a block in her movement" (Dosamantes-Alperson, 1974a, pp. 212-215). Sessions generally last for two hours. At the conclusion, the patient is asked for verbal comment and expression. In this way, the patient connects his or her own words, thoughts and images to the movement experience.

In summary, in Dosamantes-Beaudry's discussion of the receptive mode of movement she is describing West Coast ideas growing out of her training with Hawkins and Whitehouse. These ideas center on concepts of attending to the body, bodily felt experiences and felt movement and the process of connecting these bodily experiences to imagery and finally dance movement action. On the other hand, when she describes the active movement modality, one detects more of a Schoopian tone. Dosamantes-Beaudry's major contribution to contemporary dance therapy has been clarification of the psychotherapeutic process as it pertains to the dance movement experience.

Part B. Diane Fletcher: A Psychodynamic Orientation

Fletcher was strongly influenced by her dance therapy training with Whitehouse and Hawkins and was also trained in the Chacian approach. Like Dosamantes-Beaudry, Fletcher's work focuses on the bodily-felt experience or as Fletcher calls it, the "body experience." In her article "Body Experience Within the Therapeutic Process: A Psychodynamic Orientation" (1979), she states:

> ... the very process of focusing on body experience tends to draw out the psychological content and the dynamic organization to which the body experiences are linked. Such is the basis of the use of body experience as a means toward intrapsychic reorganization. (p. 137)

In Fletcher's view, internal events are represented physically as sensations, while the body itself is represented mentally as an image or series of images. When psychic disturbance is present, the images may be distorted or blocked. Through intense integrated body experiences, the individual's distorted body image can be altered and this, Fletcher believes, is one of the roles of dance therapy.

Fletcher discusses four different aspects of experience. The first is subjective experience, the "immediacy of one's own perception of self and ... quality of being" (1979, p. 137). More specifically, subjective experience is the "receptive capacity of allowing into consciousness both sensory data from the external world and internal perceptions such as sensation, image, fantasy and thought" (Fletcher, 1979, p. 137). It is important for the dance therapist to discover how the client perceives his or her sense of self.

Distortions in perception and experience may occur when parts of the self are fragmented or projected outside the body. These distorting mechanisms are usually not consciously experienced, but they may result in anxiety and a feeling of being lost. Therapy can enrich the capacity to experience through the process of association. "In this process, both physical and mental elements of experience are brought into association with each other... There is an inner dialogue" (Fletcher, 1979, p. 138).

The second aspect of an experience is identifying and reflecting on its content. One must be able to recognize and think about what is happening. This process differentiates between internal and external stimuli and reactions and "in this way, the objective and subjective aspects of the self are integrated" (Fletcher, 1979, p. 139). Verbalization becomes important in this phase. The experience is broken down and reorganized into a pattern that the individual is able to handle. This prevents the patient from becoming overwhelmed with raw emotion.

The third aspect is identifying the actions and/or mechanisms that are used to make an experience happen or prevent it from happening. It refers to "the self as the *doer*," (Fletcher, 1979, p. 139) and "relocates the responsibility and control back inside [the] ... person so that events do not ... 'just happen'" (Fletcher, 1979, p. 139).

The capacity to modify one's immediate experience is a survival mechanism, dating back to infancy. For example, we commonly try to avoid unpleasant sensations or experiences, often through unconscious physical action. Therapy can increase one's awareness and thus "many... defensive motor mechanisms can potentially be brought under more conscious control and the underlying feelings can thereby be more readily tapped" (Fletcher, 1979, p. 140).

The fourth aspect of experience is linking, "the process by which the elements of experience are internally connected in meaningful association with each other..." (Fletcher, 1979, p. 141). A person comes to know the self and the world by "linking up" various aspects of experience. When reality is too painful or overwhelming, the linking process is disrupted. "The internal destruction of these links which connect the various internal signals, associations and sensory impressions result in the destruction or alteration of the perception of reality" (Fletcher, 1979, p. 142). Linking is the first step toward self-knowledge and freedom of choice.

Fletcher describes her work with Mr. C., a successful professional in his early forties. He expressed feeling inadequate and uncomfortable in relating to others. He felt cut off from his body. Spontaneity was unnatural to him and he dreaded sinking into an inert state, which he feared was his real self.

As he spoke, Fletcher asked him to become aware of his body and to pay attention to what it was doing. What became apparent was the

> ...continual and alternating efforts of tightening and pulling in his shoulder, across the chest, arms and the whole torso ... fairly small but actually quite effortful tensions that were inhibiting not only any possibility of a more relaxed or easy state, but were constraining and covering any spontaneous motions toward action. (Fletcher, 1979, p. 148)

As Mr. C. focused on his body, he could feel the efforts he was making to hold himself back. Once he began to let go of some of the constriction, he experienced twinges of sensation. Gradually, the impulses became more defined. Over several sessions, his movements became larger and more forceful, but still not without constraint. As he became more aware of his bound energy, he began to feel frustrated. He no longer wanted refuge in inertness, but he did not know what to do.

With the physical breakthrough, he was able to feel and develop his body experiences. Mental associations were much more difficult. However, Fletcher notes,

> ... even the very process of having to articulate about his immediate experience was developing in him the capacity to find a language for his inner experiences and helping him to link his subjective experiencing self to his objective observing self. This also helped to develop his capacity to take council with himself and to communicate his inner self to the outside world. (1979, p. 149)

Once Mr. C. was able to identify his behavior, he could begin to experiment with changing it. Further breakthroughs occurred in later sessions. He became more able to use mental imagery and allowed himself to focus on memories he had previously repressed. Fletcher sums up the case by saying:

> This case illustrates some of the values of focusing on the body and following the cues and impulses so minutely. So much of Mr. C's experience was threatening, repressed from consciousness and partially expressed through the body in unconscious behavior and incipient action without being linked to awareness, self-perception or thought. In such a case, when the body information is so divergent from his self-concept, the body experience assists in the process of reclaiming some of what had been repressed. As the material was becoming more articulated and linked coherently to image, thought, memory and emotion, it began to have more meaning.... Each new linkage and integration brings about a slightly new constellation from which the next experience emerges. (1979, pp.153-154)

In discussing the therapeutic uses of body experience, Fletcher states that most body-oriented techniques can be included in one or more of the following five categories:

1. *Discovery*—referring to new experiences and to increasing and enriching the movement repertoire and range of response. This begins at a very basic level—learning about body parts, sensations and the different ways in which the body can move. New experiences must take place and there must be new awareness and new sensory perceptions if there is to be any change.

2. *Reconstitutional body work*—working on the body to help the individual "let go" or "get rid" of anxiety or negative feelings. Relaxation techniques and other forms of anxiety reduction, as well as movements that can express or discharge energy, are often used to facilitate a patient's freer response. Besides the immediate aim of momentary relief, there may also be long-term educational goals.

3. *Restructuring*—physical restructuring of movement and posture at a neuromuscular level. These techniques can have the effect of "relieving tension, of reconstitution and sometimes, of assisting intra-psychic change" (Fletcher, 1979, p. 143). However, if the client's body awareness is very limited, such techniques can result in redistortions.

4. *Interpersonal communication*—using body experience to promote human contact and communication. Fletcher attributes this type of work to Marian Chace, who used it with groups of hospitalized patients. Though this work may include reconstitutional experiences, the stress is on socialization and group interaction. "Movement," Fletcher states, "operates as a medium, like language, by which interpersonal skills and relations can be developed and an initial feeling of self through relating to others can be found" (1979, p. 143).

5. *Intra-psychic reorganization through insight into meaning*—using body experience to bring "preverbal and undifferentiated experiences" into consciousness, thus resulting in increased understanding of the inner self. The overall goal is an integrated, cohesive union of physical and mental processes.

Fletcher goes on to state: "The goals may be to teach a person how to take care of himself, how to take charge of his condition, handle his anxiety and emotions and to help himself feel better. Such a process may be depicted as being a parent to oneself" (1979, p. 143).

However, problems are not necessarily solved simply by releasing tension and negative feelings, Fletcher notes. If techniques are too abrupt and/or explosive, the highly charged material that is brought up may further disorient the person rather than the opposite. The release process must be coupled with therapeutic work so it may be utilized and integrated fully. Fletcher emphasizes that the therapist must identify which of the above uses of body experience would be most effective for each individual. She states that her focus is

> ... to use body work for the purposes of discovering new experience, interpersonal communication and intra-psychic reorganization through insight into meaning, though some reconstitutional work may occur. (1979, p. 144)

In summary, she focuses on the following areas:

> (1) developing the capacity of attending to and identifying aspects of one's experience; (2) locating sensation and movement impulses and any other body feelings; (3) discovering the motions and dynamic movements of tensions as patterns that arise from the inner impulses; (4) ... exploring the range of body functioning and expression as it emerges in the therapy, quality of efforts, tension-relaxation, blocking and the particular function it serves in each case.... (1979, p. 144)

Part C. Janet Adler: The Witness/Mover Relationship

Adler is another dance therapist who carries on the work of Mary Whitehouse. Originally well known for her work with autistic children, Adler today specializes in working with adults using "authentic movement." One of her particular interests is the role of the therapist as "witness" (the empathic observer role) in the therapeutic relationship. This concept, brought forward from her training with Whitehouse, has been a major area of study for Adler.

The witness, Adler (1985) explains, initially

> ...carries a larger responsibility for consciousness as she sits to the side of the movement space [and watches]. She is not 'looking at' the person moving. She is witnessing, listening, bringing a specific quality of attention or presence to the experience. (p. 2)

As in the work of Whitehouse, Adler asks her patients to move with their eyes closed. This, she believes, helps the individual to expand and deepen his or her awareness of unconscious and superconscious experiences. Most important in Adler's work is her emphasis on the relationship between the mover (patient/client) and the witness (or therapist). While the therapist's witness role can be generalized into the category of empathic observer role, it should not be confused with a passive experience. The relationship is an extremely active and interactive one, although the interaction may not be immediately apparent. In short, through the verbal and nonverbal interactions of the witness and mover, Adler believes that both can reach new heights of self-observation, awareness and insight. Ultimately, Adler believes that the awareness achieved has the potential to be transpersonal, that is, to go beyond the personal conscious and toward a universal unconscious (Adler, 1985).

While Adler discusses the transpersonal aspects of the witness-mover relationship, she is also cognizant of the similarities of the witness/mover relationship with that of the analyst/analyzed relationship and notes the importance of understanding the transference and counter-transference phenomena that occur.

In 2002, at the American Dance Therapy Association's 37th Annual Conference, Adler was a keynote speaker. She gave a dramatic speech comparing the essence of her work with adults in authentic movement with that of her work with children with autism. She drew a parallel between *Looking for Me* (1970) her well-known film about a child with autism that she mirrored, nurtured and reached emotionally through dance interaction and her work with healthy adults utilizing witnessing and improvisational movement.

In her speech, she poignantly and poetically integrated these seemingly disparate parts of her work. The audience stood up and, in a heartfelt response that included raising their arms up and out to the side, as Adler's child had done in the film, expressed their appreciation for the vivid connection that Adler was making.

Adler was identifying the universal need to be seen and heard. The particular methods used, be they mirroring or silently experiencing another and honoring another's dance, result in a similar effect and fulfill a deep human need.

Part D. Joan Chodorow: Whitehouse and Jung

Chodorow, formerly known as Smallwood, is a leading dance therapist and a Jungian analyst who practices on the West Coast. Her dance therapy training was with Whitehouse and Schoop. She discusses her use of a Jungian approach to dance therapy in her article "Dance Therapy and the Transcendent Function" (1978). The "transcendent function," a Jungian concept, is an "innate, dynamic process that serves to unite opposite positions within the psyche," thus facilitating "a transition from one attitude to another" (1978, p. 16). Chodorow quotes Jung who described it as "a movement out of the suspension between two opposites, a living birth that leads to a new level of being, a new situation" (1978, p. 16).

In an earlier paper "Philosophy and Methods of Individual Work" (1974), Chodorow differentiates two approaches to dance therapy, one moving toward the conscious and the other toward the unconscious. The former, Chodorow believes, is usually more appropriate for the disturbed/psychotic patient, who needs a sense of conscious, everyday reality and movement experiences that strengthen ego boundaries. This approach, Chodorow states, may include:

> ... use of structured rhythms, ... clearly organized spatial patterns, [and] intentional use of weight [which] will help the person develop a more realistic body image and strengthen his or her conscious viewpoint. (1978, p. 17)

The second approach, using movement "as a means of opening to the unconscious" (1978, p. 17), is usually more appropriate for the fair-to-well functioning individual whose ego is more intact (referred to earlier as the "normal and neurotic" by some of the pioneers).

This delineation of therapeutic approaches corresponds to Whitehouse's differentiation between "I move" and "I am moved," as well as Dosamantes-Beaudry's differentiation between the active and receptive modes of perception and behavior. Chodorow's purpose in proposing the two approaches is to gain clarity and better theoretical understanding of varying needs in different personalities. It is important to remember, however, "in reality, there is often a constant interchange, an ebb and flow back and forth between the two" (Smallwood, 1974, p. 26).

Chodorow works primarily with "relatively stable individuals who possess a... strong ego viewpoint" (1978, p. 18). The focus of her work is the use of movement to give form to the imagination. Her therapeutic approach to exploring the unconscious and integrating it into consciousness is based on Jung's method of "active imagination." (a process that was discussed by Whitehouse).

In a 1986 interview conducted by dance therapist and clinical psychologist Nisha Zenoff for the *American Journal of Dance Therapy*, Chodorow made many illuminating statements about her studies with Mary Whitehouse and Trudi Schoop and also about her clinical work. The following excerpts from this interview center around Chodorow's clarification and expansion of the Whitehouse work.

> NZ: Would you talk about how you use movement in analysis?
>
> JC: Movement is not essential for everyone, but it is essential for some. And it's helpful for most people. Yet there are people I work with who rarely feel the need to leave their chairs. They're able to enter the imagined world without getting up to move. I'm comfortable with that because that's their way. I think what's more important to me nowadays than whether someone moves or not, is whether we're able to open to the imagination or not. There are many ways of opening to the imagination and each person has to find his or her own best way.
>
> NZ: You said for some it's essential. How do you or they know that it's essential? What are your clues?
>
> JC: In my experience, people generally know when they want to move. They know that in order to go into the world of the unconscious, they've got to ground it in the movement of their own body. Some people are able to just imagine by leaps and bounds. You don't know how they get from here to there. For myself, I'm not quite connected when I imagine in that way. That kind of fantasy feels disembodied. But when I move my body through the images, then I've truly entered into that world. The people who come to work with me want to do analysis and most of them want movement to be part of it. So we do analysis. That means we talk about dreams, fantasies, life experiences, what's going on between us. We sit in chairs or we sit on the floor. We do sandplay and use art materials.
>
> Whenever there's a feeling of wanting to move, every person seems to approach it differently. There are some people who'll come and talk for fifteen minutes and then move for twenty, thirty minutes and then talk a little bit toward the end. Others will come in and before anything is said, they'll close their eyes and begin to move. They simply go into that world and see what comes. After they're through, they'll bring it to an end, make a transition and we may or may not talk about the movement that just happened. They're just as likely to be quiet for a while and then say, "Where's the clay?" and then form an image. Then we might sit down and talk about dreams. People often remember their dreams or early childhood experiences while they're moving. Or we might talk about how it felt between us while they moved, how they were aware of my watching the movement or what it stirred up in me as I watched the movement.
>
> It's different for every person. Some people just move from what their own bodies want to do. Other people will see a specific image, sometimes like a guide person who appears in their imagination. The inner guide moves and the mover mirrors or follows or interacts with the imagined figure. For some it's primarily a rite of entry into the analytic hour, where you get into your body and you separate from the everyday world. Movement and attending to the body experience can simply be a way of opening to the unconscious and then we'll sit down and talk about dreams or something else. There's no particular form.
>
> Whether we're talking or moving or engaging the symbolic process some other way, there's a kind of awareness that goes on. For me, whatever comes up from the unconscious usually has four aspects: one aspect is how is it happening here between us; another aspect is how is it happening in the person's life right now; the third aspect is what are the earliest memories from childhood of that same kind of experience; the fourth aspect brings in universal or mythic images.

In one of his letters, Jung described active imagination as his analytical method of psychotherapy. Active imagination clearly includes dance movement as well as all of the other art experiences. But it also includes imagining around transference and countertransference issues and possibilities of what the symbolic meanings might be of complexes that erupt in everyday life. In its most basic sense, active imagination is opening to the unconscious and giving free reign to fantasy, while at the same time maintaining a conscious viewpoint.

NZ: In your writings you've talked about the presence of the witness, the analyst. What is that presence?

JC: It's holding a particular kind of tension, because you bring your total being and total attention to the relationship. This is true whether you're sitting in chairs or whether the person is moving. But the experience is often more powerful when the person is moving and you're not distracted by words. Movement goes so directly to the emotional life.

I feel it's important to bring who I am and not try to clear myself or make myself too centered. When I've put a high value on being centered or receptive, I've found that I tend to split from the parts of me that are not like that. To the degree that I foster any particular attitude, its opposite tends to get constellated in the unconscious. So I've learned to just let myself be how I am and contain it.

What we're talking about now has to do with deliberately opening to the unconscious, yet not identifying with it. In other words, opening to the imagination doesn't mean merging with the images and off you go. Opening to the imagination means being yourself, with all your strengths and weaknesses and noticing what you're imagining.

There are so many different levels of witnessing. You notice what the body is doing. You're curious, interested in what the body is doing. You're noticing that. But you're also noticing the emotional tone and if there's an infantile quality to it, something of a parental caretaking, nurturing feeling may come up. Or if there's a family history in the mover of being neglected or being mistreated in some way, those kinds of indifferent or rejecting counter transference responses can also erupt.

Then there's the whole realm of what does this person's movement stir up in me from a larger cultural perspective? How has this attitude or movement sequence appeared in art, how has it appeared in literature or mythology? What paintings come to mind, what poetry or music comes to mind as I watch the person move? In what way does this express a universal human experience? So it ranges from questions about what is this body doing—to imagining all kinds of possibilities about the person's life history, particularly the early history that tends to come up so often in movement. It's all there while you're watching, but most of it is like a dream world: you can't retrieve all of it. Some of it stays, but you don't remember everything. In a sense it has a ritual quality. It's as if we enter sacred space.

NZ: Is the sacred space that you're talking about related to what you've referred to in your writing as "participation mystique"?

JC: The "participation mystique" is a phrase that Jung used to describe what we might call merging. It's when we are able to drop our boundaries in the presence of another. Sacred space is kind of like the inside of the magic circle. It's like the therapeutic container. Dora Kalff described a "free and sheltered space."

There is a tension we have to hold as we witness movement. On one hand, we deliberately open ourselves to the possibility of merging, *participation mystique*. It's like what Mary spoke of when she described a quality of movement with the word "inevitable." The witness is so connected to what the mover is doing that you feel you know what's going to happen next. (Zenoff, 1986)

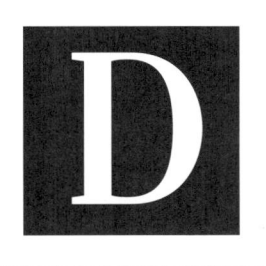

Discussion

Comparing East and West Coast Trends

Chapters 14 and 15 examined East and West Coast trends in dance therapies that emerged during the 1960s and 1970s and continue today. These trends grew out of the influences of the major pioneers. Some interesting trends and patterns emerge when comparing East Coast with West Coast influences, which will be discussed below. This chapter concludes with an account of Sharon Chaiklin's historic visit to the West Coast in 1972.

Broadly speaking, many East Coast-influenced leaders stress alternately the psychic structures of id, ego and superego, the roles these play in body movement, psychosexual stages of development and other psychodynamic and psychoanalytic concepts, including self-psychology and object relations theories. In addition, tools for the description of movement behavior and diagnosis, specifically Laban Movement Analysis, have received greater attention on the East Coast. On the other hand, many dance therapists influenced on the West Coast discuss their work with a greater focus on the immediacy of the movement experience itself, that is, the bodily-felt experience and the psychic material it evokes. These therapists tend to stress the concepts of being fully in the here and now, "attending" to the physical and mental self and finding one's "authentic movement."

There is also a greater West Coast emphasis on the exploration of the individual psyche, in contrast to the East Coast psychoanalytic, interactional and community orientation. This is not to imply, however, that all therapists trained by a West Coast leader stress only the immediacy of the movement experience while all those trained by East Coast leaders are psychoanalytical and/or interactional. Nor does it imply that one excludes the other.

These differences in East Coast and West Coast trends can be traced back to the work of Marian Chace and Mary Whitehouse. According to the Survey Results (see Unit V), most of the dance therapy leaders on the East Coast were trained or influenced by Chace and the majority of West Coast leaders were trained or influenced by Whitehouse.

These two major pioneers differed not only in theory, but also in practice. Chace worked with hospitalized psychiatric patients primarily in groups, with a major emphasis on the therapeutic movement relationship (a Sullivanian interactional approach) and the group rhythmic relationship. Whitehouse specialized in the more healthy population, often dancers were seen in her dance studio and she stressed a transcendent aspect of dance that carries individuals into another realm of consciousness and unconsciousness. The clinical differences between these two most influential leaders were, to a large degree, influenced by the needs of their patients and the setting individuals were seen in, as well as their dance backgrounds and of course temperamental differences.

However, there were also many less obvious trends that were set in motion by the other major pioneers. For example, in contrast to Chace, East Coast pioneers Evan and Espenak were working with a healthier population, while Schoop and Hawkins were doing hospital work on the West Coast. In addition, Adlerian and psychoanalytic concepts influenced Evan and Espenak, while humanistic psychology influenced Hawkins. Schoop stressed community and society. She moved with her patients and always brought movement back to conscious control and "performance." Evan and Espenak explored the unconscious through improvisation in ways quite similar to Whitehouse. All three were influenced, either directly or indirectly, by Wigman's improvisational work.

Two features that tie all approaches to dance therapy together are 1) establishing empathic rapport and 2) engaging the patient at his or her level of readiness to work. The latter has been referred to as starting where the patient is and in fact, it implies a genuine empathic relationship and an understanding of developmental needs. The therapist cannot truly intervene at the patient's emotional level unless he or she is deeply attuned to the patient. Empathy is the ability to "get inside" the other person and see, feel and think the way that person does without judging, censoring, or criticizing. This seemingly simple but actually most difficult challenge is at the root of all dance therapy theory and practice and overlaps with much of the current thinking in fields of psychotherapy as well.

What can sometimes confuse the student's understanding of basic similarities in theory, methods and goals is the use of varying terminology to say often the same thing. This is a well-known problem in many professional fields and definitely in psychology.

It is also important to recognize that while dance therapy students will initially utilize the ideas of their original teachers, they will eventually pursue therapeutic techniques that fit most comfortably with their own expressive styles and, of course, those methods that are most suitable to their patients. Tapping into the therapist's expressive potential and bringing this out fully deepens the therapist's strengths as a healer. This will be discussed further in Chapter 17.

Part E. Sharon Chaiklin Was There—1972

Chaiklin has a unique and personal historical perspective on the early acknowledgement and acceptance of the differing East and West Coast trends in dance therapy. Her own training was with Chace in the 1960s. At that time, the ADTA was based in the East Coast and little was known about dance therapy in the West. In 1972, Chaiklin was sent to the West Coast to meet dance therapists from that part of the country. The following was written by Chaiklin (personal communication, 2003), describing those early days and the poignant beginning of dialogue between East and West Coast dance therapists, a dialogue that has continued into the present but now includes, as seen in this and the previous chapter, additional branches of theory and practice. Here is Chaiklin's perspective:

> In the beginning, there began to be an awakening of the importance of dance and movement within the therapeutic process. There were a few circles of innovative people and their followers who had already begun to develop their ideas and theories in the 1950s and 1960s, but there were no bridges of communication amongst them. There was Marian Chace in Washington, DC, Blanche Evan and Liljan Espenak in New York City and Alma Hawkins and Mary Whitehouse in Los Angeles and Trudi Schoop in northern California. There was also Irmgard Bartenieff in New York City, who was known primarily for her understanding of Laban's work in the study of effort and shape, now known as Labananalysis.
>
> In my experience, creative innovators in the process of developing their ideas must have a strong belief in what they are doing and thinking. There was no one else leading the way and no peers to discuss their thinking with, few to support what might seem radical and only a few students trying to understand these new concepts. Although I met others who were creative and unique, my most involved and direct experience was with Marian Chace, who was my mentor and teacher and serves as an example.
>
> In order to trust the validity of her discoveries and theories, there was a strong need to discount or ignore others on similar paths. There may be several explanations for this, but it takes a great deal of strength and strong ego to tread where others have no understanding and offer little support. For Chace, it was a combination of strength and conviction that covered her insecurity. Likely each pioneer had a different attitude or self-doubt, but the need for totally believing in one's work was paramount to innovation. None of those mentioned made any real effort to communicate with any other. In looking at the work of these pioneers many years later, it is notable that each therapist had a different aspect of theory and technique to offer and none seemed to contradict any of the others. Each understood through her body the power of dance, having used it in varied ways. Because of their different life experiences, each found the psychological theorists they preferred or with whom they were more familiar and therefore described their findings using different words or focused on different parts of the therapeutic process.
>
> The American Dance Therapy Association was formed by a group of developing dance therapists primarily connected with Marian Chace, who desired communication with each other and with those related to other pioneers. When the ADTA was formed, it was hoped by those involved that forming an organization might start the process of sharing ideas as well as eventual recognition by the mental health world as a new profession. As beginning therapists in a beginning profession—not yet a profession actually—we

were all struggling to understand what it was we were actually doing, it felt like holding onto the tail of a dragon and not knowing if we could ever tame it. People remained suspicious of each other, again based on the insecurities of being with the unknown. Gradually it became clear that the gulf between the east coast of the United States, primarily those surrounding Marian Chace and the west coast, primarily those who had studied with Mary Whitehouse, had to be bridged. We were so naive about the work at that time that it took a while for the realization to take hold that the populations we were working with were mostly different and therefore it partly explained the differences in how we worked.

Chace's work was primarily within psychiatric institutions and focused on group work and trying to restructure those whose psyches had been shattered. She was in the midst of those who were first creating group psychotherapy after the Second World War and she was studying with the psychiatrists in the area who happened to be Henry Stack Sullivan and Frieda Fromm-Reichmann. Mary Whitehouse had gone to Zurich and studied at the Jungian Institute there. Her work focused more on individuals functioning in the community and she made use of her Jungian learning to work in-depth with the unconscious through movement.

Those on the east coast gradually began to understand the other innovators in New York City and those on the west coast began to study with all those in California. It was all a matter of geography! Keep in mind that travel was more limited at that time, comparatively expensive and that most of those involved had limited finances.

In 1972, the dance therapists in California had their first regional meeting under the auspices of the ADTA. It was decided that it would be important to start bridging the gap between coasts so that we could be unified as an association and assimilate new ideas. As president of the ADTA at that time and as a figure who represented the east and those involved with Chace, I was fortunate to be able to attend the conference held in Santa Barbara. It turned out to be a significant time for both those in California and for the ADTA. Many of the Californians who attended were meeting each other for the first time. There was an air of excitement and expectation as people began to share their work with each other. There was mutual understanding that each was in a state of flux and growth and therefore each workshop was accepted as a work in progress. It was also significant to those there that there was representation from the ADTA itself. It was a symbolic recognition of the validity of the dance therapy work being done in California and that our association was truly a national one.

After that and over time, there was a push from both coasts to further integrate our shared knowledge and participate in developing the profession in all its possibilities. The sense of east and west, of one way of working or another as being more valid, began to dissipate. Practitioners realized that there was much to learn from one another and the divisiveness faded. Much needed to be done, such as supporting each other through writing, giving workshops, opening new positions, developing programs and promoting our professionalism in the larger world of health and education.

My own clinical work became richer and was informed by varied perspectives as a result of the ongoing search for understanding. I remained working in hospital settings for over 30 years and what I learned initially from Marian Chace at St. Elizabeth's in Washington, DC, remained a firm base to that work. Group process and the trust in the body and rhythm and metaphorical expression became stronger and clarified in meaning over time. However, I also absorbed how to work with those with better ego strengths and that while working toward organization and ego was a goal with psychotic patients, it was softening the defenses and getting to the unconscious that became the work in private practice.

I became more adept at recognizing the immediate needs of individuals and this allowed me to have a range of ways of working in both situations so that neither became a rigid technique but rather a way of conceptualizing. At times I could fly with my schizophrenic friends and at other times the better functioning clients needed my more direct presence to support and sustain them through hard times. New information continually made its way into my personal learning, but the beginning was the integration of the east and west coasts' way of thinking about dance therapy, through understanding both in my body and through experience.

The beginnings of new things all have a process that must take its course. Our early teachers had so much to offer and the insights they were working on left little time or energy to think about others working differently. Their students began with the same parochialism but gradually realized there were many more truths to discover. The end result is that dance movement therapy did indeed become a recognized profession and that those who enter the field are the continuing source of new energy to build on our understanding of the complexity of dance movement therapy based on the early revelations put forth by those first dancers and thinkers from one coast to the other. (personal communication, 2003)

Sharon Chaiklin was actively involved with her colleagues in forming the American Dance Therapy Association. At its incorporation in 1966, with Marian Chace as president, she was elected vice-president. She followed Marian Chace as the next president and served for two terms from 1968 through 1972. She has served as the president of the Marian Chace Foundation; Jane Wilson Cathcart and Ann Lohn have served as secretary and treasurer, respectively. The foundation is a nonprofit organization formed to serve the needs of education, research and scholarship related to dance movement therapy.

Many East and West Coast pioneers joined forces in 1966 to create the American Dance Therapy Association (ADTA):

American Dance Therapy Association
73 Charter Members

Dian Averbuck
Irmgard Bartenieff
Beate Becker
Miriam R. Berger
Ruth Bernard
Ruthanna Boris
Nitza Broide-Miller
Mary Ann Buben
Judith Bunney
Marian Chace
Sharon Chaiklin
Pei-Fen Chin
Susan Constable
Martha Davis
Laura DeFreitas
Wynelle Delaney
Mildred Dickinson
Leslie Dinsmore
Francis Donelan
Liljan Espenak
Blanche Evan
Mary Fee
Joseph Fischer
Genieve Fox
Doris Fredericks
SuEllen Fried
Raoul Gelabert
Jane Ganet Sigel
Sally Fitzpatrick Hanes
Alma Hawkins
Mildred Hill
Doris Hinton
Hawaii State Hospital
Beth Kalish-Weiss
Stephanie Katz
Annie Kemna
Susan Kleinman

Julianna Lau
Ruth Lauterstein
Mary Ann Lloyd
Sherry Martin
Diana B. McCarthy
Peggy Mitchell
Constance Moerman
Hilda Mullin
Joan P. Orr
Ruth Panofsky
Marjorie Pasternack
Catherine Pasternak
Forestine Paulay
Elizabeth Polk
Catherine Reisman
Irene W. Reiss
Dian Rosenfeld
Gloria Simcha Ruben
Susan Sandel
Maxine F. Schapiro
Lilian Schayer
Claire Schmais
Roberta Schlasko
Arlynne Stark
Dorothy Steigerwald
Alice Bovard-Taylor
Deborah Thomas
Barbara Weiner
Barbara Weintraub
Joyce Weir
Elissa Q. White
Griselda F. White
Mary Whitehouse
Minnie P. Wilson
Mary Jane Wolbers
Louise Yokum

16 | Integration of Different Trends

The melding of influences among contemporary dance therapists is inevitable.[1] Most of today's leaders have studied the work of at least two pioneers and many of these leaders are now teaching throughout the United States and abroad. Some dance therapists now blending East and West Coast influences are also integrating aspects of other action-oriented psychotherapies, for example psychodrama, art and Gestalt therapy.

Three registered dance therapists known well for their integration of a variety of influences, including East and West Coast trends, are Marcia Leventhal, Penny Lewis and Fran Levy. Leventhal's and Lewis's work will be discussed in the following pages. Levy's work on multimodal treatment is the subject of Chapter 17. Her chapter also illustrates the unwitting integration of East and Eest Coast influences by Levy's college dance professor approximately 35 years ago.

Part A. Marcia Leventhal: Dance Therapy as Primary Treatment

Marcia Leventhal (1980), former associate professor and director of New York University's Graduate Dance Therapy Program, is widely known for her work in dance therapy among children with autism. Her extensive training in psychoanalytic psychotherapy, Gestalt therapy and psychosynthesis was complemented by her dance therapy studies with Hawkins, Whitehouse and Valerie Hunt. Hunt, retired professor of Kinesiology and Movement Behavior at U.C.L.A., was director of the Bio-Energy Field Lab in Malibu, California. Other influences on Leventhal include East Coast pioneers Evan and Bartenieff. This unique combination of training and influence drew Leventhal toward dance therapy with adult populations.

Since her retirement from New York University, Leventhal has been instrumental in developing postgraduate training for dance therapists. She co-founded the Dance Therapy Institute of Princeton with Barbara J. Harrison. During this time she developed a model for teaching, "Dance Therapy as Primary Treatment." She also developed training models for dance therapy teaching institutions in countries as diverse as Greece, Japan, Tobago and Australia.

From her work with Hawkins and Whitehouse, her main mentors, Leventhal became committed to the study and exploration of the therapeutic benefits of rhythm, both as a structure inherent in movement and in conjunction with the movement interaction between patient and therapist. This, one of the major themes of her work, has also been the subject of her numerous lectures around the world.

Leventhal (1999) believes that "with dance movement experiences, an individual has the opportunity to uncover the root of an old pattern and to modify it if it has become outgrown or outdated." Through therapy, an "individual is able to release or undo parts of patterns in which s/he is entangled." Like other therapists in the field, such as Lewis and Levy, Leventhal uses a multimodal approach. She states that "Dreams, verbal discourse, imagery, art work and music are supporters of the [therapeutic] process," but that these elements should only be used to support the key role of the dance therapist (1999).

For Leventhal, each individual has a unique essence and this essence gives shape and form to aspects of the self. She believes that dance can give individuals direct access to their essence and that rhythm and

---
[1]This is evident in the survey results section, Unit V, *Chapter 28*.

movement strengthen the ability to get in touch with one's deeper feelings (Leventhal, 1999). She believes that dance and movement "lead eventually to the acceptance and strengthening of the core essence" (Leventhal, 1999). "As we begin to move spontaneously in a purely non-competitive, self-expressive way, authentic qualities of the deepest core of our essence begin to be discovered and realized. Dance movement therapy goes beyond the spoken work ... allowing us ... to have a [n] ... integrative experience" (Leventhal, 1999).

The dance therapist meets the individual "on the developmental level most foreground for the individual at the time of interchange" (Leventhal, 1999). This level translates into what Leventhal calls "flow readiness." "Flow readiness" includes those qualities of motion that the client exhibits in his or her use of rhythm, space and degrees of energy.[2]

As noted by Avstreih in Chapter 14 and again here by Leventhal, the ability of dance therapists to adjust their movement qualities (force, time, space and flow) to match or mirror those of their clients enables clients to re-establish and possibly work through early developmental experiences (Leventhal, 1999). Dratman (1967) likened the use of mirroring in the establishment of a therapeutic relationship to having a substitute mother. Many therapists working with children, as will be seen in Chapter 18, also stress the importance of mirroring and work in dyads.

Leventhal emphasizes the importance of introducing movement that has boundaries and structure. Structured movement expression is the organizing basis of the relationship between the client and the therapist. The dance therapist helps to create these structures through the creative use of dance dynamics such as time and space. These dance dynamics become experiences with definite parameters that the client can depend on and repeat (Leventhal, 1999).

Leventhal gives the following case as an example of her work with an adult cancer patient and how she helped this patient to connect with her own essence and how she then used this connection to fight her cancer. This example illustrates the healing power of connecting with one's essence in movement.

> Mrs. G. sought assistance when her previously in-remission cancer reappeared and metastasized to her liver. She came to therapy to help her adjust to the illness, but also to try to use alternative healing modalities (whilst continuing her standard medical treatment). After several sessions of working with dance movement, visualization and various Shamanic healing practices, Mrs. G. was able to identify a strongly negative voice in her that seemed to be fighting her determination to recover her life and free herself of the cancer. During this same session, while moving expressively, she uncovered an energy quality which she was able to describe as her "healing channel." While she moved this energy quality, Mrs. G. was able to visualize this quality as light and as energy surrounding her diseased organs as well as "patching up" her personal energy field. She was able to contrast the two polarities in movement and work towards releasing the negative voices and strengthening what she felt were the healing aspects of her self. She learned to strengthen her defense against cancer by using her soothing, healing rhythm/energy flow as an antidote to high levels of stress, fatigue or fragmentation of energy. Shortly after this pivotal session, her cancer appeared to go into remission again (Leventhal, 1999).

Through the use of dance and other creative modes, Leventhal's work emphasizes the importance of healing and transformation through structured movement experiences. Therapy is aimed at helping clients to integrate their experiences and connect with their essence (Leventhal, 1999).

Part B. Penny Lewis: An Eclectic Approach

Lewis (formerly Bernstein), a dance movement therapist, author and clinician as well as editor of several books in the field, studied originally with Chace and Bartenieff and has been strongly influenced by Jungian psychology and Object Relations Theory. Although she has worked with other populations, her current work centers on the normal and neurotic adult population.

Lewis believed early on that the term dance therapy should be broadened to include the word movement in its title. She worked actively for this change, entitling her original book, *Theory and Methods in Dance Movement Therapy* (Bernstein, 1972). This was followed by *Eight Theoretical Approaches in Dance Movement Therapy* (Bernstein, 1979), which Lewis edited and contributed chapters to.

---

[2] This approach is reminiscent of Chace's Therapeutic Movement Relationship, which is discussed in Chapter One. While different leaders have trained therapists and different language is used to describe their work, interventions and goals are often similar.

At the time of the publication of her first book, Lewis was in her early twenties. Her thoughts on the field and its connections with other areas of psychological and spiritual thought have continued to grow, expand and mature throughout the years.

Lewis has always been an extremely eclectic dance therapist, integrating art, drama, sound and writing in her work. She is a registered drama therapist and a registered dance therapist. In addition to using the creative arts, Lewis uses a variety of theoretical frameworks such as Gestalt and Jungian therapy. Her choice of a Gestalt therapy approach or a Jungian approach depends on "whether the client is more of a sensation or an intuitive perceiver" (Bernstein 1980, p. 46). With the former, Lewis generally believes the Gestalt approach is more appropriate while with the latter intuitive, introverted Jungian approach is more suitable.

The Gestalt therapy approach, like psychodrama and dance therapy, stresses the importance of individuals being actively involved in an experience instead of merely talking about it. Growth in therapy, according to Lewis, is more likely to come about when the individual can participate in and achieve a "full identification with the process" (Lewis, 1986, p. 109).

This process of allowing individuals to become immersed in the expression of the unconscious affords them direct contact with parts of their being that they may have previously disowned or of which they had been unaware (Lewis, 1986, p. 112). In a supportive environment, patients can allow symbolic expression to become real without fear of the consequences.

The therapist's role is that of a guide and facilitator, assisting the patient as he or she journeys inwardly toward increased self-awareness. Empathy and sensitivity are essential (Lewis, 1986).

Interestingly, Gestalt therapy originated by Frederick Perls developed in popularity in the 1960s on the west coast. In Lewis' discussion of its relevance to dance therapy, one can hear familiar west coast themes of sensing, attending and intensified individual self-expression.

Aside from this article by Lewis, little has been written on the integration of Gestalt therapy and dance therapy. Leaders like Linni Deihl (formerly Silberman), however, are doing important work and, like Lewis, are active in synthesizing many contemporary dance therapy trends (personal communication, 1990).

Through her studies with Judith Kestenberg, Lewis also pioneered the integration of Laban's work with Dance Movement Therapy. Along with Susan Loman, Lewis has written and taught extensively on the topic of effort/shape and its correlation with psychosexual stages of development. Several dance therapy concepts have grown out of both Lewis' early studies and her more recent endeavors (personal communication, 2002).

Two concepts that Lewis discusses extensively in her writing are the choreography of object relations and somatic countertransference.

Choreography of Object Relations

This term, Choreography of Object Relations, coined by Jane Wilson Cathcart (formerly Downes) describes a dance movement therapy technique. Lewis has built on this concept and defines it as follows: "through the choreography of object relations, the dance therapist ascertains the developmental level of the client, works through any trauma associated with that level and through movement-based re-parenting gives the client the needed relationship to reach their chronological age" (Lewis, personal communication, 2002).

Lewis's method of working with object relations was developed through the integration of Kestenberg's interpretation of effort/shape with Anna Freud's theory of developmental stages and Margaret Mahler's object relations theory. Working in this manner enabled Lewis to move from doing adjunctive group dance movement therapy to in-depth primary dance movement therapy. Lewis realized that by observing movement through the Kestenberg movement profile the dance therapist could assess the dysfunctional aspects of the personality and developmental arrests. The dance therapist can also observe various tensions within the body through the language of tension flow and shape flow[3] (Lewis, personal communication, 2002).

Lewis, like Avstreih, emphasizes the Chacian concept of empathic movement reflection—entering the patient's world, picking up on the positive and negative points, feelings and transference and responding with dramatic movement, which Lewis refers to as the "re-choreographing of object relations." (Lewis, 1975a; 1982; 1990; 1993; 2000). As the effects of early deprivation are reduced through the therapeutic

---

[3]See Unit II, Section A for more information on Laban and Kestenberg.

movement relationship, new movement interactions are developed that attune to the ever changing developmental needs of the patient. Often the process begins with symbiotic movement interactions that "evolve into stages of separation and individuation. Individuals gain a sense of self through attunement, holding, rocking and visually connected love" (Lewis, personal communication, 2002). While the language varies from that of Leventhal, discussed above, the overlap in Lewis and Leventhal's thinking is apparent.

Somatic Countertransference

According to Lewis, somatic countertransference is a depth psychotherapy technique in which the dance movement therapist somatically receives feelings, sensations, images or thoughts from the body and unconscious of the client. These feelings or sensations are held, reflected verbally or sent back to the client through images or actions (personal communication, 2002).

Lewis's work with Chace and Kestenberg taught her to attune to the inner realm of the client—particularly with clients who were mute or were functioning at a preverbal level. Lewis began to realize that it was possible to receive material from the unconscious of a client through nonverbal communication. Somatic countertransference also describes the dance therapist's empathic physical response to the patient—a kind of intuition that guides the dance therapist's interventions.

Somatic countertransference can be described as an unconscious to conscious connection between the client and therapist in which the therapist may receive feelings, sensations or thoughts that the patient has split off from his or her conscious mind (Lewis, personal communication, 2002). As a result of dance therapists' sensitivity to bodily clues and ability to use their bodies to communicate, they can reflect patients' emotions (affect) back to them and in this way help them to reclaim their feelings. If the patient is not ready, Lewis explains, the dance therapist can "hold" the affect for patients so as to help them manage the intensity, or possible overflow, of their feelings (personal communication, 2002). In this way, patients are helped to contain their expression.

Lewis believes that tuning into one's bodily responses to a patient can help the therapist make a diagnosis. For example, the therapist can physically sense the borderline patient's conflict between the desires for symbiosis or for pushing the therapist away. This can result in an appropriate dance therapy movement response, says Lewis (personal communication, 2002). These internal responses or somatic countertransference feelings help to create meaningful and useful imagery that can be enacted in order to work through conflicts such as the separation/individuation conflict noted above. Imagery leads to movement work, which can creatively enact and resolve developmental conflicts (personal communication, 2002). An example of this type of creative imagery that is shared between patient and therapist is illustrated in Fran Levy's (1995) chapter "Nameless: A Case of Multiplicity."

Interestingly, this concept of diagnosing a patient through the therapist's internal response to the patient has been expressed by verbal therapists for years and is often referred to as the therapist's intuition. It seems that Lewis is describing what is most commonly referred to as a gut response—a somatic reaction. Through the eyes of a dance therapist, Lewis has attempted to identify and broaden this concept.

Collaborating with Others in the Creative Arts

Lewis worked at the Pittsburgh University Medical School's model Pittsburgh Child Guidance Center in the 1970s (Lewis, personal communication, 2002). Here, art, drama and dance movement therapists worked actively in collaboration with each other, creatively moving from one art form to the other.

The following quote is from the opening pages of Lewis's book, *Creative Transformation: The Healing Power of the Arts* (1993):

> The dance between the conscious and unconscious is choreographed in the magical place of the imaginal realm. Here is where children play and heroes and heroines come alive in spontaneous creative dramas. Here is where remembered dreams live to pull us from our misguided paths. Here is where all the creative arts emerge: painting, sculpting, singing, dancing, acting, composing, writing. Here is where inventions spring forth and spurts of intuitive insight erupt. Here is where a culture's unconscious is brought forth in the form of myth, fairy tales and stories of gods and goddesses. Here is also where our histories live, where childhood emotional patterns and early relationships with primary care givers hang

out and influence our present lives, distorting the moment by recreating the past in an imaginative "pretend" drama of which we are unaware.

In this transitional space exists all that impedes us from our growth and wholeness, but also all that can serve to heal the wounds, bring us to balance, transform inner relationships and direct us on our unique life journeys. (p. 3)

Lewis integrates a variety of modalities in her therapy and often refers to her work as Interpersonal Improvisational Dance-Drama and Intermodal therapy. A more extensive examination of the integration of the arts in therapy will be discussed in the following chapter.

Early Childhood Trauma

Lewis's work has also centered on early childhood trauma and its influences on the development of the brain. She writes:

The brain can be seen as developing hierarchically (LeDoux, 1996). The sensorimotor level of experience is seen as the most basic followed by the emotional level and finally the cognitive level. Individuals who experience physical trauma such as sexual abuse, battering and other energetically and physically invasive violation early on in life receive this information and store it on a sensorimotor level. (personal communication, 2002)

The sensorimotor level includes the parts of the nervous system that control unconscious bodily functions, the emotional center of the brain as well as elements of the body's peripheral nervous system.
Lewis continues:

D.W. Winnicott has said that often "early memories are pre-verbal, nonverbal and unverbalizable" (Lewis 1994). Those who suffer early childhood abuse are riddled with the repetition of isolated, fragmented and incomplete sensorimotor somatic responses which can be triggered by outside stimuli such as sounds, smells, bodily sensations, touch and images and inside stimuli such as thoughts, feelings and internal sensations. Individuals who experience sensorimotor flashbacks often feel that they have no cortical control over the occurrences or their sympathetic autonomic nervous system responses to them. And they don't. Frequently, these responses are just as fragmented as the stimuli that produce them. More often than not, there is an inability of higher cortical levels to modulate and modify these more primitive stimuli-response reactions. Thus, purely cognitive cortical interventions may not be able to touch these lower circular sensorimotor level responses.

Dance movement therapy approaches that tap into sensorimotor processing and experience are effective in altering and regulating the responses of individuals who have suffered physical trauma. Movement therapists have been able, through an awareness of the significance of sensorimotor somatic held memory, traumatic flashbacks and primitive responses to danger, to facilitate the client's ability to have choice regarding their responses thereby helping them to alter their previous sensorimotor responses (Lewis, 2000). This is carried out by slowing unraveling triggers and by separating the triggers from the sensations, from the feelings, from the images and from the self-damaging thoughts. (Lewis, 1994; 2000; personal communication, 2002)

In handling early childhood trauma, Lewis notes the power of touching and holding. She draws from the writings of Pert (1997): "From my research with endorphins, I know the power of touch to stimulate and regulate our natural chemicals, the ones that are tailored to act at precisely the right times in exactly the appropriate doses to maximize our feelings of well-being" (p. 272).
Further, Lewis states:

Body movement is the most primary means of communication with the infant. The mother, through the observation of the baby's movement, begins to attune to the needs and wants of her child. If the attunement is successful, the infant will experience the world as safe and need-satisfying rather than depriving and abusive. The movement ministrations of the primary caregiver are crucial to the development of the child. Deprived baby's brains are 20-30 % smaller. (personal communication, 2002)

These more recent thoughts from Lewis concerning the emotional part of the brain and the interaction of infant and mother further expand her thinking about the choreography of object relations and somatic countertransference.[4]

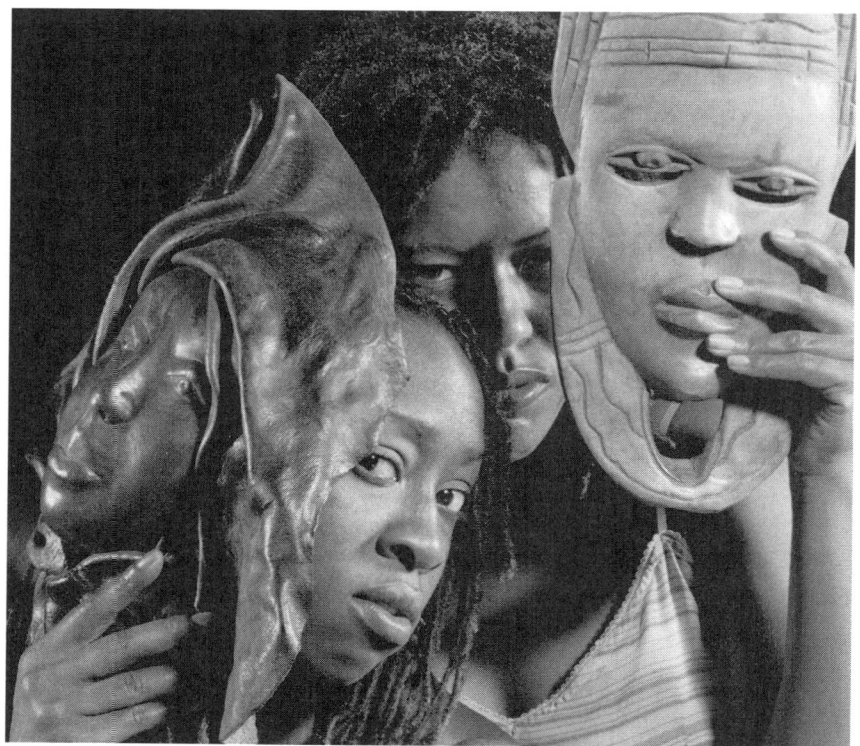

Dancers Tamara Thomas & Nadirah Rahman collaborate in the creative arts (Photo courtesy Steve Clarke)

---

[4]To further understand Lewis's thoughts on child development and dance therapy, one should consult the following references: Mahler, M. (1968) *On human symbiosis and the vicissitudes of individuation*. New York: International Universities Press; Kohut, H. (1971). *The Analysis of the Self*. New York: International Universities Press; Winnicott, D.W. *Playing and reality* (Out of Print); St. Clair, M. (2000) *Object relations and self-psychology*. (3rd Ed.). Stanford, CT: Brooks/Cole Publications.

 Fran Levy's Multimodal Approach: Theory and Practice

In the process of revising this chapter, I inserted new, more personal material and so I have rewritten it in first person. This, I feel, allows for a more intimate portrayal of my experience and that of the people with whom I work.

The chapter is divided into three parts. The first part recalls a profound personal experience in dance class that influenced the rest of my life and directed me toward a career in dance therapy.

The second part describes the integration and theoretical basis for interweaving psychodrama, art, dance, music and writing into clinical practice and particularly into dance therapy. This work is with adults, individually and in groups. The section includes case examples that are particularly illustrative of the multimodal approach and show the need to integrate various forms of creative expression when working with certain types of problems and individual expressive preferences.

Dance Classes with Melissa Laughman: Integrating East and West Coast Dance Therapy Trends

When I was at Goddard College in Vermont in the sixties, I had the good fortune to study dance with an extraordinary teacher, Melissa Laughman. Goddard was known for its creative, experiential program that honored nonverbal experience and the arts. Through my studies with Laughman, an empathic and courageous dance teacher, I discovered what was, for me, the true meaning of dance.

At the age of 18, I was a shy college student, away from home for the first extended period of time and anxious. Movement had always been my salvation and many creative dance classes had helped me through my childhood struggles with dyslexia and the resulting depression and anxiety. At 18, I was no longer a child and there were academic expectations placed on me that I was afraid I couldn't handle. Goddard was a progressive school and much of the pressure I felt was self-inflicted, but it paralyzed me with fear. I was majoring in psychology with a minor in dance and art. My stress was apparent and expressed itself in my dance classes. I performed dance technique but without feeling.

Melissa (that's what we called her) had a different way of teaching dance and her approach had a significant impact on me. She began class by instructing us to lie on the floor and not to move until we felt a feeling so deep inside that it forced us from our spots on the floor and not a moment sooner. She played all kinds of music while we lay on the floor: *Bolero, Appalachian Spring*, Pachelbel's *Canon* and more. Melissa gave us images to help us relax; we breathed deeply and imagined a large mound of sand being gently washed away by the ebb and flow of waves until the mound of sand was flattened.

Like a teacher of meditation, she helped us give up our daily worries, transporting us into our feeling-moving selves. This process of waiting to be moved as opposed to consciously pushing ourselves to move was, I later discovered, the Wigmanian approach to dance and subsequently, the Whitehousian approach to dance therapy.

At first, it was hard for me to completely let go and move from my core. I was afraid I'd never move and tended to prematurely push myself. I struggled painfully to let go of my dance technique. Melissa saw my struggle; she danced close to me and caught my eyes with hers. She looked at me with a warm smile and said, "Get dirty, Fran, get dirty." I will never forget those words. She yelled them at me over 30 years ago and I hear them as if it were yesterday. Aside from the melting mounds of sand, I remember little else that

Melissa actually said. It wasn't her words that pulled our inner dance out; it was her movements and complete comfort with her body as an expressive, communicative tool. She was fully present and available whenever she danced.

Melissa danced next to me and shared with me her incredible energy and I "got dirty." I began to dance like never before, kicking my feet, swirling around, gyrating, screaming, jumping, stretching and collapsing. Before I knew what was happening, I was telling the story of my life and my feelings in dance. When the session ended I felt as though I had found a part of myself that had long been repressed, my spirit.

To end the groups, after our emotions were released through dance, Melissa took the time to close the session with a circle ritual in which she danced around the room reaching out with her arms, hands and eyes to everyone until we were all together, back from our unique, separate experiences. We often moved in

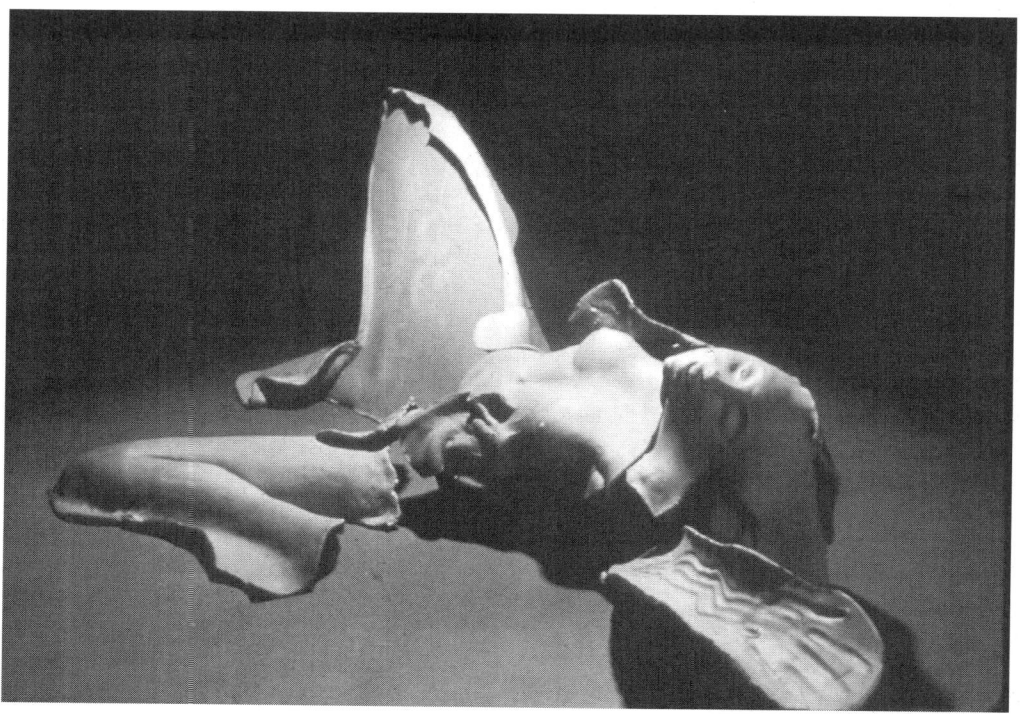

Persephone sculpture by Mary Frank, 1985, private collection (Photo courtesy D. C. Moore Gallery, NYC)

unison at this time and were reassured by the group rhythmic experience. It brought us back from deep individual places that were often filled with intense thoughts and feelings. We needed the closing ritual to put us back together. This was also a method used by Chace, Evan and others.

Melissa reached out to all of us in what came to be called, in dance therapy terms, the therapeutic movement relationship, a Chacian approach. In retrospect, I see that Melissa, who knew nothing about the formal world of dance movement therapy, was brilliantly (albeit, unwittingly) integrating east and west coast trends. I studied with Melissa between 1964 and 1966. The American Dance Therapy Association was formed in 1966 and communication between east and west coast dance therapists was just beginning at this time. My formal work as a dance therapist began in 1970.

Melissa said she wasn't familiar with dance therapy. She saw herself only as a dance teacher. The Goddard dance students referred to her in their own ways, psychic, wizard, psychotherapist, good witch, dance therapist, shaman, etc., but she would have none of it. She told us over and over that she was just teaching dance. We knew differently.

Melissa kept a low profile about her work and rejected giving it esoteric labels. There were no dance performances and she used no fancy language to describe what she did. She didn't try to couch her work in elaborate theories. She knew one thing and believed in it with a passion. She believed that everyone was a dancer and could dance from the heart if given the chance. She created a life and work that remained true to her passion.

Melissa's impact, especially on my desire to become a dance therapist, was undeniable. I wanted to do for others what she had done for me, but I knew I had to find my own style and it would be very different from Melissa's. What she did was unique to her and an expression of a gift she had that came from, if you will, her soul. I had yet to find my gift, the part of me I'd use to best connect with and reach out to others.

My own background eventually had a great impact on my career choices. My mother was an artist and dancer. Through her, I learned to express myself through the arts. In addition, both of my parents loved to write. Luckily, their approach to the arts was a creative, expressive one in which the process was more important than the goal. Because of the frustrations I experienced with learning, I thrived on the freedom they had given me and on creative expression. Art, dance and writing were all modalities that I had a passion for and eventually I felt comfortable enough with myself to use them.

In Social Work school at Hunter College in the seventies, they taught us over and over again to use ourselves in the treatment. What a strange and simple statement! It was so simple that it took years to fully appreciate its meaning. It's the kind of statement that gets clearer as you mature. Now I believe that the process of discovering oneself and using oneself in the treatment goes on forever and so, as professionals, we are always using ourselves in newer and broader ways.

Similarly, as our expressive potentials are realized and strengthened, our styles of therapeutic interaction also expand. The more ways that we can interact with our patients and the more open we are to ourselves the richer and fuller the therapy will be. Each of us has unique expressive gifts that need to be discovered in order to give the most to others and after learning the essentials from our teachers we must all go on to discover our own expressive and interactive preferences. It is widely accepted today and openly discussed among psychotherapists that the patient's continued growth is deeply and often unwittingly, intertwined with that of the therapist.

I began integrating dance therapy with psychodrama and art into a creative approach to psychotherapy in the early seventies. I combined my training with Blanche Evan, who used dramatic enactment and creative imagery, with my training in psychodrama with Robert Siroka and in art therapy with Jean Peterson. Also, the pioneering research in animal and figure drawing analysis of my mentor, psychologist Sidney Levy (1950, 1958), had a major influence on my work (F. Levy, 1995). Originally, I called the work psychodramatic movement therapy (F. Levy, 1979; 1988), but as I found myself using more and more of the visual arts and other art forms, I felt the name needed to be broader and so I chose multimodal psychotherapy and multimodal dance therapy. Other titles that therapists use to describe the integration of the arts in therapy are expressive arts, intermodal and creative arts therapies.

The cases that follow illustrate the integrative art therapy approach.

Theory and Practice of Multimodal Work

What follows is a discussion of the combined use of the arts in dance therapy. The incorporation of drama can be traced back to several of the early pioneers. The introduction of dramatic enactment by Franziska Boas and Blanche Evan, dance-drama by Elizabeth Rosen, characterizations by Trudi Schoop and role-playing by Marian Chace and Shirley Genther demonstrate the early integration of dance and drama noted in Unit I.

At the heart of this approach is the concept of reaching people through the medium that they find most expressive. Some individuals are verbal and feel most comfortable with verbalizing their thoughts and feelings. Others find verbalization alone inadequate for expression. It is not uncommon to hear people say that they feel they are hiding behind their words. When they speak they feel as though they are not really telling the truth or conveying a genuine feeling. This leaves them feeling empty and alone. They have a deep yearning to be seen and heard but feel that their words have failed them. These individuals often come to me with a request for some form of physical and/or visual art experience. Some people are more in need of action as in drama and dance, while others may need the tactile or visual, as in the visual arts.

Individuals can have different needs at different times and may require unique combinations of creative experience in order to access their thoughts and feelings. For example, a tactile individual might respond best by first creating sculptural forms and then becoming aspects of the sculpture through dance, maybe creating a dance story about their creation and from the story developing a dramatic movement dialogue. A more physical person might benefit most from starting immediately with the freedom of improvisational dance and then decide to delineate aspects of the dance into movement conversations in which the individual acts out various roles discovered during the dance. This experience might best be concluded with drawing, writing or talking, depending on individual needs. Each person paves his or her own course of creative expression.

Incorporating Psychodrama and Other Dramatic Techniques into Dance Therapy

Typically, when used in psychotherapy, a dance or visual art experience will provoke emotions and loosen the tied-up energy connected to conflict. This leads individuals to bring forth associations and images that can be put into dance/dramas. A dance/drama can be stimulated in a variety of ways. For example, an improvisation stimulated by a color choice, let's say the color red, could help one get in touch with feelings of anger. This could lead to images of specific people in life toward whom the individual has unresolved emotions. In this way, the patient moves from the visual (color) to content (images of specific people). The conflict then can be explored more deeply through psychodramatic movement. This would involve the playing out of the individual's feelings verbally and nonverbally. Some individuals might rely on pure dance to express themselves, while others might prefer to combine expressive movement with verbalization.

Drama is a medium ideally suited for dealing with unresolved emotions and inner conflict. Inherent in dramatization is a division of roles and an interaction among them. Drama is also helpful to individuals who are both verbally and physically oriented in that it actively combines both forms of expression. Drama organizes an individual by giving shape to the many sides of one's experience and in this way bringing out conscious and unconscious conflict. Our emotions are often projected onto a cast of internalized characters. Some of these are "significant others" (J.L. Moreno and Z.T. Moreno, 1975a), that is, influential people in the person's life. Their influence can be highly emotional as in the case of an abusive parent or spouse. Other internal characters can be different parts of the individual, representing various selves that have not been given adequate attention and expression (Levy, 1995). These characters assert themselves in all of us from time to time, often making us feel "tied up in knots" or "torn apart." The diverse needs and demands of these internal selves reflect emotions that need to be explored. It is the conflict among one's internal cast of characters that often brings an individual into treatment (Levy, 1979; 1995).

Role-playing provides a vehicle through which individuals can access their inner dramas. Dramatic action or dialogue connects individuals to inner conflicts that they may have not been aware of and in this way releases and transforms the energy tied up in these conflicts and allows them to be expressed through controlled and structured action. The stories of patients that follow will illuminate this process and how it works in combination with dance, visual art and writing. Also the case of "Nameless: A Case of Multiplicity," which was published in *Dance and Other Expressive Art Therapies: When Words are Not Enough* (Levy, et al., 1995) is an in-depth, long-term study that depicts many aspects of this work. A brief look at this work can be seen in Chapter 20.

Methodology and Case Material

This work paves the way for 1) the recognition of thoughts and feelings, 2) self-expression, 3) catharsis and 4) insight. The following illustrates how a multimodal approach to dance therapy might develop.

After a thorough movement warm-up, the therapist might encourage the exploration of contrasting movements that express opposing feelings, such as push/pull, heavy/light, gather/scatter or hard/soft. The therapist would then help individuals to explore further the set of opposing movements that seemed most compelling or meaningful. This could be done by trying several combinations and then broadening and embellishing the movements to which the person responded most intensely.

Drama is the product of role-playing, what Moreno (J.L. Moreno and Z.T. Moreno, 1975a), the founder of psychodrama, described as "the personification of other forms of existence through the medium of play" (pp. 140-141). During this phase, the therapist encourages spontaneous role change between the two contrasting themes. For example, in dance movement one might first become the role of "the push" and then that of "the pull," continuing back and forth in a spontaneous role-reversal. In group work, role-playing usually involves two or more people in dramatic dialogue, moving back and forth between roles. However, this can also be done in individual work where the person plays all roles themselves.

At times, the therapist can help by taking on roles and interacting with the individual. But, when the therapist takes on roles of significant others, it must be done with great caution. It can stir up feelings that are traumatic and retraumatize an individual. When such feelings, like rage and helplessness, are projected onto the therapist, the patient can lose touch with reality. He or she might suddenly see the therapist as "the enemy" and feel that there is no one in the room who can be the protector. This is a dangerous situation for the patient and therapist. The following examples illustrate how provocative something as simple as contrasting movements can be and why all of these methods must be used carefully.

Through role-playing, one is permitted to express emotions in new ways and through this to clarify the emotions attached to inner conflict. While one explores feelings through dramatic dance movement dialogue, free association and spontaneity are encouraged. To facilitate this, the therapist asks questions such as, "How does this movement feel?" or, "Do you want to add sounds or words to your movements?" Individuals are asked if they have any associations to the movements (thoughts, feelings or images)? If so, can the associations be described in terms of their color, movement, shape, rhythm, etc., and can they be danced out? Such questions and suggestions help focus and organize the underlying material. This, in turn, promotes clarification, catharsis and insight.

Another approach could be to ask if "the pull" has something to say to "the push" or, "Would you like to assign names to 'the push' and 'the pull'?" One might be asked to create a dramatic story using these contrasting roles.

During this process, individuals frequently become aware that the movements chosen represent significant people in their lives or conflicting parts of themselves. For example, in one of my groups, when I used the theme of contrasting movements, a young woman, Diedra, became aware that "the push" was her father who was ill all of her life and always pushed her away, while "the pull" was her mother who she felt pulled on her to meet her own needs but was never genuinely interested in Diedra. The drama that followed exposed and confronted her feelings of never being truly seen or appreciated by either parent or the deep sense of emptiness that this created in her as a child and as an adult.

Another individual, Sara, became aware that "the gather" movement represented the mother she wished for but never had and the "scatter" movement depicted how she actually experienced her mother. Sara's experience brought to light just how angry and frustrating it was to grow up in her mother's chaotic house and how much she longed for order and tranquility. This insight helped her to understand why she was so intolerant of her sister and others, who she thought lived haphazard lifestyles. It also helped her to straighten her own home so that she would stop living, she said, "in my mother's house."

Finally, Jennifer, a young mother, became aware that her decision to explore the push and pull sequence stemmed from her ambivalent drives toward her husband and children. She had always tried to be the perfect wife and mother but lately she was feeling extremely anxious. Through her movement, she discovered that she had mixed feelings about her roles. She wanted to have her family close to her while also wanting to push them away. She desperately needed space for herself, but took her roles very seriously and didn't allow herself to have down time. Acknowledging that she had mixed feelings about the demands of her life and being reassured that her feelings were natural and not something to feel guilty about helped her to become more realistic in her expectations of herself. This unburdened her.

From individuals' responses the therapist can assess on what level they are able to focus their thoughts and feelings. Can they focus on early memories, for example, mother, father, siblings, etc., or do they need a more emotionally removed association like a teacher, client, boss or friend? Some individuals may need to express thoughts and feelings entirely symbolically, as in the use of a metaphor. Others may rely on a purely dance form without associations or images. Self-expression can take place on many different levels and through countless forms.

The structure of drama complements the freedom of dance. Dance frees thoughts and feelings in pure unburdened form. Drama then organizes this into polarized action. This organization helps to clarify areas of conflict. Individuals are helped to make the transition from form (dance) to content (drama). The therapist helps to set up scenes for dance improvisation within a dramatic format. It is the therapist's ability to empathize with the patient that paves the way for choosing levels of intervention. Empathy, the ability to get inside another person and see, think and feel as that person does, without judgment, is the most important ability the therapist needs. The following cases illustrate a variety of methods determined by patients' needs and expressive preferences.

The Case of Elly

The following case of Elly, a financial analyst in her late forties, further illustrates the clinical application of dance and drama in a multimodal dance therapy group. Elly was one of eight women in a group that had been working together once a week for approximately 18 months. She was a fragile woman with suicidal tendencies.

Elly began one session with the statement, "I'm crazy today, I've been crazy all day." When asked what "crazy" meant, she replied, "Well, I just feel torn apart." I then asked her to describe this feeling of being torn apart more specifically, for example, identifying how many parts of herself there were and whether they had any particular shape, form, color or texture or did the parts have names or voices. She replied, "I feel torn into four parts," but could not describe them verbally.

I then suggested that Elly become these four parts in movement, giving each part its own place in the room. As Elly moved to the first place, her posture changed and she began to gesture angrily, as if scolding someone. This time, when asked whether this part had a name, she replied, "My mother." After exploring this figure in movement with some verbalization, she moved to a second place in the room. Again, her posture changed and she took on a sexually provocative and aggressive attitude. This time, without prompting from the therapist, she identified this part as representing her stepfather. Elly took a little longer to decide on her third place in the room. She looked scared. It also took her longer to start moving. When she did, a very tough, teasing and ridiculing person appeared. After doing the movements, she realized she was portraying her sister. As she moved into the fourth part, her posture immediately collapsed and she looked suddenly beaten down, acknowledging this to be herself. It was as if her body had given up, succumbed to her family's anger and provocation.

Upon seeing her withdraw, I encouraged her to allow a movement dialogue to develop role reversing, as she desired between herself and each member of her family. Through enacting the role-reversed positions of mother, father and sister, she was able to manifest a great deal of her own anger. (Frequently, a client is more able to express certain emotions through role-playing significant others than in his or her own role.) The emphasis was on Elly expressing the movements as well as the language of family members. In this way, Elly was helped to externalize her own aggressive feelings and gradually to organize these feelings verbally and nonverbally.

As Elly's drama continued to unfold, various group members spontaneously took on the role-reversed positions of mother, stepfather and sister, according to what Jacob Moreno called "sociometric choice." Sociometry, applied to group therapy and psychodrama, refers to the measure of relationships and networks within the group, as well as to each individual's own network of significant others or relationships outside of the group (Siroka, personal communication, 1980). The group members who chose to participate in Elly's drama were drawn in on an emotional level to play the role(s) they identified with. For example, one man, who had a ridiculing father, took on the stepfather role. This helped group members to release some of their own feelings, while also providing a dialogue for the protagonist. In this way, members of the psychodramatic audience (i.e., the group) become spontaneously involved in the drama. The role-playing acts as a springboard not only for the protagonist's (Elly's) feelings but also for the feelings of other group members.

This session provided a major breakthrough in Elly's therapy. Through the release of her own aggressive feelings in the role-reversed positions (i.e., mother, stepfather and sister), in combination with the group's participation in all four parts, Elly's strength and confidence were boosted and she was soon able to respond assertively, using gesture and words, to each family member. She shook her fists, told them off, declared her independence, stamped on the floor in defiance and released a great deal of pent up emotion.

The problem had been that Elly was out of touch with how upset she was with her family. She knew intellectually, but could not feel it. It was locked up inside. Only after she externalized her internal cast of characters could she really unravel the knot that she experienced in the pit of her stomach.

The language an individual uses often helps to structure a movement experience. In this case, Elly said she felt torn apart. The arts lend themselves well to the exploration of different parts of a person, unresolved parts, conflicting parts, sick parts, etc. (F. Levy, 1995). Elly gave the therapist a huge verbal clue as to how to approach her chaotic, upset feelings. Using Elly's own words to structure her experience paved the way for her to gain insight into the content that underlay her confused feelings. What had once been experienced as chaotic and amorphous and therefore menacing, was now organized dramatically into posture, gesture, rhythmic movement and words. Combining these elements led to the psychodramatic appearance of Elly's family. The accompanying movements were so rich and expressive that Elly could no longer hide behind her usual intellectualizations. The psychodramatic structure supported her emotional expression and revealed the complexity and turmoil of her internal life. This experience marked the beginning of freedom for Elly. As a result, her suicidal thoughts decreased significantly and Elly was eventually able to create better boundaries for herself with her family.

Incorporating the Visual Arts with Dance/Drama and Psychodrama

A multimodal approach begins where the client works with unresolved emotions at the level most comfortable and accessible for the client. Individuals vary in the level at which they are ready to cope with emotions and in the medium through which they can best express their emotions. A multimodal approach can incorporate several different expressive media that, when used creatively and empathically, enable the therapist to help individuals approach the unapproachable. These expressive media include dance, drama, music, verbalization, writing and the visual arts. In this section, stress will be placed on the various ways in which the visual arts complement the other art forms.[1]

The visual arts (drawing, painting, sculpting, etc.) are a natural medium for the expression of inner conflict. The visual arts require that individuals make choices. These choices are often symbolic projections of unresolved emotions. Even if asked to draw something specific, one still must choose colors, shapes, textures, etc. Even the rhythmic action of the individual's hand on the drawing board is a choice, for example, soft curved lines, dark heavy lines, dots, etc. Each choice an individual makes externalizes a unique aspect of the self.

Art can facilitate expression in a variety of ways. It is a projective technique that provokes psychological material and manifests it in a visual and concrete form. This enables one to step back from the finished product and reflect on it. While viewing one's own artwork, the individual is visually taking in that which was projected. In this way, one is given an opportunity to reclaim one's own projections and try to understand their meaning. If advisable, individuals can portray or embody their artwork through movement in the form of dance, play and/or dramatic action. In this way, they are supported to experience projected aspects of themselves on physical, as well as visual, levels. As individuals find creative ways to embellish and reclaim their projections they are supported to probe deeper into their internal experience. The creative modalities should be used with the intent of helping individuals to organize and express aspects of the self previously out of reach. Like all of these techniques, this must be done carefully and only with an in-depth knowledge of the personality of the patient and the ability to analyze the patient's art work. The case of David that follows illustrates the importance of knowing your patient's psychodynamics and knowing when to limit the use of movement with art.

The Case of David

David, a bright young professional, was one of my earliest patients and I learned a great deal from my work with him. A psychiatrist referred him for individual therapy sessions. The psychiatrist said that David was extremely intelligent, creative and would benefit from interventions that involved the arts. When David arrived he said he was upset with the traditional verbal therapy he had been undergoing. David felt that he

---

[1] Fran Levy is a protégé of Sidney Levy, Ph.D. (not a relative), the founder of the Levy Animal Drawing Story Test (LADS), a projective technique used widely in diagnosis and treatment. In addition, Fran Levy's training with Jean Peterson, a registered art therapist, clinical social worker and psychodramatist, was most helpful to her in the development of her use of art therapeutically. She was also influenced by the literary contributions of leading art therapists including Art Robbins (1980) and Edith Kramer (1971). The creative work of Robert W. Siroka and Ellen Siroka have also been extremely influential in the development of these creative techniques.

was lying to his therapist, not on purpose, but because his words could not express his real feelings. When he was with his therapist, he felt invisible. He said, "He doesn't really see me. He listens to my words as if they were important but I deceive him. Not on purpose, I just can't find the right words to really say what I feel. It's all just words. I don't really feel anything."

After several weeks in treatment, I asked David to draw an animal. The animal that he drew looked like a person more than an animal. It had long sharp fangs for teeth and there was no delineation between head and body in that the neck was very wide and received the same heavy stroking as did the rest of the body. It looked like a monster that held a large sharp knife. With its dark, excessive lines, the drawing encompassed the entire sheet of paper. All of these graphic indicators pointed in the direction of a serious problem with impulse control. In the drawing, mind and body (thoughts and feelings) were interwoven with no ability to censor emotions and control behavior. David's small build, 5' 2", and seemingly calm and soft-spoken manner masked the rage that smoldered inside. He was ready to burst. David came to me because he knew something was very wrong, but all he was in touch with was his emotional isolation, not his rage. This made it all the more dangerous. He hoped that creative/expressive work would break through his defenses. Initially, though not in touch with his anger, he pushed me to structure movement exercises for him to release his aggression. After seeing David's drawing, I felt that this was not safe; he was a walking time bomb.

It was clear that something was provoking David's rage and feelings of helplessness, but I wasn't sure what. What was clear was that David should not try to embody (physically portray) his drawing and that emotional expression would have to start in small doses and be projected onto safe objects that were not overly charged with emotion. A lot of probing had to be done, but gently, to find out what was really making David tick.

In one session, after four months of having David draw and talk about his feelings, he seemed unusually agitated and then, matter-of-factly, reported a memory of being raped by his uncle when he was nine and being sexually humiliated by his father. In subsequent sessions, along with these memories came David's rage. He wanted to kill.

Now that David was in touch with his rage, there was real concern about how he would handle it. The issue was how to continue helping him to express his feelings without destroying his very delicate hold on reality. Together David and I worked out creative avenues of expression that I hoped would be safe for him. This included an emphasis on drawing and role-playing.

It was openly discussed with David that he could and should talk about his uncle but not dance out his feelings. David's drawing of the monster made it very clear that the freedom and unstructured quality of dance tore him open. Since a part of David wanted this to happen (i.e., to kill his tormentors), I had to be extra vigilant during sessions. Before starting expressive work, time out signals that meant to stop all action were designed so that he would not spin out of control. Also, emphasis was put on David's expressive use of drawing. He liked to draw and was good at it. The boundaries of the page, his representational expression and tenacious attention to detail all helped him to bind, while simultaneously expressing, his feelings. Working with David was at times like walking an invisible tightrope. I will always remember the lessons David taught me as a young therapist, to go slowly and stay deeply attuned.

The cases that follow will shed more light on the issues of control and expression and the use of the arts. These cases also illustrate how one art form can help to harness and modify, as well as deepen, broaden and clarify another.

The arts, in general, allow individuals to express themselves in many ways, including: abstraction, symbolism, realism and fantasy. They also pave the way for a variety of experiences: physical, verbal, visual, tactile and auditory. Everyone has his or her own way of experiencing the world and organizing this experience. A multimodal approach allows for, accepts and encourages the uniqueness of the individual.

The Case of Chris

Chris, a small blonde sexually repressed woman in her late thirties, walked into the office slowly, almost ghostlike, with no sense of body weight and a blank expression on her face. She began to speak in an almost inaudible voice. Chris had come for individual therapy, seeking a therapist to work with her through art and dance, her favorite activities along with writing. I saw Chris for approximately three years. She had previously been hospitalized for a psychotic episode in which she had taken off her clothes in a subway car in a sexual frenzy. She had since then disguised her sexual feelings and the guilt these feelings provoked and projected them onto the image of a cloud, which she visualized sitting on her head. She described the cloud as heavy, stiff and constricting, with many layers. Arieti described this type of perception, known as "misplaced concreteness," in his classic book, *Interpretation of Schizophrenia*. His theory describes the manner in which patients with schizophrenia defend against feelings (Arieti, 1974).

Chris was the first patient I worked with who had these symptoms. Looking back, I see that my initial attempt to help Chris displayed my naiveté. Not completely understanding the concept of misplaced concreteness, a form of somatic delusion, I suggested that Chris role-play by attempting to step away from the cloud and try to create a dialogue with the cloud. Chris was able to project the image of herself with the cloud on her head across the room. She became angry and physically tried to remove the cloud using pantomime movements.

While this simple attempt at role-playing did help to free up some of her aggression, she could not remove the cloud. The cloud was symbolic and as I gained a deeper understanding of the meaning the cloud played for her (i.e., the containment and representation of her sexuality) I was better able to make suggestions that would bring her closer to her real sexual feelings. Until she got in touch with those feelings the cloud would remain.

In the 5th session, with a greater understanding of Chris's dynamics, I asked her if she could choose one part of the cloud and interpret its meaning in movement. In response, she moved her arms gently and sensually, resembling a Hawaiian dancer. The rest of her body was essentially still except for a very slight, almost disguised, hip motion. When she finished I asked her how the cloud felt, she replied, "It feels lighter and more flexible." Now that Chris was being given permission to uncover the meaning of the cloud through creative movement, she was helped to tap into her repressed sexuality without having to label it as such. This safe and very modest display of sexual feelings marked the beginning of her freedom from overwhelming constriction and physical bondage.

In a subsequent session, I suggested that Chris draw her feelings. Knowing that Chris enjoyed drawing, I felt that she might benefit from interpreting her drawings through dance. Chris proceeded to draw pictures of flowers that clearly held secret sexual symbolism. She then explored the movements and feelings that the drawings elicited and this allowed for an increasingly rich release of her sexuality.

After several minutes of sensuous movements, Chris had a sudden feeling that her mother was in the room with us, watching her and shaming her. Chris became angry. I asked her if she wanted to express her feelings to her mother through role-playing. She said yes. Keeping in mind that Chris had had several psychotic episodes, I made sure that she understood that her mother was not actually present. She said she did. We agreed that if at any time Chris started to feel that her mother was actually in the room, she would tell me. She agreed. While setting these boundaries is not a guarantee that the patient will stay in touch with reality, it is still important to build in as much safety as possible.

I also made sure that Chris did not cast me in the role of her mother. In the event that she had trouble differentiating between us, no one in the room would be safe. Through role-playing, Chris entered into a symbolic dialogue with her mother. In that dialogue, in the role-reversed position, Chris ridiculed her own sexuality. Her "mother" called her a tramp. When Chris reversed back to herself, she expressed anger at her mother by yelling and showing off her newfound sexuality through dance. Chris had now challenged her mother's right to control her.

In the third month of treatment, she had a particularly intense session where her sexual expression through dance provoked an acute awareness of her Oedipal feelings. The veil of symbolism she had projected onto the flowers had broken and a flood of sexual anxiety and feelings of shame had surfaced. Chris called me late in the night and came to the office in a panic. Her body shook and she cried as she verbalized the feelings of wanting to have sex with her father and wanting to hurt her mother. I comforted her by helping her to understand that her feelings were not unnatural and that little girls had such feelings. I explained to her that feelings are not the same as actions. We can't control our feelings. The only things we can control are actions and she had not hurt anyone or done anything wrong.

Talking helped Chris to relax and lifted her harrowing sense of guilt and disgust with herself. She was able to continue with the work but what was left in my mind was the incredible power of the arts, particularly movement, to release repressed feelings and how important it is to cautiously navigate the depths of a patient's thoughts and feelings. While Chris's feelings still left her uneasy, the panic and paralyzing shame were gone. She now had creative avenues of expression for her sexuality and a verbal understanding of her fears and feelings of shame.

Chris was much more relaxed in subsequent sessions and eventually was able to bring in artwork that was overtly sexual and to talk about it. She also began to write stories and illustrate them with watercolors and pastels. She would then playfully act them out in sessions. Chris began feeling like a "whole person," happy and content with herself for the first time, she said, since she was a little girl.

This case is not meant to imply that the arts can cure schizophrenia, but that creative expression can provide essential relief from and insight into one's psychodynamics, in addition to and most importantly, a deep feeling of being accepted and understood.

The combination of movement and art was particularly powerful for Chris. She lived in a nonverbal, symbolic world with an intense fantasy life that she discussed with no one. The visual arts, like drama, can act as an intermediary step connecting the intellect (words) with the body (movement). The inherent limitations of artistic materials (paper, crayons, etc.) place a natural boundary around the psychomotor aspect of the experience, restricting the expression largely to finger, arm, shoulder and upper body movement in a defined space, the paper. These limitations can be helpful to individuals for whom complete body action may initially be too threatening. Limiting movement expression to upper body action allows individuals a measure of muscular release that is safe. The artwork safely frames the individual's experience (Robbins, 1980). This can later lead to more complete physical expression through dance movement or if contra-indicated, can simply enhance and deepen verbal expression.

The Case of Brenda

The case of Brenda, a 23-year-old research assistant, illustrates the use of art as an intermediary experience as a bridge between movement and words. Like David, Brenda came for dance movement therapy as a result of her frustration with traditional verbal therapy. She felt her intellect was a barrier against her feelings and she hoped that expressive movement and dance would free her. However, it soon became clear that for Brenda, movement was too exposing and terribly frightening. Brenda was hiding from something but she didn't know what it was. Each time she tried expressive movement she panicked, dropped her head and sat down as if trying to hide in the huge pillows on the floor of the studio. As a result of her rigid, repressive orthodox upbringing, Brenda had internalized taboos that prevented her from expressing herself. These taboos were largely in the area of physical movement. The inhibition of her feelings was apparent in her awkward speech and severe psychomotor restrictions. She appeared to be tied in knots. Initially even very modest movements, those that are often part of a general warm-up, would throw her into a panic.

The one thing that Brenda loved to do as a child was draw. Her parents had discouraged her from majoring in art in high school by telling her that she had little real talent. While this was an extremely painful memory for Brenda and one that needed to be addressed, it did not stop her from enjoying drawing in our sessions. When I suggested that she just let her arm relax and allow her hand to move freely on the page, not worrying about the results, but just enjoying the interaction of colors, shapes and textures, her previously withdrawn body became animated and expressive. Her movement repertoire expanded as she drew various rhythms, creating a textural mosaic of shapes and colors. Larger pieces of paper were introduced as she became ready to handle more space.

After releasing a wealth of feelings, Brenda said she thought she was ready to experiment with small movements. Brenda tried head rolls and leg and arm swings but still with embarrassment and trepidation. At times she asked me to not look at her while she moved. When I asked her what she was afraid of she said that I would see that she was ugly. Brenda was very upset as she spoke about her fears of being grotesque. I was still mystified by the cause of these paralyzing feelings.

Brenda was discouraged. Her parents had been harping on her to learn to dance, not because of their love of dance, but to get her to go to socials and meet men. But Brenda was so ashamed of her body that she couldn't get herself to move in ways that might appear sensual. Despite her anxiety and the negative feelings that dance was bringing up, she pushed me angrily to make her dance. Her drive to have me force her had a cruel quality, as though her feelings didn't matter. What mattered was that I whip her into shape, fix her. I soon realized that she was trying to get me to behave toward her as her parents had, with a punishing type of control and aggression.

The message from her parents was that she was not okay; she had to be more, be better and not be herself. I couldn't do this to Brenda. I felt that she was using me to act out aggressively against herself. Instead, I reassured her that she was doing just fine and I explained to her that I didn't want to take on the critical, controlling role of her parents. Brenda responded first with anger toward me, but as we talked more she began to cry. Brenda needed to know that she was all right just the way she was and that what she felt really mattered and that her feelings would be paramount in our sessions.

Interestingly, coming from an orthodox family, Brenda always felt that her parents put their beliefs before her in importance. This feeling was now being transferred to me. Because my role was that of dance therapist and in fact her parents were pushing her in this area, Brenda was sure that dancing in the sessions was more important than what she felt and what she wanted to do. This negative transference, the identification of me with her parents, had to be discussed and worked through. Also, the feelings that provoked this deep sense of shame still had to be uncovered.

We continued to draw in the sessions. By this time, Brenda and I had been working together for about four months. One day, at Brenda's suggestion, she and I painted a mural that included a group of kids playing baseball. We playfully pretended to throw the ball by painting a ball in motion and similarly, batted the ball and ran the bases. Since this had become a drawing in motion, I suggested that we act out the mural together, using the entire studio as our baseball field. Brenda was game. To warm up, we began to throw an imaginary ball back and forth and than began to bat the imaginary ball and run the bases. We tagged each other out and yelled a lot and all together had a great time.

I had never seen Brenda so animated and fun loving. Her previously very soft, child-like voice became deep almost husky and her passive, defensive demeanor became assertive and tenacious. She bullied me around and I fought back. "I tagged you." "No you didn't." "I'm home free." "No you're not," etc. When we finished, Brenda was still laughing. She said, "I haven't had this much fun since I was a child. I loved to play ball."

I asked Brenda to tell me more. She said, "I was a real tomboy but I hated to be called that. I was a good athlete and loved playing football with the boys in the park but when I reached puberty my parents stopped me from all of the physical activities that I loved. They made me stay indoors or go to my cousin Jewel's house, but she was into makeup, clothes and boys. And when her friends came over they made fun of me. I had to stop the roughhousing and be a lady they said. I felt like a misfit. I felt awkward and disgusting, grotesque. I was miserable. I think I've been depressed ever since."

After this breakthrough, Brenda recalled that at the same time that she was going through puberty, her family became more involved with their religion and, in her mind, turned their attention away from her. "That was how they controlled me. They shamed me by saying I was really a boy in a girl's body and they turned away from me." Brenda and I discussed the concepts of male and female. I told her that girls loved to roughhouse and play ball just as much as boys and it didn't mean that they were not really still girls and that it was terribly sad for a girl to have to give up all that fun to become some false image of being a lady. I also told Brenda that I loved playing ball with her and that we would do it again if she wanted. In the next session, she suggested we play imaginary basketball. We did and Brenda laughed as she moved around me quickly, stealing the ball from me and jumping in the air to make baskets.

What was clear was that Brenda as a child had felt a great sense of freedom, joy and mastery when it came to sports until, in adolescence, she was made to feel guilty and ashamed of what she came to call her masculine side. She remembered her parents forcing her to wear conservative dresses that covered her whole body and she began to feel grotesque. Eventually she shared with me her biggest secret, a secret she herself had not previously been aware of: she feared that under her long orthodox dresses and between her legs she was hiding a penis and that was why she had to wear clothes that covered her from head to toe. Part of her knew this was "silly" but yet the fear was real. Brenda was experiencing a painful confusion over her sexual identity.

Brenda's depression stemmed from many things. She felt like a misfit and as if she was unlovable. Her sexual confusion over male and female identifications, along with her parents' ridicule, was tearing her up inside, undermining her every move. In addition, the energy that had once been released through sports and competition now had no place to go and had in effect turned against her. Her "masculine, tomboy" energy, the part she secretly felt was really her, had become the enemy. What had brought incredible joy to her as a child now threatened to embarrass and humiliate her. Finally, the secret was out. She was deathly afraid that her masculine side would suddenly resurface, jump out when she moved. Now, in the sessions, she was reliving and reclaiming her playful, aggressive and physical self. Brenda laughed and cried and together we enjoyed Brenda's reunion with her "little tomgirl self."

In future sessions, Brenda frequently spoke of her parents' negative reactions to her during puberty. She also remembered both parents trying to inhibit her artwork, an activity that had also been very meaningful to her. Luckily, their ridicule in the artistic area, though destructive, did not leave her as severely impaired, as had their restrictions on her physical self. Before Brenda could move, she had to spend time liberating her ability to draw and her aggressive, sexual and tender feelings. Drawing brought forth memories and emotions that were later developed through dramatic play and dance movement. Through these games, Brenda was able to act out her competitive and aggressive feelings without shame and guilt.

In Brenda's case, destructive parental restrictions had left her impaired in many areas of expression, most profoundly in expressive movement. The artwork accompanied by dramatic movement served as a bridge between dance expression, which was too threatening and verbalization, which left her feeling frustrated. My work with Brenda spanned three and a half years and included first individual and then group dance therapy. She joined the group when she started to feel more comfortable with her body. She received a great deal of support and affection from group members and this was deeply healing. Of course, in the dance therapy groups she was most animated and happy when she got the group to "Play Ball."

For some individuals, body action may generally be safe and manageable, except for certain highly charged topics or memories. Movement can unexpectedly provoke memories that are too powerful for a person to handle. In such cases, the psychomotor limitations of the visual arts may serve as a safety valve, diminishing the intensity of highly charged thoughts and feelings. This enables a gradual release of emotions without overwhelming fragile defenses and paves the way for more intense expression and the eventual exploration of underlying material. This doesn't mean that artistic imagery is not equally provocative; it can be. Careful choices regarding all forms of expression must always be made.

The Case of Karen

Karen, a petite 33-year-old actress, was someone who normally had no trouble expressing her feelings through dance movement. She loved to dance and felt most alive during the improvisational part of the dance therapy group. However, in one session, something frightened Karen so much that she began to tremble out of control and abruptly stopped moving. A group member was expressing anger at her abusive father and this triggered a fury in Karen so penetrating that it shook her to the core. She began to breathe heavily and became paralyzed with fear, complaining that she felt nauseated.

I suggested that she sit down. The other group members stopped dancing and moved close to Karen and in various ways expressed their concern and desire to help. I knew that Karen had been abused and felt that her sudden paralysis was her way of keeping her rage and memories from exploding out of control. I approached her and asked her to sit down with me. I handed her a large piece of paper and a box of oil-based crayons and suggested that she choose colors to draw with that would best express her feelings. I was worried about Karen. I didn't want her to lose contact with her emotions, but I also didn't want her memories to tear her apart. Sitting, I thought, would anchor her and make it easier for Karen to express herself. I stayed close to her and watched her, ready to intervene if necessary.

I hoped that drawing would help to slow Karen's emotional expression down while also providing some structure and form to her feelings but I was aware that the opposite could also occur and the drawing could further exacerbate her distress. The only thing I knew for sure was that I had to stay close to Karen and that the group's empathy and support was of vital importance.

Karen took the paper and chose a deep red oil-based crayon. She drew but the rapid breathing that seemed to be triggered both by fear and anger continued. Several group members sat near Karen and put their arms around her. Karen's body was stiff at first but gradually she allowed her rage out in dark red, intense lines that filled the entire page. No other colors were chosen. During this process her face, which had been distorted by the flood of feeling, gradually changed to a look of determination. She was taking back control of herself and her feelings. The nausea lifted.

Karen was finally able to look up and acknowledge the other group members, but she was not yet able to comfortably verbalize what had happened. She knew she was experiencing panic and rage but could not talk about any thoughts or memories. It was still a huge blur of feeling with very little shape or content but

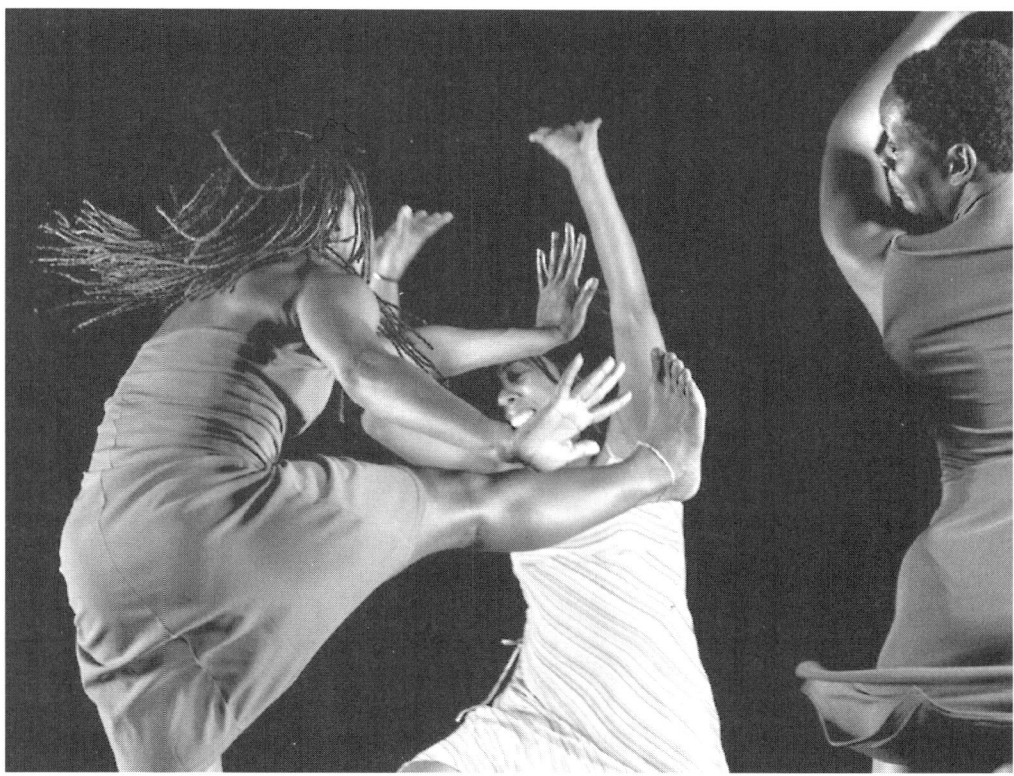

Models Tamara Thomas, Nadirah Rahman and Stephanie Hope dance with intense expression (Photo courtesy Steve Clarke)

she seemed stronger, more in control. I asked her if she could write the things that she could not say out loud, again hoping to give structure and clarity to her nonverbal experience.

Karen took a new sheet of paper and in large letters, also written in red, she wrote, "get off of me you bastard, get off ... I'll fucking kill you...." Karen was referring to her ex-husband who had humiliated her for years and physically abused her. She had discussed him in the group before but had never expressed her feelings about him through dance movement. Her father had also emotionally and physically abused her. In this session, the dam had broken and her feelings about both her father and ex-husband had flooded into consciousness.

Drum music was playing softly in the background while Karen was writing. Some group members had returned to their own dance improvisations and Karen, after about ten minutes of writing, decided to join them. She appeared more in control and more related to the other group members, more in the present; however, she still needed a lot of structure and support. Her rage could still mushroom out of control. She immediately began moving with great intensity fueled by feelings of fury and humiliation. I moved with her and reminded her often and vehemently to stay with the rhythm of the music, " Listen to the beat, keep the beat!" The rest of the group moved with Karen and all stayed intensely with the beat.

The rhythmic beat of the music was extremely important at this point. It signified being oriented in time, staying connected to the group and her surroundings and in this way it provided a frame in which she could safely express herself. The music, like the boundaries of the drawing page, served to organize, limit and clarify her expression, keeping her in the present while still uncovering unresolved issues from the past. Karen emerged from the dance experience feeling stronger, in touch with her past but no longer reliving it as though it was the present.

Now that Karen was back in the driver's seat, she was ready to handle some of the underlying issues. She spoke about her ex-husband at length, describing the way he incessantly put her down and undermined her. She spoke of his threats to physically abuse her and the time he did. She also spoke about her father and her memories of his abuse. After she spoke, she expressed a desire to dramatically act out some of her feelings toward her ex. Her emotions were still very intense. The group members cared about Karen and were familiar with her past, so with little direction from me they were able to spontaneously interact with her through dramatic dance movement and role-playing.

One group member began expressing Karen's ex-husband's abusive behavior by throwing insults and shouting at her. In so doing, the individual provided stimuli that Karen needed in order to interact with the ghosts of her past.

Karen was having trouble standing up to this abuse. One of the group members (Pia) most attuned to Karen moved closer and supported her emotionally by joining her in synchronous movement and together, in gesture and words, they fought back: "This is my house. Get away from me, you can't push me around," etc. In coming to her support, Pia became what is called the psychodramatic double or auxiliary ego. "The auxiliary ego becomes the link through which the patient may try to reach out into the real world" (Z. Moreno, 1966, p.8). The auxiliary ego uses dance therapy techniques of kinesthetic empathy to connect with the protagonist.

With Pia's support, Karen was able to continue her expressive movements with increased conviction, declaring her independence, indignation and wrath at how she had been treated. A division within the group followed this revelation. Those who identified with the aggressor stayed in the position of Karen's ex and those who identified with Karen joined her and Pia. Others moved back and forth between roles and in this way worked on their own issues while still reflecting Karen's drama.

The action in the group gradually wound down and came to a natural end. Group members sat in a circle and shared verbally their own experiences with Karen and their support of her. All of the members had found some part of themselves in Karen's experience and all seemed to feel empowered through their participation in her drama.

During this session, sociometric choices were spontaneously made. The initial decision by the group members was made when Karen naturally emerged as the protagonist. She was handling an overload of feelings with which the group readily identified. When the group split, another choice took place. Those who at that moment identified with the aggressor remained in the role of the ex, while those who empathized with the rage of the victim moved toward Karen. The sociometric networks within the group and each individual's own sociometry influenced these choices. These dynamics were also discussed in the final sharing part of the group session.

The group had been together for many years. The techniques of role-playing, role-reversal, doubling, sharing and sociometric choice had all become a natural part of their interaction. This helped the process to unfold with little direction from me.

In my use of the multimodal approach, the therapist rarely assumes sole "directorship," preferring to relinquish leadership as much as possible to the individual whose drama is being explored and to the group. In this respect, the work differs from traditional psychodrama. In psychodrama, the director usually decides on the basis of client cues when to reverse roles. In contrast, this approach encourages people to make their own decisions spontaneously. The goal is to help individuals trust their own psychomotor responses.

The psychodramatic director also traditionally plays a significant role in helping to set the scenes and guide the dramatic action with clarifying questions such as, "How old are you now?" "In which room are you sitting?" "What do you see in the room?" "Is anyone with you?" and so forth. In this way, the director focuses the protagonist, bringing memories and feelings from the past into the present.

These psychodramatic methods can be used in the multimodal approach but often they are used in an abbreviated manner. For example, when a scene is set it is usually to help individuals begin their movement exploration. Once the scene is set and the dramatic movement action has begun, participants are encouraged to direct their own experience through a form of free association via dance movement. Individuals often decide independently to reverse roles or may incorporate all roles through an integrated dance improvisation.

The goal is to pave the way for meaningful expression directed as much by the individual and group as by the therapist. This creates an empowering atmosphere in which individuals are trusted to design their own experience. These methods can be used individually and in groups. The degree to which a multimodal group can be self-directive is usually determined by the amount of time the group has worked together and the degree to which they are able to be empathic to each other.

The Case of Katharine

Some individuals who seek dance movement therapy have been dancers and have learned to use movement in a controlled way to defend against, rather than to express, their feelings. The case of Katharine, a tall, dark-haired physical therapist in her mid-forties, provides an example. Katharine first came to me as a dancer seeking training in dance therapy. She began her work with me by participating in a dance movement therapy group but was unhappy. She recognized that she was unable to be spontaneous and expressive. Katharine appeared to be depressed. I invited her to work with me privately.

Katharine had her body under excellent control through years of practicing yoga, dance and figure skating. She moved in an elegant fashion, always keeping her head extremely high and her shoulders straight. When I encouraged Katharine to use movement expressively she became frustrated and could not break away from rigid dance patterns.

Feeling that drawing might help to release Katharine's inhibitions, I asked her to draw an animal. Animal drawings provide a rich source of psychodynamic material. Katharine drew a turtle that she described as living in the sewer. Then, when asked to make up a story about the turtle, she explained that he accepted the filthy, smelly sewer as his home and never experienced daylight. The turtle, she said, "feels helpless and ashamed. He was born in the sewer and has remained there; though he doesn't like it, he doesn't fight to get out." Through her drawing and story, Katharine was expressing her real feelings about herself and her world.

I asked Katharine if she would like to do a dance improvisation about her drawing. She was reticent but wanted to try. She lowered her head and spine and walked around the room slowly with shoulders drooped for the first time and suddenly fell to the floor in a womb-like position. Eventually, she drew one arm forward, palm up and reached toward me in a gesture of asking for help. She began to cry, deep sobs heaved in her chest. She could no longer hide her loneliness, despair and frustration.

For Katharine, the drawing brought out the most vulnerable aspect of her personality. She had been hiding her despair from everyone, including herself. After exposing her feelings through her drawing and then verbalizing them indirectly through her story, she was finally able to let go and just give in to her depression. The weight of her shell, with its high personal price of loneliness and isolation, finally came crashing down. From the ground, in a pile of long overdue tears, she reached out and said, "I just want to be me. Is that okay?" Kneeling down next to her, I was deeply moved. I took her outstretched hand and, fighting back my own tears, said, "Yes, absolutely."

Katharine talked about the experience. She said that she had lived forever in a quandary, one part of her struggled to remain detached and aloof, to appear superior and special, while the other part wanted to be real and connected to others, but she was deathly afraid to let go. What emerged from our discussions was that her true feelings about herself were that underneath it all she was just ordinary, nothing special and this created a sense of shame. Her parents had been extremely successful and they conveyed to Katharine that appearances were everything. Hence, Katharine had worked hard to mask what she believed to be her very ordinary, inadequate self. Katharine's constant hiding left her so distant from others and lonely that she became jaded and sarcastic about the world (the world was a sewer). Her perception changed when she felt it was safe to let down her guard.

Conclusion

The multimodal approach to psychotherapy and dance therapy incorporates a variety of expressive media. Decisions as to which medium to use and in what order are based on the therapist's ability to intuit the needs of the individual and on creating a milieu that allows for self-direction, spontaneity and creativity. The success of a session is not determined by the number of modalities used or the order of their use, but rather by the communication between therapist and patient or therapist and group during the creative process. It is the empathic therapeutic relationship, the interventions and interactions that emerge from this that provide the foundation for a safe healing environment.

These methods, as illustrated, can be powerful and must be used conscientiously and respectfully. It is important to note that not all sessions will be as outwardly dramatic as the case illustrations presented in this chapter. These have been chosen from years of experience and were selected specifically because they depict the methods and rationale of multimodal work. Patient growth can also take place quietly. This kind of growth is not immediately obvious but must be respected.

UNIT III

Dance Movement Therapy with Different Populations

The field of dance therapy continues to expand, focusing on specific types of problems, new patient groups and the clarification of theory and practice for these groups. In this third edition of *Dance Movement Therapy: A Healing Art*, a separate unit has been created for areas of specialty. This was done through the written contributions of contemporary dance therapists who work with specific patient groups, such as children and adolescents, the physically handicapped, patients who have suffered sexual, emotional or physical abuse and patients with dissociation or eating disorders. The following is an outline of the changes in this edition.

Section A, Chapter 18, discusses dance therapy with children and includes more detailed material on work with sexually abused children and current work in the area of autism and other children with special needs. The chapter also discusses violence prevention, work with adolescents and William Freeman's work with Dianne Dulicai and Elise Billock Tropea on movement assessment with children.

Section B discusses specialized work in dance therapy with adults. There are three new chapters in this section. Chapter 20, Adult Victims of Physical, Sexual and Emotional Abuse discusses the work of several contemporary dance therapists, both in private practice (individually and in groups) and in the hospital setting. Unique uses of dance therapy and case examples of dance therapy with patients with multiple personality disorder (known today as dissociative disorder) are also discussed in this section. Susan Kleinman and Terese Hall wrote chapter 21 that covers work with women who have eating disorders. There is little written on dance therapy with this population, yet dance therapy is particularly useful in helping women with anorexia nervosa and bulimia. Susan Sandel updated the last chapter in the section, Chapter 22, dance movement therapy with The Elderly.

In Section C, Chapter 23 was written by Cathy Appel and discusses the theory and practice of dance therapy for rehabilitation of patients with serious physical limitations. Appel begins with an extensive discussion of the pioneering work of Norma Canner with children. While Canner never referred to her work as rehabilitation, Appel demonstrates the importance of her contribution to working with patients with a range of physical disabilities. Appel then goes on to discuss the work of contemporary leaders who specialize with this population. Appel believes that dance therapy has a unique role in rehabilitation, which she poignantly addresses through case discussions.

Finally, in Section D, Chapter 25 includes a new dimension to the field, dance therapy in corporate settings and describes the innovative work of Virginia Reed at J. P. Morgan Chase.

SECTION A

Children

18 Children with Special Needs

This chapter illuminates the work of individuals who have pioneered dance movement therapy with children and youth in a variety of settings. The chapter is broken into seven subsections. Part A discusses dance movement therapy with young children and includes the work of Suzi Tortora and Jane Wilson Cathcart. Part B discusses Rena Kornblum's violence prevention strategy in an elementary school setting. Part C focuses on work with adolescents in schools and includes the work of Diane Duggan and Nancy Beardall. William Freeman's work on movement assessment of students in schools is discussed in Part D. The last three sections discuss major therapists who have worked with children: in psychiatric hospitals (Part E), with autism (Part F) and those who have suffered sexual abuse (Part G).

Part A. Young Children: Social, Emotional, Physical and Cognitive Goals
Suzi Tortora

The *Ways of Seeing* program, developed by Suzi Tortora, utilizes nonverbal movement observation, dance, music and play for the assessment, intervention and education of children and their families. The program is run privately in Tortora's clinical practice. Children are seen individually and with their families when indicated. Tortora frequently acts as an advocate for the child and family in the school system. Her program is based on the principles of Laban Movement Analysis (LMA), dance movement therapy practice and early childhood developmental theory. It is particularly used with children from birth to 10 years old. The following information on Tortora's work was received as an unpublished paper and is the subject of her forthcoming book.

The program is called *Ways of Seeing* to emphasize that there are many ways to look at and experience our surroundings and to receive information about the self. The key elements in the *Ways of Seeing* program include observation, perception, experience and interaction between the child and others. The program has been influenced by the notion that seeing is at the core of how one senses oneself and interacts with others. It implies that each individual desires to be known and acknowledged. Tortora uses the term *seeing* both in the literal and metaphorical sense; for her, the idea of seeing goes beyond what we see with our eyes alone.

The child's nonverbal body cues are observed and used as the primary tool for intervention. Tortora uses these cues to set up meaningful communication between the child, therapist and the family. She creatively plays with the various movement patterns presented and intertwines these patterns into a social and emotional relationship.

Regardless of the child's diagnosis, treatment always starts with the same focus—establishing a social/emotional relationship. As the *Ways of Seeing* program is relationship-based, a strong bond is primary, supporting all other levels of development. Parents are always involved, within the actual session or separately through individual sessions.

Using the LMA system, the dance therapist is able to describe how a movement occurs using a set of movement-based parameters. These include what parts of the body are used, the spatial path of the actions and the feeling tone the action creates. A Laban analysis-based observational tool called *Movement Signature Impressions* (MSI) was developed by Tortora to note these observations.

During treatment and observations Tortora continually asks three questions: 1) How does the child's way of relating and moving color the child's experience? 2) What does it feel like to experience the world through the child's movements? and 3) How can I structure an environment that enables the child to experience his or her own way of relating and functioning, while simultaneously enabling the child, through that experience, to explore new ways of interaction with the environment?

The answer to these questions is found in experiencing the child's movement style. Tortora describes a four-part procedure for this therapeutic process:

1. Match-feel the movement qualities through attunement and mirroring;
2. Use these movements in dialogue with the child;
3. Use interaction to explore/expand these actions and
4. Move the communication from nonverbal to verbal exchange.

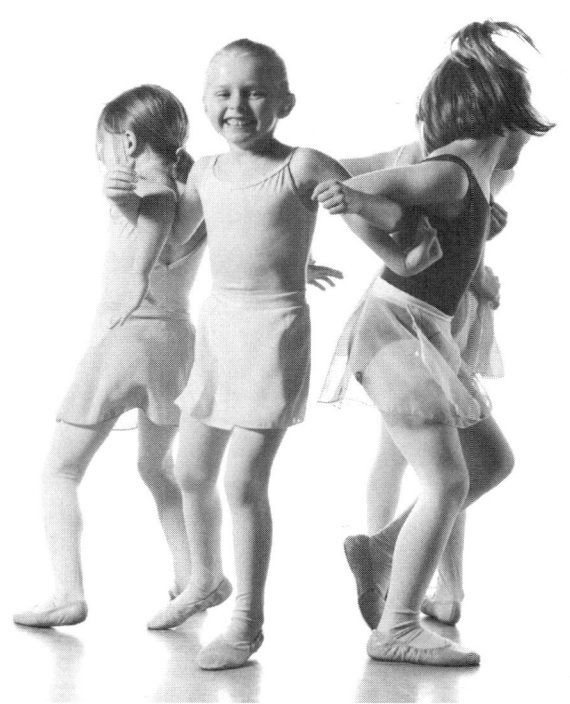

Dancers at play, Ballet & Performing Arts Center/Winston-Salem
(Photo courtesy Steve Clarke)

While engaging in the four-part method, the therapist monitors his or her own experience through self-observation. This includes witnessing, which is an awareness of the therapist's personal response to movements of the client. Witnessing includes kinesthetic seeing and kinesthetic empathy. Kinesthetic seeing[1] is a form of self-observation of one's bodily and sensory responses to the child and family. Tortora stresses the importance of kinesthetic seeing and explains that dance therapists must be aware of changes in their breathing pattern or tension level as they observe and interact with their clients. These self-observations allow therapists to determine what is happening inside them, before effecting change in the treatment. Kinesthetic empathy refers to therapists' awareness of their emotional reactions to the moving client.

In an open space that enables free unencumbered mobility, a variety of modes of nonverbal communica-

---

[1] Tortora again uses the word seeing in the metaphorical sense and includes all of the senses.

tion are used including movement, dance, touch, sound, music, rhythm, breath, eye contact, conscious awareness of how the participant moves in the space and self-observation. Materials used in that space such as music, pillows, scarves, balls and blankets promote movement awareness and foster the child's own imagery. The following case study is an example of Tortora's work with a young child with a disability.

The Case of Brianna

Born with agenesis of the corpus callosum, a rare congenital abnormality of the brain in which the part of the brain that connects the two hemispheres is absent, Brianna demonstrated severe delays in all areas of development. She displayed a marked lack of eye contact and overall poor social relatedness. Her most prominent behaviors were to stare at her hands, shaking them in a quick short pulsing action or to gaze into space with a glazed look in her eyes. She showed no recognition of her parents, although her father attended the sessions with Tortora. Tortora was very aware of her kinesthetic response to Brianna—a deep sense of isolation and self-containment came over her. Tortora sat on the floor opposite Brianna to share her spatial orientation.

Using touch, Tortora first attempted to engage Brianna by shaking her leg, matching Brianna's pulsing hand rhythm. Brianna stopped her hand actions and turned her head toward Tortora. Encouraged, the therapist shook Brianna's leg, stopping each time Brianna ceased moving. Tortora followed Brianna's lead so as not to impose her own eagerness for contact. Brianna became excited; shaking her hands with more vigor and began to squeal as she maintained a steadier gaze in the therapist's direction. Tortora increased her actions and vocalized with gleeful affect. Over the next few weeks Brianna continued to extend her interaction, maintaining her gaze toward the therapist when shaking her limbs.

Next, Tortora played music with a steady medium rhythm, darkened the room and encouraged Brianna to follow a pen flashlight as she glided it up and down and side to side to the beat. In pace with this rhythm, Tortora intermittently focused the light on her own smiling face, attracting Brianna's attention. As Brianna followed the gliding action with her eyes and head, her movement repertoire expanded, enabling her to experience fluid movement in contrast to the pulsing she did on her own. Brianna was delighted and held Tortora's gaze for a longer time.

Sensitive to Brianna's short attention span, Tortora moved the flashlight away from her own face when Brianna looked away. Tortora demonstrated to Brianna's father the importance of following the child's waxing and waning of attention as a way to slowly start to build rapport.

In the next few weeks, with the lights on, Brianna began to reach her arms out purposefully towards her legs as Tortora shook them in rhythm with the music. Sensing that Brianna was welcoming more interpersonal contact, Tortora mirrored Brianna's reaching arms with her own, lifting them up and then down and forward toward Brianna's extended body, verbalizing "Here I come!" Brianna giggled and tracked Tortora with her eyes as Tortora rocked backwards and said, "Here I go!"

This dance-play turned into a game of coming towards and pushing away. Tortora encouraged Brianna's father to join in. Lying on his back, Brianna's father rolled towards Brianna, who watched him intently and shook her leg, "pushing" him away. Brianna's father immediately exclaimed and rolled away with exaggerated vigor as Brianna watched his actions with laughter.

Through these interventions, Brianna was able to connect with Tortora and eventually with her family.

Other Work with Young Children
Jane Wilson Cathcart

Jane Wilson Cathcart (formerly Downes) has worked with children and adolescents with learning disabilities and mental illnesses since 1971. Her clinical work at Manhattan Children's Psychiatric Center spanned 20 years. In 1988 she also began a dance movement therapy program at Little Meadows Early Childhood Center, where she continues to work with preschool children and their families.

Cathcart sees freedom of expression as a basic tool for the healthy development of full selfhood. The goals of her treatment model are to enable children to become aware of their own resources, to perceive themselves as worthy beings, to communicate ideas and emotions and to experience their own senses as an active force in their lives.

In Cathcart's work (Downes, 1980), movement forms are chosen by the child from the repertoire of everyday actions and from the actions inspired by creative imagery as directed by the therapist:

> By using her body movement as a structure ... the movement therapist supports, enhances, mirrors, absorbs and otherwise participates in the meaningful movement expressed by the ... child. The movement therapist becomes the catalyst for change ... [by] afford[ing] the child the opportunity to move through the external environment as well as his internal one in a purposeful, exciting and achieving manner. Much of this is spontaneous. (p. 17)

Tortora's and Cathcart's interventions are supported by theoretical work on nonverbal interactions between mother and baby by Stern (1985), Sanders (2000) and Beebe et al. (2000). This work has focused on observing the nonverbal interactions between mother and baby to analyze how each member of the dyad contributes to and affects the baby's early bonding experience and overall sense of attachment.

Cathcart, like Tortora, uses mirroring as one of the central elements in her work. Therapeutic mirroring often matches movement interactions that are found in early stages of healthy childhood attachment with a loving caregiver. The dance therapist, at crucial junctures in the child's treatment, revisits this early mirroring experience to re-establish trust when trust is threatened (Cathcart, personal communication, 2002). "It is this mirroring which lessens the sense of lonely isolation, then extracts and imbues each person in the dyad with a sense of the other" (Downes, 1982).

Cathcart described her work with Joshua, a four-year-old boy who possessed receptive language but babbled in response to questions. He played by himself at a much younger level. His solitude was not purely by choice, since other children at the school shunned his dirty, unkempt presentation. This child arrived at school with infrequently changed diapers and often wore the same clothing for a week or two. Staff interventions with the home met with little or no success. He initially appeared to be of low intelligence. In dance movement therapy sessions Cathcart observed:

> Interspersed with Joshua's activity and contact was a quality of gaze that was almost dissociated—he did not appear to focus on the external world. His lack of focus was accompanied by a decreased focus on his body as well. In working with him, it appeared that no one was "there"; Joshua did not appear to recognize the therapist or objects. As work with Joshua progressed, he at times caught eyes with the therapist in the mirror, then traced his steps over to her, bringing blocks. He soon included the therapist in the play, building towers and knocking them down, as he waited and listened for her running commentary to continue. Cathcart gradually became more active as she joined his search for himself in the mirror.

> One day as he searched for her eyes in the mirror, he visibly relaxed with a smile and a sigh as he saw Cathcart seeing him. This was quickly followed by a collapse on the floor in distress as he discovered his release of tension had brought on a rush of urine. When he looked ashamed, Cathcart verbally minimized his accident and brought him back to class. The therapist and others, who celebrated him in the most basic way, quickly tended him to: touch. They washed him and taught him to wash himself. This affirmation of his boundaries, without punishment, found him fully present for the first time in his 18 months at the center. He joined his classmates in session with a dance specialist who at first did not recognize him. He began to speak in full sentences and revealed a keen sense of humor and intelligence. The sense of belonging he felt at school, with staff and children alike, only partially mediated the rejection he felt at home. By graduation, however, Joshua learned to smile from within and was eager to see himself while being seen. (Cathcart, personal communication, 2002).

In this case study, the dance movement therapist acted as a mediator between the inner and outer realms, the self and other dance and showed the ability to be available to recapitulate and rework significant moments. As a nonverbal communication specialist she also provided a model context for staff. This facilitated a wider holding environment for the development of positive self-concept, expression and healing in children.

Cathcart believes that the use of systematically explored movement dynamics, as discussed in the work of Bartenieff and Laban, enables the dance therapist to foster a full range of communicative expression in the special child. The child gains a stronger sense of self as his or her inner drives and states of being are manifested through expressive movement. The therapist regards the themes and issues that emerge empathically. The dance therapist's modulated and empathically connected use of movement becomes a model of functional adaptive behavior for the child, who is still in the process of learning how to use his or her internal regulating mechanisms. Ultimately, for the young client, "individuality and identity will emerge from deep levels of the self" (Downes, 1980, p. 17).

In 1982, Cathcart referred to her work as the choreography of object relations. This creative juxtaposition of words grew out of her integration of the work of D.W. Winnicott (1971) and Margaret Mahler (1968) with her dance background and clinical work as a dance therapist (Cathcart, personal communication, 2002). Penny Lewis (1982) picked up this terminology as the title of her book to which Cathcart contributed a chapter.

Part B. Children at Risk: Violence Prevention
Rena Kornblum

Kornblum has been active as a dance movement therapist since 1978, working with children who are coping with learning disabilities, autism, emotional disabilities, ADHD, sexual and physical abuse, neglect, domestic violence, attachment disorder and foster care and adoption issues. She has worked in individual, group and family therapy. Currently, Kornblum is employed at Hancock Center for Movement Arts and Therapy in Madison, Wisconsin, where she coordinates outreach and provides movement-based therapy and prevention sessions in the public schools.

Kornblum's work combines perceptual, cognitive and psychosocial approaches. Her therapy sessions start with a movement and/or verbal warm-up in which each child is recognized and accepted by the group. Children then have skill-based, structured movement activities that deal with socialization, body image and boundaries, energy modulation and attention span. A more client-initiated time follows, encouraging

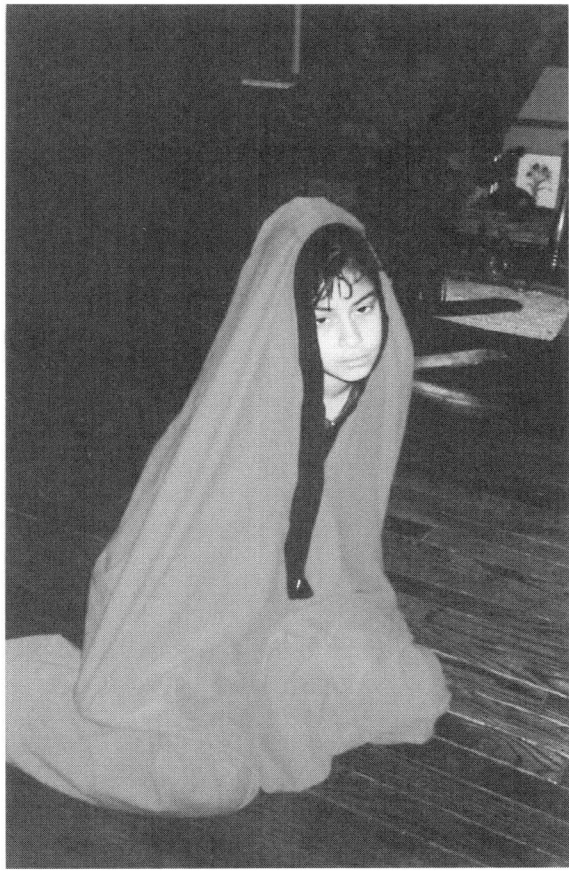

Contemplative model Stephanie Class demonstrates Bodysox from Kimberly Dye/Dyenamic (Photo courtesy Fran Levy)

creative and dramatic expression. Sessions end with a closing circle that involves sharing and processing (personal communication, 2002).

Kornblum began working with classrooms of children after an experienced physical education teacher approached her for help with a group of students. In this class, there were two very disturbed children for whom six weeks of classroom movement was not enough and three dominant students whose negative leadership affected other children. Movement work began by using movements that expressed strength in fun, safe ways, allowing the notion of positive leadership to emerge. Children experimented with matching each other's intensity and being able to both lead and follow. Kornblum discovered that the movement experience helped students to ignore provocation, redirect aggression, assert themselves appropriately and support one another and resulted in a significant increase in the overall safety and control in the classroom. The positive impact of six weeks of movement work with one class led Kornblum to undertake work in other classes as well (personal communication, 2002).

Preventing violence requires three major skills: the ability to be pro-active, the ability to manage anger and the social skills necessary to get one's needs met without hurting others. All three of these, in turn, call for the integration of the mind (the decision of what to do in a tense situation) and the body (the implementation of that decision) in order to be successful. Kornblum believes that too many prevention programs overlook the importance of body awareness and movement skills. Physical experiences of moving with others in synchrony, while respecting personal (spatial) boundaries, are body level skills that help children learn to peacefully get along.

From teacher and student responses, she developed: 1) a curriculum called "Violence Prevention through Movement" described in her book *Disarming the Playground: Violence Prevention through Movement* (2002), 2) an introductory video, *Moving Toward Peace: Violence Prevention through Movement* (2001) and 3) two training videos.

Case Study: Violence Prevention in the Second Grade

Four second grade classes received the Violence Prevention through Movement program for twenty weeks. These classes had more than the usual number of children, around 30 to 50 percent, who were impulsive, distractible, emotionally vulnerable, had learning disabilities, etc. There were frequent fights and much agitation. The behaviors were extreme enough that the teachers felt that they could not teach and a few of them went home crying regularly.

After working on spatial and body awareness and teaching respect for personal boundaries for a month, Kornblum shifted her attention to the ability to self-settle and focus, spending several weeks working on energy modulation. The children practiced moving from low energy to high energy and back again. Kornblum divided the room into energy zones and used animal imagery. They explored what body cues they felt while in each energy state. This helped them realize when they were getting excited and how different the feeling of excitement was from the feeling of calm. This marks the beginning of body awareness and the rudiments of control.

The students also learned to be connected to their bodies in stillness as well as in action. This supported them to feel comfortable and safe even if they were not moving. This was a new and significant experience for many and helped them to maintain control and calm even when anxious. An exercise that Kornblum used involved asking the students to plant their feet firmly on the ground, then move wildly in place and then freeze or stop short and do deep abdominal breathing, while remaining aware of their feet on the ground.

Kornblum also practiced relaxation techniques with the children and tried to have them sustain feelings of calm, but alert energy over longer and longer periods of time. They learned to distinguish between high energy that was under control versus high energy that was dangerous to them. This was done through playful activities, self-observation and group discussion. The culmination of the unit was learning "The Four B's of self-control," a four-part movement phrase that was developed by Kornblum to help children learn to calm down. The phrase consists of:

> *Brakes*—catching the energy with your hands and doing an isometric push to contain it;
> *Breathing*—lifting your arms overhead and doing deep abdominal breaths;

Brains—resting your hands on your head and using self-talk to tell yourself to calm down; and
Body—put your hands on your chest and feel your body get calm.

Kornblum challenged the classes to practice the 4B's outside of movement class. They reported several successful incidents. One was during a school tornado drill. It was very loud and many children were having difficulty maintaining control. One of the second grade students called out to her classmates, "Let's use what Rena taught us." Everyone from that class did the 4B's and calmed down immediately.

One teacher picked the three times during the day that her class frequently had problems and began using the 4B's to prevent these problems. All classes reported success with this approach.

While these classes showed significant improvement in many areas, they still had problems in others. It is important to note that not all behavioral problems were solved by the 4B's. On an individual basis, however, children reported using the 4B's to help them calm down at home and at school. One child reported that he now knew that when his face started to get hot or he started knocking into things, it was time to do the 4B's (Kornblum, personal communication, 2002).

Part C. Adolescents in the School System
Developing a Model for Peaceable Schools: Nancy Beardall

For the last twenty years, Nancy Beardall has implemented the dance movement therapy program in Newton Public Schools, Newton, MA. The program has been integrated into the school day through a dance elective in the Arts Department and through Comprehensive Health, which all students take.

Within the Comprehensive Health curriculum, Beardall incorporates body movement work in the interactive and expressive movement activities of the "Creating a Peaceable School" curriculum. These activities are directed toward social, emotional and relational learning and allow for integrating experiences where emotional intelligence is reinforced through dance, movement and the arts and a mutual connection between students is established. The Peaceable School program helps students develop an individual "body sense" as well as a positive attitude toward individual differences while contributing to a school climate where students feel respected, encouraged to participate and are important members of the community (Beardall, personal communication, 2002).

Beardall asserts that creative dance is a therapeutic experience for young women, citing a 1992 AAUW (American Association of University Women) report. Many studies have found that body image is inexorably linked to self-image in young women. Not only is physical appearance extremely important to them but also young women feel increasingly more negative about their bodies as they go through puberty. Harvard's Carol Gilligan (1982) speaks of girls developing differently from boys. Gilligan's belief is that girls are more relational and more concerned with connecting to their peers. Gilligan and Brown (1992) refer to early adolescence as a time when girls silence their voice, "separating themselves or their psyches from their bodies as to not know what they are feeling …" (p. 217). Beardall's dance elective helps middle school students, primarily girls, express their feelings through movement, encouraging them to stay in connection with their bodies and psyches at this developmentally challenging time.

Beardall explains that Marian Chace's basic technique has influenced the development of her creative, therapeutic approach to dance. Like Chace, Beardall uses a warm-up with mirroring, expanding movement repertoire, theme development such as nonverbal clues, verbalization and imagery and lastly the ritual closure through coming together in a circle. In addition, the Bartenieff Fundamentals and Laban's use of effort and space/shape allow students to experience their basic anatomical connections and sense of alignment as well as experience a broad-based movement repertoire.

Beardall uses an eclectic approach to dance technique (jazz, modern, ballet, ethnic, yoga) along with the Laban vocabulary, which allows students to experience and understand a range of movement possibilities. This exploration allows girls to express their own movement patterns and style.

In Brown and Gilligan's (1992) book, *Meeting at the Crossroads*, their last chapter is entitled "Dancing at the Crossroads." Beardall interprets this phrase literally, stating, "It is in 'Dancing at the Crossroads' of girls' development, that teachers, parents, community and children come together to dance, connect, support and reflect. Through dancing, girls' voices are individually and collectively expressed and their voices are clear and powerful" (personal communication, 2002).

Dance therapists have much to offer educators where education and therapy meet in the integration of

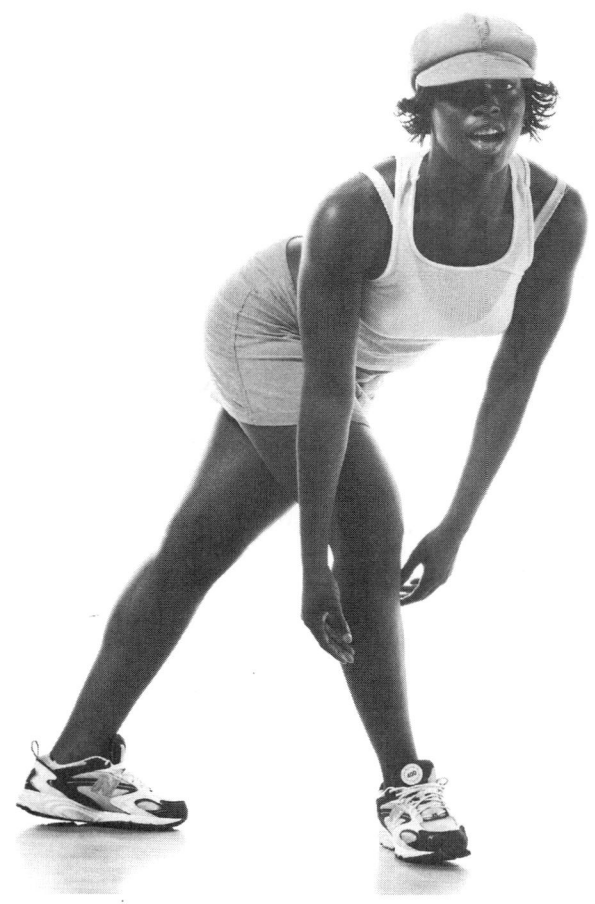

Dancer Melissa Jackson (Photo courtesy Steve Clarke)

social and emotional learning for each student. Through Beardall's innovative public school curriculum this dialogue has begun.

Dance and Movement with Troubled Adolescents: Diane Duggan

Since 1973, Diane Duggan has worked in the field of dance therapy as a clinician, supervisor, teacher and author. She conducts dance therapy and theater groups in public schools with adolescents. Her students typically have emotional and learning disabilities. She also teaches in the Dance Education program at New York University.

Parts of this section have been extracted from Duggan's chapter, "The '4's': A Dance Program for Learning Disabled Adolescents," which appears in *Dance and Other Expressive Art Therapies: When Words are Not Enough*, edited by Fran Levy with Judith Fried and Fern Leventhal.

Duggan (1995) finds that structure is essential in the dance therapy process:

> [Structure] 'holds' the client providing an environment in which he or she is safe and free to respond. This promotes the trust that is crucial in a therapeutic relationship. Structure also 'holds' the movement. Because movement is transitory it is easily lost; structure enables movement phrases, images and

insights to coalesce, preventing their energy and meaning from dissipating. This allows for the acknowledgment of the client's experience as well as for the possibility of further exploration and development of what has transpired." (pp. 225-226)

Duggan (1995) notes, "structure is a dynamic, interactive concept" which "develops within the interaction between the therapist and the client and should be flexible enough to accommodate a range of possibilities in this relationship" (p. 226)

The "4's": A Dance Therapy Program for Adolescents with Learning Disabilities

Duggan began the dance therapy program described here in 1979 at a public high school for adolescents with learning disabilities. The school was composed of approximately 250 special education students, most of whom were male (Duggan, 1995).

Duggan (1995) first used the Chacian circle with this group. However, when the adolescent group members persisted in forming lines, she recognized the importance of their nonverbal communication, attributing it to adolescent ambivalence towards self-display and the group members' need to be differentiated from her. The circle was uncomfortable for the teens because it exposed everyone to everyone else and was inclusive and nonhierarchical. "I was asking the adolescents to risk something new involving body movement and self-disclosure in full view of their peers and in full collaboration with me" (Duggan, p. 227).

Duggan recognized the need for an alternative, viable structure for her groups, "not to restrict them but to set them free. An ideal structure would engage and organize them and address prominent adolescent issues ... It would be definite enough to support them but also flexible and responsive to their needs" (1995, p. 228).

While dancing with the teens, Duggan spontaneously came upon a simple movement structure, which captivated their attention. It was a symmetrical, four-beat pattern that derived from her study of Haitian dance with Jean-Léon Destiné. Christened the "4's," the pattern proved to be compelling but challenging for the teens because it required impulse control. "In order to execute the step properly they had to bind their flow, ... suspending the impulse to commit their weight on the final beat. The inability to do this was in fact an embodiment of the most pervasive problems in the group, poor impulse control. The 4 steps required them, not to deny the impulse to move, but to channel it into a gestural 'lightness'" (Duggan, 1995, p. 129), thereby preserving their options and becoming more flexible. "It took some reflection and effort ... to achieve this. The challenge was real, but limited enough to overcome. Their mastery of it was a genuine accomplishment" (Duggan, 1995, p. 129).

In the early stages of her program, Duggan adopted the linear 4's pattern as a structure for group dancing with the adolescents. "The most compelling and meaningful aspect of the 4's was that it enabled them to move in unison, submerging individual fears and doubts in the certainty of group action. It was the perfect manifestation of the peer group: accessible but exclusive, "hip" but conforming" (Duggan, 1995, p. 229). The 4's pattern provided a rhythmic and spatial structure, but the shape and dynamics of the movement within this structure were open.

Duggan worked with the teens to develop vocabularies of 4's movements that were unique to each of her groups. The adolescents offered stereotyped dance steps in this process. Duggan accepted these steps as valid expressions of subculture, gender identity and self. She noted that it is important to begin where clients are, rather than requiring them at the outset to attempt something unfamiliar. "The use of adolescent dance steps is in some ways analogous to mirroring the stereotyped gestures of an autistic child. It establishes a bridge to the clients while permitting them the security and gratification of familiar movement patterns during the early, difficult stages of establishing a relationship" (Duggan, 1978; Duggan, 1995, p. 230).

Within the 4's structure, the stereotyped dance steps became a means of self-expression and relating to others.

> The paradox that structure and stereotyped movement can permit freedom and authenticity mirrors the paradox that formalized roles can facilitate real relationships... The external order permits the expression of emotionally charged impulses because it contains the impulses and permits their control. Interaction is facilitated because attention is initially focused on form and roles rather than on personalities, thereby reducing self-consciousness and anxiety. The structure is both an organizing factor and a tem-

plate for interaction ordering experience and affording a safe opportunity for self-expression and satisfying contact. (Duggan, 1995, p. 230)

Although Duggan uses various other means of providing structure in her groups with adolescents, the 4's pattern she used early in her career is illustrative of how the specific structures that dance therapists use in sessions should be appropriate to the needs and interests of their clients and flexible enough to accommodate a wide range of expression and interactions. Duggan's serendipitous 4's "succeeded because it engaged [the adolescents] and provided a secure, age-appropriate structure with which to begin the difficult, rewarding work of self discovery and change" (Duggan, 1995, p. 240).

Part D. Movement Assessment in Schools

A protégé of SuEllen Fried, Norma G. Canner, Carolyn Grant Fay and Barbara Mettler, William Freeman has designed and directed innovative programs in movement and expressive arts education and therapy for children, youth and adults for the past 25 years. In this field, he founded, developed and directed both a professional development and demonstration program with the Kansas State Department of Education and, subsequently, Accessible Arts, Inc., a not-for-profit educational organization in Kansas to make the arts accessible to all people, including individuals with disabilities. Since 1999, he has conducted professional development and parent education programs with the Center on Disability and Community Inclusion at the University of Vermont, where he directs the Expressive Movement Project. In direct service and teaching of providers and parents, Freeman extends his work in movement by employing other expressive media, including voice and sound, color and clay, words, story and dramatic action. In his school-based practice with students with significant disabilities, he works collaboratively with voice-movement therapist Anne Brownell to assist students in increasing vocalization and interaction through voice and movement.

During the 1980s, Freeman, with support from Carole Weiner, Sally Totenbier and Fried, ensured inclusion and approval of dance movement therapy as a related service by the Kansas State Department of Education. As a result, Kansas was the only state known to recognize and approve four arts-related services in special education (art therapy, dance movement therapy, music therapy and special music education) as listed and defined in a state plan for special education and state administrative regulations.

Since 1990, Elise Billock Tropea, Dianne Dulicai and William Freeman have worked to develop a movement assessment instrument for school children (William Freeman personal communication, 2002). The assessment procedure aims to evaluate students by assessing their nonverbal behavior in developmentally appropriate settings. For the past six years, Freeman, in collaboration with Dulicai and Billock-Tropea, has developed a comprehensive service delivery model for movement assessment and intervention with children and youth with various disabilities in Vermont public schools. Dulicai indicates that the results from this study will then be compared with standard school assessment tests. While this study is still in progress, it is hoped that movement assessments will identify students at risk of poor performance or students who need further help (Dulicai, personal communication, 2002).

In addition to working together to develop a movement assessment procedure, Freeman, Dulicai and Billock-Tropea work collaboratively with members of the Evaluation and Planning and Individualized Education Program (IEP) Teams, which include parents, administrators, educators and related service providers, to coordinate and support services for children with disabilities and those who serve them.

Part E. Children with Severe Disturbance: Inpatient

Dance Movement Therapy with Children in a Short-Term Inpatient Psychiatric Setting
Tina Erfer and Anat Ziv

Tina Erfer is the coordinator of the Hospital Schools program in the Department of Child and Adolescent Psychiatry at Mt. Sinai Hospital in New York. For the past 20 years, she has worked as a dance movement therapist in special education settings.

Anat Ziv is a dance movement therapist with additional training and certification in family therapy. Ziv's professional experience includes working with adults in a psychiatric outpatient setting and working with children and adolescents in an inpatient psychiatric unit.

For three years, Erfer and Ziv led dance movement therapy groups for children with severe emotional disturbance. The following section includes extracts from an unpublished paper by them, describing their work as dance movement therapists with children in a short-term inpatient psychiatric setting.

There is a high patient turnover in this psychiatric unit and children with a wide range of diagnoses and behaviors attend the same dance movement therapy group. Treatment is geared toward resolution of acute problems and/or crises. For these children, the goal of short-term psychiatric hospitalization is "to ameliorate the patient's problematic behaviors so that he can once again function outside the hospital" (Yalom, 1983, p. 53).

Erfer and Ziv work actively towards promoting group cohesiveness and state that a "present moment" attitude is essential due to the abbreviated time available for treatment. They cite Yalom (1983), who states that "a group focusing on the here and now, on its own interaction, is almost invariably a vital, cohesive group" (p. 48). Yalom postulates that cohesiveness is a "necessary precondition for effective therapy" (1985, p. 50). Since dance movement therapy with children in this setting is anchored in the present moment, it is highly effective in promoting group cohesiveness.

Erfer and Ziv (2002) emphasize the importance of body image and self-concept:

> A child who has an impoverished body image and sense of self may not be able to interact effectively and meaningfully with others. It would be difficult for a group of such children to become a cohesive group, unless those issues are addressed.
>
> ... [In dance movement therapy] with these children, sensorimotor and perceptual motor development and integration are fundamental aspects of the work; [they] help to build body image and develop positive self-concept. (Erfer & Ziv, 2002, unpublished paper)

Erfer and Ziv quote Schilder (1950) who states, "We do not know very much about our body unless we move it" (p. 112). They see the development of body or self-awareness as the first step towards establishing awareness of others. This further helps patients become tolerant of differences between themselves and others. Without self-awareness and tolerance it is difficult to achieve group cohesion.

Group cohesion is an essential foundation and helps children work toward other goals. Like Kornblum, Erfer and Ziv's work ultimately aims to improve children's socialization skills, sharing, cooperation, communication and self-expression. Through dance movement therapy, they help children to control their impulses, improve their attention spans and maintain appropriate boundaries. In further explaining the process of treating children, they state:

> [Therapy] leads to more effective interactions with others and with the environment. Essential to the treatment are expansion of movement repertoire orientation to time and space, focusing, balance, sequencing and following directions. As these develop, they are often accompanied by release of tension and more creative problem-solving and expression. Whenever possible, verbal processing of the movement experience takes place in order to develop cognitive awareness (unpublished paper, 2002).

As in Duggan's work, Erfer and Ziv maintain that a clear structure is extremely important with children who are severely emotionally disturbed. They state, "when the structure is predictable and secure, with a clear beginning, middle and end, group members can begin to feel safe and free enough to take risks in movement exploration and in social and emotional expression" (Erfer & Ziv, unpublished paper, 2002). Kernberg and Chazan (1991) also emphasize the need for a predictable structure:

> Adequate structure is not used to keep the children under control but to help reduce their anxiety to a tolerable level so that the children's chaotic, intense feelings and impulses can be expressed and shared in ways that are not overwhelming for the individual child and other group members. (p. 188)

The goal of Erfer and Ziv's work is to help the children internalize a sense of structure so that it becomes their own. Ultimately, this allows disturbed children to rely on their own bodies for control. As children become more able to internalize a sense of structure, they are able to express themselves better and are given more opportunities for creative expression. Despite the necessity for structure in Erfer and Ziv's group work, they emphasize the importance of freedom of choice and self-expression.

Part F. Children with Autism

What is Autism?

Much controversy has centered on the diagnosis of autism, as well as the etiology. It is not a disease, but a behaviorally defined developmental disability that affects language, ability to socialize and various brain functions. Tina Erfer (1995) cites the clinical observations of Leo Kanner, which still form the basis for many subsequent theories about the condition. Kanner wrote:

> The common denominator in all these patients is a disability to relate in the ordinary way to people and situations from the beginning of life. The case histories indicate the presence from the start of autistic aloneness, which shuts out anything that comes to the child from the outside (p. 717).

A wide range of behaviors are demonstrated by children with autism, including self-stimulating actions, difficulty in understanding or using language, abnormal sensory responses and intense resistance to change (Erfer, 1995). In these children, skills and abilities in some areas can co-exist with gross impairments in others; therefore level of intelligence cannot be predicted. The autistic pattern of behavior can be associated with mental retardation, average intelligence or even (more rarely) with above-average intelligence. According to Victor (1983), autism is more accurately described by the term "pervasive developmental disorder," since it seems to be a general adaptation or personality organization that affects all major aspects of life.

Children with autism are often described as living in their own world. They shun human contact, are unable to relate meaningfully to others or to the environment and frequently engage in idiosyncratic movement patterns. While approaches vary, the dance therapists whose work is reviewed here stress the need to reach these children at their own developmental level, which is the primitive sensory-motor level. Through the use of techniques such as reflecting, sharing and mirroring the child's movements, the dance therapist creates "... a dance which is reassuring in its familiarity and implicit acceptance of the child" (ADTA, p. 5). This leads to the development of trust and the formation of a relationship between therapist and child.

The following sections review the pioneering work of Beth Kalish-Weiss and Janet Adler. Although Kalish-Weiss and Adler's work was done more than 20 years ago, it is interesting to note that the theoretical underpinnings of their work is similar to more recent work done by Erfer in the public school system. Erfer's work is discussed at the end of this section. Although she uses different terms to describe her work, all three therapists stress the importance of reaching children at their developmental level and work towards similar goals.

BRIAAC and the Case of Ana: Beth Kalish-Weiss

Beth Kalish-Weiss received her original dance therapy training in New York City with Marian Chace at Turtle Bay Music School in the 1960s. Like other early leaders in that class, notably Schmais and White, Kalish-Weiss went on to study with Irmgard Bartenieff. However, whereas many of the early Chace disciples went on to broaden and clarify the Chace technique with hospitalized psychiatric patients, Kalish-Weiss was particularly concerned with the psychodynamic make-up and movement behavior of the child with autism. This interest led her to pioneer as a dance therapist with this special group.* Her theoretical, practical and diagnostic contributions to this population are the topics of the following discussion.

In the mid-1960s, Kalish-Weiss explored her unique interest in the movement characteristics and treatment of autism, believing that these children could be reached most effectively through nonverbal means. Feeling there was a need for a systematic way of measuring the nonverbal communications of the child

---

*Today Kalish-Weiss is a training and supervising psychoanalyst. Her BRIAAC scale can be further understood by E-mailing her at bkalishweiss@mindspring.com.

with autism, she set out to create a movement scale, "which could be learned and applied by anyone on a regular basis, in a clinical setting, for use with nonverbal, 'untestable' psychotic children" (Kalish, 1976, p. 126).

In 1971, Kalish-Weiss introduced the Body Movement Scale (BMS), one of the eight scales of the Behavior Rating Instrument for Autistic and Other Atypical Children (BRIAAC).[2] Each of the eight scales, including BMS, notes the successive behavioral changes in a child's progress towards more adequate psychological functioning. The overall goal of BRIAAC is to provide a universal language of movement terms (Kalish, 1974a). The knowledge of atypical behaviors gained through the use of BRIAAC can guide the therapist in assessing the needs of a child and in planning therapeutic intervention. Today, more than ever, Kalish-Weiss views BRIAAC as supporting and clarifying, not only behavioral theory but also psychoanalytic theory in that the unconscious is revealed through behavior (personal communication, 2003).

Kalish-Weiss (Kalish, 1976) developed and designed the body movement scale using effort/shape terminology and incorporated many of the theories of Laban and his protégés concerning how to observe movements. The theoretical basis of BMS also includes: Kestenberg's tension-flow system; Freud's body movement theory of function and adaptability; the works of Ruttenberg, Dratman and Teitlebaum concerning the delayed, slow motion development of children with autism; as well as the theories of Hunt and Allport (Kalish, 1974a). It was her assumption, as well as her motivation for developing this scale, that "movement behaviors would reveal developmental data about the nonverbal child if a method could be found to measure these behaviors reliably" (Kalish, 1976, p. 126).

The goal of the body movement scale is to specify body movement patterns in autism and qualities of those patterns, which are significant in the process of maturation. BMS "attempts to place the 'pure movements' in a developmental framework based on empirical observations of both normal and atypical (autistic) children and how they move" (Kalish, 1976, p. 6).

Kalish-Weiss stresses three important demands placed on the dance therapist: 1) to observe the child's nonverbal communications; 2) to know his or her own nonverbal communications and 3) to find a point at which his or her own body movements can communicate with the child's body movements, hence promoting communication and interaction on a movement level.

The following quote from the Kalish-Weiss 1967 article written with Dratman (one of the originators of BRIAAC) demonstrates how the therapist uses her own body movements to relate to the problems of autism. One sees here her stress on the developmental progression from the early symbiotic phase, when the child is merged with the adult, to the separation-individuation phase (Mahler, 1968).

> She [the therapist] takes the child where she finds him and tries to become one with him. She mirrors and imitates what he does until the child is comfortable with her—and she attempts to be his body double—with all his disturbance and his withdrawal—his autism. She practices blendsmanship, to coin a phrase. Then slowly she changes just one small part of the space and rhythm around him. (Dratman & Kalish, 1967, p. 44)

At this point, the separation-individuation phase is introduced.

> Where he ends and she starts he doesn't know and after many weeks or months she [the therapist] slowly disentangles herself—very slowly.... Gradually he recognizes her as an entity, sees where he begins and she starts. In the same way as a mother feeding her child—or holding her child—does with a movement, a look, a sign, a touch, which impinges on her child a thousand times during a day.... The dance therapist also does it thousands of times with the child until he is within her narcissistic milieu and a transfer of emotions ... takes place from her to him. This allows the child to slowly become aware of his own arm or finger or leg in a way much different from before. (Dratman & Kalish, 1967, p. 44)

Once trust is established by reaching the child at his or her developmental level, Kalish-Weiss (1968) stresses the need to build the child's body image. She believes the child with autism, who has never formed an intrapsychic representation of his or her body, can develop more normally once a sense of self is achieved.

Kalish-Weiss' (1982, unpublished) case study of Ana illustrates aspects of her approach. A genetic disorder, Di George Syndrome, discovered shortly after Ana's birth, forced doctors to perform

---

[2]The other seven scales of BRIAAC are: relationship, communication, vocalization, speech and sound reception, social functioning, psychosexual development, and drive for mastery.

several life-saving surgical procedures during the postnatal period. Her labored breathing was relieved somewhat by a tracheotomy and she had to be fed through a tube leading to her stomach. She was rescued from heart failure. Her thymus gland was missing and thymus substance had to be surgically implanted.

When Ana was finally taken home, her mother soon noticed that she didn't smile, respond to sounds or demonstrate normal four-month-old playfulness and curiosity. When Ana was picked up, she would stiffen her body and arch her back or go completely limp. She made no eye contact with others.

Her parents, suspecting autism, had her evaluated. She was immediately discovered to be profoundly deaf. She was fitted for bilateral hearing aids, but would not tolerate them.

Enrolled in an infant-toddler program for children with disabilities, Ana did not interact or make eye contact with anyone and spent most of her time lying on the floor, flipping her hand rhythmically against the side of her head. She scrupulously avoided physical contact or proximity to others, pushing them away or rolling away from them. Her parents and teacher were very discouraged.

At two years and four months, Ana was referred to Kalish-Weiss for body movement therapy. Kalish-Weiss hypothesized that the active quality of Ana's resistance to people and things was a sign of ego-strength. She hoped to use movement and play to offer the child more pleasant experiences than she had had thus far. If the child could be motivated to crawl, roll and play hand games in interaction with others, she might develop a sense of her own mastery and ego controls and move out of the autistic-like stage to the next stage of symbiosis with her mother.

With Kalish-Weiss' support and guidance, Ana's mother became her co-therapist during therapy sessions and at home. Ana's mother experimented with new ways of holding and positioning the child to encourage greater physical mastery and more eye contact. She played actively with Ana, but also learned to hover over her less, encouraging the child to actively seek out her mother when she needed or wanted her. She moved Ana out of the master bedroom into a separate room equipped with an intercom so that Ana could be heard if her tracheotomy needed suctioning during the night.

After a few movement therapy sessions, it became clear that Ana was learning to differentiate between her mother and the therapist. Ana was also becoming more inquisitive about her environment and smiled briefly when she was moved using her own rhythms. Interestingly, during this period, her tracheotomy needed suctioning far less frequently than before.

As sessions continued, Ana's face would brighten when she approached the therapy room. She would wriggle out of her mother's arms and study herself in a large three-way mirror, moving her head from side to side. She crawled eagerly now and was delighted when Kalish-Weiss crawled with her. Her mother and the therapist both began to suspect that she was hearing sounds. (Children with autism frequently lose their "deafness" as they learn to seek out and make rewarding contact with the people and objects around them.)

The therapist's modeling of how to play with Ana was instructive and encouraging for the mother. She was gratified to see someone having fun with her child. She learned to relax more with her daughter and to enjoy interacting with her. These attitudes and skills were carried back into the home environment and contributed significantly to the overall success of the therapy.

After three months of therapy, Ana's functioning was evaluated using the BRIAAC scale. Although the assessment clearly showed that Ana had made progress, she was still functioning primarily in the autistic range performing at about one-half her age level.

Kalish-Weiss subsequently decided to try working alone with Ana, feeling that the child might feel comfortable and secure enough with her to allow the mother to leave for a while. The experiment was successful. Ana's attention span increased and her movement behaviors were more directive. She would indicate what games she enjoyed the most and direct the therapist to repeat them.

One day, Ana was missing her mother. She crawled over to her mother's handbag, pulled out the car keys and brought them to Kalish-Weiss as if to say, "Where's mom? I'm ready to go now." She was learning to communicate.

A second BRIAAC rating was done shortly thereafter and showed marked progress since the previous assessment. An audiology test showed that Ana was, in fact, beginning to hear. She would now tolerate hearing aids for short periods.

A third BRIAAC rating, done about six months after the second, showed continued, encouraging progress, especially in the areas of body movement, sound reception and relationship building. There can be little question that movement therapy intervention was one of the primary factors in stimulating Ana's developmental gains over a ten-month time span. And the BRIAAC scale provided a valuable tool for assessing her functioning and documenting her progress.

In another case study, Janet Adler (1968) describes how the development of a three-year-old autistic girl named Amy during two months of therapy corresponded with the developmental stages in an infant's first nine months of postnatal life. That is, first she began to explore the therapist's body as the infant explores the mother's body. Later, she began to explore her own body and finally she started imitating the therapist.

By allowing the child to regress during sessions, Adler helped Amy to move through the early stages of infancy and toward a more developed style of interaction. As Amy was able to tolerate more physical contact with Adler she demonstrated a simultaneous reduction of autistic gestures. Adler's work with Amy, similar to the work of Kalish-Weiss, focused on the use of reflection and synchronous movement interactions. Both dance therapists emphasize the importance of responding empathetically to the child, that is, experiencing what the child experiences.

Adler's work with Amy and the well-known film, *Looking for Me*, depicting this case have become landmark contributions to the practice of dance therapy among children with autism.

Treating Children with Autism in an Educational Setting: Tina Erfer

Erfer, as mentioned in the previous section, works in a short-term inpatient psychiatric hospital. She has also worked as a dance movement therapist in the New York City Public Schools for the past 20 years and she is certified in special education. Much of the information below is extracted from Erfer's chapter, "Treating Children with Autism in a Public School System," in *Dance and Other Expressive Art Therapies: When Words Are Not Enough*, (Fran Levy et al., 1995).

Erfer states that dance movement therapy is ideally suited for working with autism. She refers to Leventhal (1981) who wrote that dance movement therapy for the special child "deals fundamentally with sensory motor and perceptual motor development and integration; ultimately building the body image and developing the self-concept" (p.1). Sensorimotor activities combine full-body movement and the sensory input that such movement provides. Perception refers to the meaning the brain gives to the sensory input, through the process of organizing or interpreting the raw data obtained through the senses. Perceptual-motor integration involves the interaction of the various channels of perception (visual, auditory, tactile and kinesthetic) with motor activity.

As in work with children with mental illness, Erfer stresses the importance of the body image, seeing it as one of the most fundamental concepts in human growth and development and one that appears to be lacking in children who are autistic. She cites Schilder's (1950) definition of body image as the three-dimensional picture or image of our own body that we form in our mind. Without a body image, a symbol of one's own body:

> ... the psychic structures necessary for symbolic representation of other things cannot be formed, since they depend on previous symbolization. Consequently, the autistic child develops no words to form ideas; he cannot make the bridge from the concrete to the abstract; [and] is functionally unaware of object, self or world. (Dratman & Kalish, 1967, p. 7)

Erfer (1995) states:

> Body image has a physiological basis. It is based on input from various systems: vestibular, kinesthetic, proprioceptive, tactile and visual. The development of body image parallels sensorimotor development, which forms the basis for the sense of self, cognitive development, the acquisition of self-help skills and many basic concepts. (p.197)

Erfer sees Schilder's (1950) correlation between movement and the body image as especially applicable. Schilder writes, "movement leads to a better orientation in relation to our own body ... [and] movement is a great uniting factor between the different parts of our body" (p.112). Schilder also says that in order to build a body image we have to know where our limbs are and we must also be aware of the relationship of different body parts to each other. Schilder maintains that movement experiences can lead from a change in body image to a change in the psyche. This has become the cornerstone for much dance movement therapy work.

Erfer further states that children with autism must be helped to understand their bodies and their capacity for movement before they can cope with the external demands of the environment. "In other words, unless there is a sense of oneself as a separate entity, differentiated from others, one cannot effectively or 'affectively,' relate beyond oneself" (Erfer, 1995, p.198).

In a similar manner to Kalish-Weiss and many other dance therapists, especially those who work with children, Erfer describes the initial goals of therapy as: reaching the child at the level at which he or she seems to be functioning (what Erfer calls the sensorimotor level); establishing a relationship; and working toward the formation of a body image. These goals are concurrent and ongoing (Erfer, 1995).

Erfer uses mirroring to establish a connection with these children. Mirroring gives the therapist valuable information about these children that might not be discovered otherwise and also conveys to them the important message that they are being accepted just as they are. Erfer stresses that mirroring is not imitation. It is a deeper and richer experience of making genuine contact and engaging the child through movement. This rapport conveys a deep acceptance. "Such acceptance often causes a child to shift his or her focus from inner stimuli to stimuli in the environment, which then leads to increased connectedness and paves the way for reciprocal interactions" (Erfer, 1995, p.199).

Erfer's group work includes activities or interventions that involve basic sensory awareness, body parts awareness, movement dynamics, locomotor movement and eventually more expressive movement. In addition, experiences that involve tactile stimulation, identification of body parts and boundaries and visual-kinesthetic awareness development (which are strengthened by having children alternate between moving and observing others move) all serve to help these children develop self- and body-awareness.

Erfer also utilizes a process called "sensory integration," which provides additional opportunities for body-image formation.

> Sensory integrative therapy includes full-body movements that provide vestibular, proprioceptive and tactile stimulation, offering pleasurable sensory experiences to otherwise overstimulated or isolated children. The goal is to improve the way the brain processes and organizes sensations, so that the various parts of the nervous system work together to enable a person to interact with the environment effectively and experience appropriate satisfaction. (Erfer, 1995, pp. 199-200)

According to Erfer, sensory integrative therapy, like dance movement therapy, starts at the child's current level of functioning. Theoretically, a child cannot progress to a higher or more complex level of functioning until the prerequisite skills at the preceding level have developed (Levy et. al, 1995).

Erfer also uses music and props. Further information about Erfer's approach and a discussion of Erfer's work in a public school system can be found in *Dance and Other Expressive Art Therapies: When Words Are Not Enough* (Erfer, 1995).

Part G. Children Who Have Been Sexually Abused

Dance movement therapy stresses the nonverbal expression of experiences and for this reason it is especially suited for the treatment of the sexually abused child. Generally, it is difficult for children to talk about feelings related to sexuality. It becomes even more difficult to discuss these feelings if the child was sexually abused in early childhood, particularly if the abuse occurred prior to the child's development of language and conceptualization and if the child has been threatened or made to feel guilty and responsible for the abusive acts.

For the child, dance therapy provides an arena for expressing feelings about sexual abuse, while circumventing the need to verbally describe the abuse. Through dance therapy, the abused individual can re-enact feelings and experiences with the guidance of a trained dance therapist, who helps to structure and direct the re-enactments in such a way as to reduce the patient's fear, anxiety and guilt over the experience. How the child or adult is helped to re-experience and reintegrate the trauma of childhood sexual abuse is key to how he or she will survive the experience (Weltman, 1986).

Case Example: Marsha Weltman

An article written by Marsha Weltman (1986) is reviewed here as an example of dance therapy with this population. In her article, Weltman describes her work with children who have been sexually abused at the Neuropsychiatric Institute in Los Angeles and reviews the special problems and specific treatment needs of this population.

Drawing from her clinical experience (five years working with sexual abuse) and her clinical studies of Finkelhor's (1985) "model of traumagenic dynamics" and Summit's (1983) "accommodation syndrome," Weltman has delineated four conflicted areas in the sexually abused child's development: sexual identity, self-esteem, relationship building and body image. In all of these areas, basic conflicts over control and power are present.

Weltman stresses the importance of establishing a relationship of trust with the children. This is essential if they are to open up and share with an adult (the therapist) the pain, fear, anger and humiliation of their experiences. In this connection, the therapist must listen to, believe and respond with empathy to what the children say, never pushing them to describe their experiences in any greater detail than they are ready for. Any form of coercion will break the trust and will be experienced by the children as an additional violation.

One key element in establishing and maintaining trust is providing the children with a sense of security. Weltman states, "It is essential to tell the children that they deserve to be protected [they are the innocent victim] and are worthy of being loved" (1986, p. 55). In addition, the therapist must make it clear from the beginning that they will not be harmed in any way. Special signals between dance therapist and child should be designed to communicate if and when touch is going to be used in the session. This gives sexually abused children the power to control their bodily experiences and exposures and provides them with the feeling of personal power and control that had been taken from them.

Because of the children's need to feel they have some control over the therapeutic process, Weltman recommends "self-directed process oriented sessions" (p. 56), in which the children are allowed the space and time to move on their own with the encouragement and empathic support of the therapist. "Concrete experiences involving body awareness and [the] free exploration of personal and interactional space can restore integrity on a body level, at the core of their being" (Weltman, 1986, p. 56).

Weltman provides several case examples that illustrate self-directed process-oriented sessions. One example is the case of Edward, a nine-year-old who had been molested by a babysitter. In a group session in which the other children were playing spontaneously with Weltman by flopping in her lap, Edward withdrew. After engaging in frequent eye contact with Edward, Weltman motioned for him to join the game. Wanting to join but at the same time afraid of being hurt, Edward was motivated to express his conflict verbally by asking the therapist, in his own words, whether she would sexually assault him if he joined in the game. Weltman responded to his fears by firmly stating "... adults don't get sexual with children around here" (1986, p. 59). This stimulated Edward to take play items and push them together, acting out sexual intercourse. To this physical manifestation Weltman responded by clarifying Edward's concerns. She helped him label one play toy the adult and one the baby and then said, "That adult must be confused. When adults are sexual with children they are confused and need help" (1986, p. 59). Here, Weltman was trying to relieve Edward of his guilt over being molested.

In another case example, she describes how Daniel, a seven-year-old boy who had been molested by an older man, was mobilized by an evocative game to act out his sexual invasion. The physicality of the game, in which the children in Weltman's group would roll up in a blanket and rock themselves, finally provoked Daniel to foist himself on one of the boys and symbolically act out his homosexual encounter. This enabled him to express nonverbally something that had been confusing and troubling to him.

Since Daniel's acting out of his emotions involved an imposition on another group member, Weltman had to step in and put limits on the movement process. She asked Daniel if anyone had done that to him. He said that someone had and indicated it was a friend. Weltman then tried to help Daniel explore other forms of expressing friendship and warmth without sexualizing these feelings. In this way, she encouraged insight and clarification in place of physical acting out and thus helped Daniel to integrate his emotions and actions in new and more agreeable ways. This was done with warmth and understanding and was further supported by the group process.

For Melissa, age seven, sexual feelings, associations and vocalizations were evoked by small movements of her toes and relaxation movements, which involved tightening and releasing buttock muscles. At the end of her first dance therapy session, she drew a broken heart on the blackboard and printed the words "Sex Ed."

Melissa was anxious to talk about "Sex Ed" when she arrived at the second session but Weltman encouraged her to move first. She began with her usual small movements, wiggling her toes and then exclaimed, "It feels weird. It feels like a banana. It feels like a nail" (Weltman, 1986, p. 61). Weltman describes what followed:

> Suddenly her movements became increasingly large, rapid and strong, as she began kicking and screaming frantically. I moved closer carefully, in order to support and focus her expression. When Melissa stopped, I asked what was happening. She replied that it was disgusting and she felt angry.... (1986, p. 61)

Melissa went on to describe the act of being forced to watch sexual acts and then being abused. Weltman listened to every detail with belief and acceptance of the child, reflecting Melissa's own feelings back to Melissa through her (Weltman's) nonverbal and verbal communications. By reflecting the child's feelings, she facilitated Melissa's obvious need to re-enact what had been done to her in a variety of movement configurations. After her re-enactments, which were guided by questions and responses from Weltman, Melissa would climb into Weltman's lap to be cradled and rocked. This emotional support and the feeling of trust and security were clearly essential to the success of Melissa's treatment.

In her work with abuse, Weltman integrates the expression of thoughts, feelings and memories provoked by movement and play with the development of a trusting, reflective and nonpunitive relationship in which she takes an actively protective role in the abused child's life.

Work with Adopted Children Who Have Been Sexually Abused: Steve Harvey

Steve Harvey (1995) is a licensed psychologist working privately with young children and their families in Colorado Springs. He teaches and consults on family issues involving abuse and adoption throughout the United States and Europe.

Harvey (1995) used expressive arts therapy to work with an adopted child who had been abused, as described in "Sandra: The Case of an Adopted Sexually Abused Child." The following extracts from his chapter in *Dance and Other Expressive Art Therapies: When Words Are Not Enough* (Levy, et al., 1995) illustrate further how dance and games can help sexually abused children learn to develop trusting relationships with others.

Harvey, citing McNamara (1989), asserts that sexual abuse of children in foster care is common. McNamara estimates that by the time foster care children reach school age, approximately three out of four have experienced some form of sexual abuse. Therefore, it is not uncommon for adopted children to have been abused in previous foster care or family situations. In addition, McNamara (1989) and Ryan (1989) point out that the practice of avoiding past issues in adoptive processes can have significant negative consequences on the adoptive family. Young children who have been sexually abused prior to their adoptive placement experience ongoing feelings of betrayal and mistrust.

Harvey stresses the importance of creative arts therapies, which can address problems of previous abuse in adopted children. Through expressive arts, the parents and child can engage in joint activities that facilitate emotional expression and interaction without relying on language. He states, "As young children begin to trust their new parents, they may also begin to identify past episodes of abuse. These disclosures are a by-product, rather than a direct goal of the therapy process" (Harvey, 1995, p. 168).

Harvey used the creative arts in the following summarized case study, in which a 3-1/2-year-old girl, Sandra, has the symptoms suggestive of sexual abuse. While Harvey did not ask Sandra direct questions, after approximately a year of therapy, which was spent on improving mother-child and family-child interactions, she made unprompted statements to a social service evaluator who later confirmed that the assault had taken place.

The following is a description of the girl's initial presentation:

> Mr. and Mrs. Robinson were referred for expressive therapy with Sandra, their 3-1/2-year-old foster-adoptive daughter, shortly after Sandra was placed with them.
>
> In the initial interview, Mrs. Robinson described a number of difficulties. Sandra constantly moved and talked and ignored almost all verbal direction. She woke up two or three times a night and was unable to go back to sleep for several hours. She masturbated in front of her parents and other children and stopped only when Mrs. Robinson picked her up, held her and removed her from the room. Sandra confided in

> Mrs. Robinson that other unnamed adults had touched her "pee-pee." When Sandra did play, however, she could entertain herself for hours without seeming to need adult attention or socialization with other children....
>
> In the following three sessions, Sandra and her adoptive mother were asked to complete movement games, dramatic play and a series of drawing activities. The games included follow-the-leader and a mirroring activity and both Sandra and her mother were to take turns leading....
>
> During both mirroring and follow-the-leader, Sandra became very distracted, darting quickly from one part of the room to another. She was unable to take turns and did not allow Mrs. Robinson to lead. Mrs. Robinson was able to engage her daughter fleetingly only by following Sandra's movements.... This resembled a game of "chase," rather than follow-the-leader and Mrs. Robinson was frustrated after a few minutes of trying to lead Sandra verbally. No positive feelings showed from either mother or daughter. (Harvey, 1995, p. 171)

Harvey used his observations on the interactions between Sandra and her mother to establish initial treatment goals. "The central idea was to help the adoptive mother and her child develop play that enabled an exchange of genuine feelings. Once interaction could be established through games, the goal would be to help Sandra and her adoptive parents express their deeper feelings" (Harvey, 1995, p. 172).

Harvey used a series of play activities to increase the ability of Sandra and her mother to communicate and connect with each other. In the game, "Sandraland and Momland," Harvey prompted mother and daughter to create two different spaces made of pillows about ten feet apart, from which they could mirror each other's movements. "When Mrs. Robinson and Sandra were in these defined spaces, activities were more successful" (Harvey, 1995, p. 173).

After the first few months of treatment, Sandra herself introduced new aspects to Harvey's games, including "Tug-of-War," in which Sandra and her mother played a tug of war game between the Sandraland and Momland and "Chasing Away the Monster." In this game, Sandra and her mother used similar gestures to chase away a ghost/monster that the therapist physicalized with the help of scarves and pieces of cloth. "In this game, Sandra and her mother developed a metaphor with which to address Sandra's underlying fears and her need for protection.... Sandra and her mother were increasing their connection to each other" (Harvey, 1995, p. 175).

As Sandra's therapy began to progress, Sandra described past abuse and chose safe games to play with her mother. During this time, Sandra frequently became afraid when talking about the abuse and asked Mrs. Robinson to hold her (Harvey, 1995).

> All the sexual assaults by both her birth mother and father described by Sandra occurred in the bathtub. Sandra reported that other adults were also involved. She spoke of threats, including kidnap and murder, to keep her from revealing these secrets....
> During this period of disclosures, Sandra compulsively masturbated at home and at school; in front of her peers or family.... Finally, just before her fifth birthday, Sandra reported her abuse fully to a Department of Social Services worker. After the interview, Sandra used the "Chase Away the Monster" game to help reduce her anxiety.... Sandra and Mrs. Robinson both experienced intense feelings during this enactment. Sandra again was fearful and Mrs. Robinson was focused, intent and serious when dancing away the monsters. (Harvey, 1995, p. 178)

Harvey used other games to help Sandra deal with how she felt as a result of the abuse.* Therapy was terminated approximately 2-1/2 years after it had begun. Harvey states that the relationship between Sandra and her parents had clearly changed and that Mrs. Robinson was able to play a more protective and nurturing role in her daughter's life. In addition, Sandra felt closer and more connected with her family. Harvey states: "Finally, on a movement level, Sandra and her adoptive parents were able to develop a matching in their interactions and some sense of calmness and relaxation with physical closeness" (Harvey, 1995, p. 180).

Summary—Acknowledging Norma Canner

In this chapter, the use of dance movement therapy with children and adolescents has been traced through

---

*For a more in-depth discussion of Harvey's treatment process, consult *Dance and Other Expressive Art Therapies: When Words Are Not Enough* (Levy, et. al., 1995).
It is interesting to note that the goals and many of the methods described in this section can also be helpful to adults, depending on their development needs. The following chapter will discuss this further.

the innovative work of practitioners in the field. From different perspectives, they have made contributions to the profession and are respected for their collaborations within schools and with families. As in work with adults, the first priority of dance therapists working with children is to establish trust and empathy, creating a safe environment where the children can relate to themselves and others in order to become more comfortable in their own bodies. Inherent in genuine empathy is the idea of starting at the child's developmental level, a general concept that is reiterated often.

Helping children develop an accurate, strong and delineated sense of their body is a major goal of this work. Many methods are used to this end, including interactions, touch, the exploration of movement fundamentals and props that broaden and embellish movement dynamics. In this chapter, a crucial theme is "structure." Some therapists use games or mirror movements, while others teach techniques or patterns of dance. Structure provides protective boundaries for children, allowing them to express themselves with ever-increasing freedom.

We must conclude this chapter by recognizing dance movement therapy pioneer, Norma Canner. She wrote the groundbreaking *...and a time to dance* in 1968, one of the earliest books on creative methods with children. Since the 1950s, she has been acknowledged as an innovator in the practice of early intervention and mental health programs for children with either physical or emotional disabilities, as well as with healthy children. Canner greatly influenced the work of William Freeman and Nancy Beardell, who were both discussed earlier. For a detailed exploration of Canner's contributions to the dance movement therapy field, please refer to Chapter 23.

SECTION B

Adults

19 Individuals in Psychiatric Care

Not all individuals can express themselves through verbal language. For some, thoughts and feelings can be processed more fully when permitted somatic expression. One often finds this when working with psychiatric patients, who frequently have been hospitalized because people could not speak with them "in their language."

As discussed earlier, Marian Chace was the first to initiate direct communication with psychiatric patients via dance in the 1940s. Other early pioneers, notably Schoop and Rosen, began working with this population in the 1950s. Today, hospitals and community mental health clinics throughout the United States are recognizing and including dance therapy as a part of their total treatment program for psychiatric patients.

The Therapist/Patient Relationship

The therapist/patient relationship is an essential part of dance therapy with all populations. With hospitalized psychiatric patients, developing this relationship can be a particularly trying process, especially for new dance therapists. Susan Sandel (1980), a former student of Chace and an important writer in the field, believes that without self-examination, supervision and peer support, the new therapist may be prone to feelings of frustration, self-doubt and emotional exhaustion.

Emotional Stress on the Therapist

Working with hospitalized patients with schizophrenia, Susan Sandel (1980) contends, is difficult and demanding, often with little to show in the way of progress and personal reward. In response to this it is not unusual for a new dance therapist to act in a defensive and/or compensatory manner to guard against feelings of anger and hopelessness. This denial is considered natural by Sandel and at times necessary if the therapist is to sustain his or her commitment to the treatment. However, Sandel warns, it is imperative that the new therapist understand how these same mechanisms may also be detrimental in a therapeutic situation.

For example, the therapist may see some glimpse of a behavior that he or she believes represents change or growth and may exaggerate the importance of this behavior. The danger here is that the therapist may think the patient is capable of more than is actually the case. These expectations often arise as a partial defense against frustration, but can in turn produce feelings of discouragement and anger when regression occurs. Sandel reminds us that schizophrenics demand intense emotional involvement and at times the dance therapist may feel he or she is being devoured by the patient's needs. Since in dance therapy the therapist and patient move together, frequently involving close physical contact, the therapist's emotional connection is a necessary part of the treatment. While empathy demonstrates an acceptance of the patient and may provide a glimpse into his or her inner world, it can leave the dance therapist feeling disoriented and depleted in addition to experiencing compelling desires, even omnipotent thoughts of curing the patient. In essence, the dance therapist may find him or herself vacillating between feelings of omnipotence and despair. All of these reactions need to be sorted out if the dance therapist is to remain effective.

One form that transference takes for the patient with schizophrenia is viewing the dance therapist as either the "good" or the "bad" mother. Sandel gives an example of each and discusses the resulting counter-transference phenomena.

In one of her sessions, issues of the "good" mother and nurturance were acted out when a patient briefly sucked Sandel's thumb. At the close of the session, the patient was reluctant to talk about the incident but did say she may have been feeling like a baby. Later, with help from her psychotherapist, she realized that she wished Sandel were her mother.

Sandel felt that by tolerating and understanding her own anxiety resulting from counter-transference feelings, she was better able to accept the patient's behavior without making it an uncomfortable issue for the patient. Hence, the productiveness of the treatment was enhanced.

There will also be times when the dance therapist is viewed by the patient with schizophrenia as the "bad" mother. At these times the patient may try to frustrate the dance therapist by refusing to dance. Sandel gives the example of one of her patients who lay face down on the floor throughout her sessions for more than a year. Nothing would rouse her. Each week the therapist would talk to the patient prior to the session asking her to join and the patient would say "OK," but then proceed to lie on the floor. One day, she stood up and began moving. After that day, still participating, she would remind the therapist of her prior behavior and say with a grin "It made you mad, didn't it?" (Sandel, 1980, p. 28). Sandel experienced intense counter-transference tensions resulting from the patient's earlier negative transference, that is, the bad mother. While she was pleased that the patient was now moving, each time the patient reminded her of her earlier resistance that had lasted one year, Sandel found herself experiencing fury. Both negative and positive transference phenomena produce stress for the therapist. Self-examination, supervision and support are vital.

Finally, Sandel believes that individuals with schizophrenia are intuitively aware of therapists' investment in their medium and the resulting feelings of vulnerability as to their effectiveness. Patients can lead therapists to doubt their own value by a verbal attack, such as "This is dumb. It isn't therapy." The therapist must guard against defensive explanations and/or putting on a show as both behaviors expose the therapist's self-doubt, confuse the transference and destroy objectivity in the treatment situation.

Joan Lavender's (1977) description of her work with Nick, a 43-year-old patient diagnosed as chronic undifferentiated schizophrenic, further illuminates the difficulties faced by new dance therapists trying hard to use their art therapeutically. Lavender's account traces not only Nick's progress, but also her "growth as a young therapist learning to trust the dance process as a most powerful enhancer of the therapeutic relationship" (p. 123).

Lavender felt her work during the first year with Nick was "artless and mechanical" (1977, p. 125) and the sessions were "either pre-structured and ineffectual or chaotic or both" (1977, p. 126). She believed she was responding to Nick's movement strengths and weaknesses rather than seeing him as a whole person. Furthermore, she states:

> I distinctly felt that I was not yet using dance, but isolated and therefore awkward movement exercises instead. I could not get Nick to stop imitating my movements; but then, neither could I stop seeing him as an incomplete person. Because we both felt this inequality, we were not free to dance. (1977, p. 127)

During the second year, the therapist-patient relationship began to grow and as a result "the dancing deepened" (Lavender, 1977, p. 128). Lavender played more of an empathic role, moving with the patient and supporting his movement style. She became familiar with his movements and gestures and with the meanings they conveyed. Later, she began to use her own variations in responding to his dance. The sessions were less contrived and Nick began to create themes of his own. Improvisational dance was a major part of the sessions and role-playing often emerged from it.

As the therapy continued into the third year and the therapist-patient relationship continued to grow, Nick's self-confidence increased and he began to stand more upright. He also, at times, began to speak more coherently. As Lavender puts it, "word thinking and movement thinking were becoming integrated" (1977, p. 128).

Throughout her account of her work with this patient, Lavender stressed the importance of allowing the dance process to unfold naturally and the patient's dependence on the dance therapist's comfort in the movement relationship.

I came to understand that dance provides its own structure, according to the thoughts and feelings of the dancer. It is the emotional context of the dance that motivates the dancer to expand his/her movement-emotional world. Nick would assume his true height when something in the dance inspired him to unfold. He would breathe deeply only when the dance demanded it. He would command the space he moved through only when our dance would evoke such commanding feelings in him. A trusting relationship would nurture these new feelings. (1977, p. 128)

Issues of Space and Separation/Individuation

Joan Naess Lewin (1982) discusses the link between the patient/therapist relationship and the developmental stages discussed in object relations theory. Although these stages are not always clear, she believes that understanding development can help to make sense of the intense feelings aroused in both patient and therapist in movement interactions. In the following case material, Lewin's developmental framework is illustrated in two ways: through the growth of the relationship between patient and therapist and through demonstration of the level of psychological functioning, which the patient had attained.

The first case described Ann, age 23, diagnosed chronic undifferentiated schizophrenic. It was clear that Ann was in the autistic stage during her first dance therapy session. Her movements at this point were stretching, rolling, sliding, crawling, climbing and collapsing. Ann made no attempt at eye contact and appeared to consider the presence of the therapist an intrusion. Future sessions appeared to be transitional. Although no eye contact was attempted, patient and therapist worked side-by-side, stretching and releasing. Ann spent months in this transitional stage, which Searles (1961) has called "ambivalent symbiosis," a period during which she wished for and yet was terrified of fusion with the therapist. The patient broke new ground for herself developmentally when she entered into the symbiotic stage, the point at which her maturation had previously been arrested. During this phase, Ann accepted eye and physical contact and began requesting back rubs. As the therapy progressed, Ann began to initiate push and pull movements with the therapist, suggesting, Lewin believed, the beginning of the separation-individuation phase. Unfortunately, this coincided with her release from the hospital to a halfway house.

In the second case study, Lewin described her work with Vera, age 21, diagnosed borderline personality disorder. Vera came from an old world "proper" background and felt isolated as she was considered a snob by the other patients. She appeared limp, depressed and frightened, with an overanxious desire to please. She felt unworthy of her relationship with Lewin whom she over-idealized.

Vera would stretch with the therapist or on her own, simply because she was requested. She was not ready to communicate the feelings underneath the compliance. Slowly, by using relaxing music and lazy stretches, rolls and curls, the facade began to fall away and Vera entered the symbiotic stage. At this time, she allowed the therapist to playfully slide her and eventually the two achieved synchronicity of movement while rocking, spinning and expanding and contracting body shapes.

Vera was comfortable in symbiosis but had to be pushed by her dance movement and verbal therapists to confront her good and bad object splitting in order to progress to the separation/individuation phase, her level of psychological arrest. Vera's entry into that phase became apparent when she began exploring her own body movements, expressing her emotions verbally and nonverbally and becoming playful in the sessions.

Sandel (1982) also writes about patients' developmental stages, referring specifically to group dance therapy with patients suffering from schizophrenia. She finds numerous examples in the dance therapy literature of therapists forming symbiotic attachments with their regressed patients, using mirroring and rhythmically synchronous movements. Less attention has been devoted, she notes, to the therapeutic relationship with patients in the separation and individuation stage of development.

Citing the work of Kestenberg, Mahler and Spitz, Sandel postulates that just as different mothering styles are required at the different stages of child development, so are varying therapeutic styles needed at different stages of patient development. However, because the early developments of the profession took place largely in work with the schizophrenic population, many "classic" dance therapy techniques are based on the symbiotic needs of this population, but are less effective or even counterproductive when used with patients not in this stage. Techniques such as the circle structure and continuous unison movement can block a patient's experiments in autonomy. Rather than signifying a "good" dance therapy session, a group of patients with chronic schizophrenia moving synchronously in a circle may indicate excessive "dependence, compliance and apathy." (Sandel, 1982, p. 13)

In order to facilitate separation/individuation, Sandel (1982) makes the following suggestions. The technique of sharing the leadership role among the patients is ideal for fostering patient autonomy. However, this too can be subverted by the therapist if not done sensitively. If the therapist interrupts with strong verbal and movement suggestions to the patient "leader," the therapist will communicate that although she has delegated the leadership, she does not find the patient capable in this role.

The therapist may also intervene prematurely in an attempt to prevent boring or anxious moments. This does not allow the patients time to struggle with mastery, so they cannot learn and progress. On the other hand, the therapist should not abandon the patient, who depends upon his or her structure for a sense of safety and caring. It is indeed a delicate operation to provide a balance of support without intrusiveness.

Sandel points out that patients may be capable of participating in extended improvisations, requiring little external structure. They may work in small groups, lines or around the entire room. They may pair off, preferring peer interaction to that with the therapist. They may ask for specific exercises for weight control and fitness. Role-playing and dramatic techniques may also be used to foster differentiation, through practicing assertive behavior and experimenting with unfamiliar situations and roles.

Sandel (1973), who stresses that the therapist must respond to the patient's need for distance after periods of intimacy, also points out the importance of personal space. Bovard-Taylor and Draganosky (1979) have also written of the importance of personal space in fostering both the therapist-patient relationship and the therapeutic process. From their clinical experiences, they make the following suggestions: 1) allow the patients to feel that they can be in control of the space; 2) be sensitive to changes; 3) be alert to misunderstandings; 4) accommodate personal space preferences; and 5) respond verbally or nonverbally to signs of comfort or discomfort.

The Case of Jay

In a case study, Arlynne Stark (Samuels, 1972) discusses how Sharon Chaiklin helped a patient to break through his isolation, express his emotions, take control of his personal space and relate to his environment. Jay was a 21-year-old male whose diagnosis was catatonic schizophrenia and mental retardation. According to tests, he was mentally four years and five months old. He attended individual sessions for three months, one hour weekly.

Chaiklin's work focused on the following physical goals: helping Jay to move with more strength and quickness; encouraging deeper breathing; improving his ability to control his body; relaxing his physical defenses; and encouraging his use of verbalization. Through the therapeutic relationship Chaiklin was attempting to bring him out of his withdrawal and reduce his emotional defenses and physical rigidity.

Jay kept his eyes closed and his body rigid and was mute in the beginning of sessions. His process in the therapy was like a puzzle being put together. Through the twelve sessions, the rigidity of each body part was unlocked, until the whole could move fluidly and in unison. The following is an overview of this process.

Chaiklin focused first on the strength and depth of the patient's breathing. Soon he initiated the breathing exercises himself and by the fifth session was able to breathe out with force and strength.

She used many props to increase the range of Jay's movements. She explained that initially she chose to use props because of his ostensibly low IQ. As they worked together, she came to regard Jay's impairment as emotional rather than cognitive in origin and exacerbated by lack of education. However, she continued the use of props because he responded well to them, creating games and increasing his use of space. A stretch rope, for example, gave him his first opportunity to stretch his arms out to each side; hoops were used to rotate and relax his tense right arm and became the basis of the "space game" wherein he and Chaiklin attempted to block each other in moving around the room. Streamers encouraged rhythmic fluid movement and balloons called attention to the grasping motion of fingers. Props also encouraged him to keep his eyes open throughout the session—he had to watch where the hoop descended in order to catch it in mid-air.

As his relationship with the therapist deepened, he allowed himself to use strength to push and pull with his hands against hers or to lean against her and sway gently to the music. Eventually (session six) he began to assert himself, not allowing her to move him further than he wished, using his weight to say "no." Chaiklin encouraged Jay to create his own meaningful space through his movement interactions with her. Her respect for his needs helped Jay to trust the therapeutic relationship. She encouraged him to express both his needs for closeness and distance.

At about session seven, pure movement gave way to affect. The patient entered the room swishing and talked during the session. In the succeeding sessions, he laughed, cried and showed a range of feelings in his facial expressions for the first time.

In the last session of the study, Jay had begun to manipulate his movements to control his feelings, realizing that when a feeling surfaced from a movement, he could change the movement to change the feeling. He no longer had to resort to totally blocking out the environment by closing his eyes and making his body rigid. With Chaiklin's help he learned that he could be in charge of himself. Chaiklin gave him room to push, pull, lean, sway, block, grasp and stretch, all forms of defining and regulating his personal space and hence himself. Individual work with Jay continued after the twelve sessions of the study. Two months later he was able to participate in a news film demonstrating dance therapy. A movement observation scale created by Stark (Samuels) and Chaiklin was used to assess Jay's progress. It is useful for dance therapists who do not have extensive LMA training (Chaiklin, personal communication, 2003).

Group Interaction

Group work revolves around interaction among group members as well as the dance therapist's relationship with each patient and with the group as a whole. Helene Lefco's (1974) work with a group of six patients in an in-patient private clinic setting provides an illustration of the group process.

Lefco begins with two group structures only, the circle formation and warm-up movements. After this the spontaneous group interaction takes over and Lefco seems to ride the crest of the group's emotional wave.

For example, Lefco describes a dramatic scene where the patients, frustrated by their own emotional needs, spontaneously began to imitate one of the group members, Laura, an obese patient. The group proceeded to act out, through dramatic movement, the desire to gorge themselves with food. Laura at first was reticent, but eventually joined in. After much aggressive exaggeration of oral needs was acted out in unison, the group settled into a more passive contented state, which included rocking and sucking movements. "The room was quiet except for the subtle sounds of the music and the hungry suck of baby's mouths" (Lefco, 1974, pp. 35-36).

The creative and spontaneous aspect of Lefco's work presents itself most potently in the simultaneous interplay of dance and dramatic action with the ongoing verbal dialogue among the group participants. Lefco also interacts spontaneously, reflecting both verbally and nonverbally the feelings group members are expressing. She quickly changes the music to facilitate and accommodate the expression of feeling. Lefco's work reflects her courage in meeting the challenge of the unforeseen moment and giving the group a great deal of latitude for personal expression without judgment. She then creatively deals with the results of her permissive group structure.

Lefco's work is unique in that it is done in a small group setting at a private clinic located on acres of farmland, where the patients and staff live together as a family unit in small trailers. At the clinic, drugs and shock therapy are not part of the patients' treatment. This is significant in that many dance therapists have experienced the reliance on chemotherapy and shock treatment in some hospital settings as a hindrance to the dance therapy process, often rendering patients so lethargic that they have little energy left for body movement or self-expression.

Structural Analysis of Group Dance Therapy

David Johnson and Susan Sandel (1977) developed a system called the Structural Analysis of Movement Sessions (SAMS), a system still used today. It grew out of their work with adult psychiatric patients in dance and drama therapy groups. Johnson and Sandel describe SAMS as "both a vocabulary of group events and a method of analyzing aspects of the group's functioning" (p. 32). It is an important and unique contribution in that it focuses on the structural aspects of the group (i.e., the patterns of group activities) rather than on the content (i.e., what the activities are). The authors believe that generally the therapist tends to determine the structure while the participants define the content. Thus, "by analyzing and categorizing these structures," SAMS "may provide the therapist with a useful framework for thinking about his/her interventions" (Johnson & Sandel, 1977, p. 33). Specifically, SAMS defines 46 kinds of structures, which are divided into task ("the observable action and sound patterns of the group as a whole" (p. 33), space ("the physical relationship which the group members have to one another, i.e., the group formation" (p. 33) and role ("the particular pattern of formal roles that the group sets up in conducting the activity" (p. 33).

Johnson and Sandel then go on to describe its use in analyzing two dance therapy groups, both consisting of hospitalized psychiatric patients. They conclude:

> While SAMS has potential as a research device, perhaps its greatest immediate benefit to dance and drama therapy may be as a system for observing and thinking about groups and how they are functioning. It is our belief that SAMS has helped us in improving our clinical acuity and it has certainly helped us in communicating more clearly what occurs in our sessions. SAMS might provide valuable data for therapists in training to use in developing their group leadership skills. As it focuses attention on disruptions in the flow of the session, SAMS may help the therapist identify when such disruptions begin to occur and decide how to deal with them.... (1977, p. 36)

Johnson, Sandel and Bruno (1984) used SAMS to compare the efficiency of different amounts and types of structure in dance movement therapy groups with three populations: schizophrenic, character-disordered and normal. The authors' previous clinical observations had shown them that schizophrenic and character-disordered patients, often grouped together on a hospital unit, responded differently to the undifferentiated structure and flexible rules of the "classic" style dance movement therapy group.

Their hypothesis was that patients with schizophrenia, who tend to "have difficulties in maintaining clear...boundaries in their thinking and interpersonal relationships," (Johnson, Sandel, & Bruno, 1984, p. 417) would show a higher activity level in a dance movement therapy session with less-differentiated structure and tasks. Patients with character disorders, who tend to have "rigid, inflexible ego boundaries," would show a higher activity level in a session with clear differentiation and structured tasks. Normal subjects, with whom most previous research had dealt, would be active in both types of session structure.

Three different therapists led one group of each population (schizophrenia, character-disordered, normal) in two dance movement therapy sessions. Session 1 was highly differentiated, using games with rules, a cloth prop and a specific order of activities. Session 2 was less differentiated, using spontaneous movement and development of images. Use of the circle and rhythmic unison movement were the only pre-planned aspects.

The videotapes were scored using SAMS. The results were consistent with the authors' expectations. The character-disordered groups responded to the less-differentiated session by dropping out, "challenging the therapist to set limits' (Johnson, Sandel, & Bruno, 1984, p. 426) or getting into conflicts with each other. They did not want to hold hands or stay in the circle. The authors believe these behaviors were motivated by the patients' fears of fusion and anxiety about intimacy.

The patients with schizophrenia became more anxious in the more-differentiated sessions. The rules confused them, while the character-disordered patients had made up new rules of their own.

The normal groups seemed most concerned with what was expected of them. Although they were bored by the less-differentiated session, they did not disrupt it.

The authors suggest that useful structures for the character-disordered population are: games with structured comings and goings from the circle; pair as well as whole group interaction; and competitive, not unison, activities. They believe that the structure of the group affects the therapist's efficiency, in that:

> Disruptive challenges to the therapist's leadership will probably be diminished if authority is located in complex rules rather than in the person of the therapist. (Johnson, Sandel, & Bruno, 1984, p. 427)

In another study, the leadership styles of dance therapists and their subsequent effects on normal, schizophrenic and character-disordered groups were the subject of a study by Johnson, Sandel and Eicher (1983). The authors do not believe that analysis of transference and countertransference phenomena alone can explain the patient's perception of and reaction to the dance therapist.

In the dance therapist's role as a group leader, he or she serves many managerial functions, including:

1. Maintaining the external group boundary;
2. Mediating the level of complexity in the group's tasks;
3. Controlling the group interaction and
4. Tolerating ambiguity and uncertainty. (p. 17)

Being in the unique position of facilitating therapy via a broad spectrum of action-oriented activities, the dance therapist is required to manage ever-changing group spatial arrangements and leader/follower roles. Thus, the individual in the dance therapy group (perhaps more than in verbal therapy groups) has a genuine reaction to the dance therapist as a group manager.

Using SAMS, the authors analyzed the reactions of the three patient groups to the management styles of three dance therapists and found a correlation between diagnostic category and preferred management styles. The findings corresponded with those of the 1984 study, discussed above, concerning the effects of different types of group structure. For example, the group with members who suffered from schizophrenia preferred leadership styles that evoked a well-defined, intimate social milieu, whereas the character-disordered patients preferred groups that avoided fusion and ambiguity. The authors speculate that the managerial style of the group leader evokes patterns of responses from participants "based on the degree to which the group corresponds to internalized configurations of familial interaction" (Johnson, Sandel, & Eicher, 1983, p. 28).

The overriding goal of the study appears to be less in establishing guidelines for dance therapy with specific patient populations than in clarifying the complex role the dance therapist plays transferentially and managerially. Johnson, Sandel and Eicher believe that "leadership style is a relatively stable configuration of behavior unless the therapist is actively and consciously attempting to alter it" (1983, p. 29). They conclude that the effectiveness of the dance therapy group can be enhanced through a deeper awareness by the dance therapist of his or her personal leadership style and its impact on different patient populations.

In another study, Sandel and Johnson (1983) examined group work with severely disturbed patients with schizophrenia and geriatric patients, believing that groups with severely disordered patients are substantially different from groups of higher functioning populations. The primary difference is a lack of group identity. Patients are so disoriented that they "often remain silent, do not know why they are there or feel that they have been forced to come for no reason" (Sandel & Johnson, 1983, p. 131). Because they do not hold an internal representation of the group, members cannot "become socialized ... to the group culture," lending their energies to help each other change. Thus, the therapist becomes the "container" of the group identity, since only he or she can connect to the participants in the group and to reality and can maintain a mental image of the group as a "group."

This places enormous pressure on the therapist who may react in a number of ways. He or she may become depressed before each group begins, knowing that without his or her presence, the group would disappear entirely! During the group, the therapist may be hypersensitive to any nuance of changing patient behavior, viewing it as a sign of progress. An outside observer would not even notice the change. After the group, the therapist may spend a great deal of time "processing" what happened, comparing it to the various theories, in order to reinforce his or her sense that the group really exists.

The authors coined the term "nascent groups" (Sandel & Johnson, 1983), connoting that their organization does not resemble groups usually discussed in the literature. They find that the group structure is stable, but that it does not develop, rarely even approaching the early formative stage of the other groups. The therapist's reactions to the group's characteristics are included as an essential part of the description of an experimental "nascent" group. The following is a discussion of the progression, of a nascent group, using SAMS.

The authors organized and videotaped a 10-session dance therapy group with 12 hospitalized patients suffering from schizophrenia. They then analyzed the sessions using SAMS, along with clinical observations obtained through the therapists' process notes, questionnaires and videotaped analyses.

The patients ranged in age from 31 to 60 and had been hospitalized numerous times for 10 to 30 years. None received intensive therapy. All were disheveled.

All forms of clinical analysis showed that the 10 sessions fell into three distinct phases. The first phase showed patients and therapists on their best behavior. The patients were compliant and curious about their new therapists. In the first session, the therapist served as the focus of attention as the patients touched her face and smelled her hair. Therapists were optimistic and enthusiastic.

In the second session, several of the male patients had responded to the videotaping by washing, shaving and dressing neatly. In the movement, aggression was expressed through kicking, with images of people upon whom the patients had been dependent in their lives.

Phase II began in the third session with the collapse of Phase I's high hopes. One patient dropped out, several resisted coming to the group; two men returned to their dirty, unshaven state. Movement included a tug of war game and unison walking around the circle with tiny steps. The second phase comprised the heart of the therapeutic work, as group members struggled to relate to each other. The authors' comment:

> Each advance toward intimacy was followed by a temporary retreat into unrelatedness, distancing and disruption of the sessions. (Sandel & Johnson, 1983, p. 136)

In session four, group members appeared to be aware of each other as individuals for the first time. They introduced themselves to each other in words and movements; they symbolically made a "fish stew," each member adding an imaginary ingredient.

Members retreated from the intimacy in session five by coming late to the session or, in several cases, refusing to come at all. The therapist felt pressured to entertain the patients. All were relieved to draw, in an exercise at the end of the session, which decreased the interpersonal contact.

The group moved toward intimacy again in session six with increased touching and a discussion of how difficult it is to maintain friendships in the hospital. One member acted out the group's anxiety over this closeness by behaving in a bizarre fashion. The author's interpretation of this was that the individual, not able to accept the group's intimacy, attempted to break up the experience and in so doing acted out the feelings of other group members as well.

In session seven, the therapists were active, pushing for greater interpersonal gains, but the patients were happy with simple synchronous movements. Several times they returned to the circle formation without direction from the therapist. The therapist initiated the image of building a sand castle; the patients changed it to a "sand pit" in which they could be buried. The authors interpreted this as the patients preferring fusion to the therapist's push for differentiation.

The eighth session preceded Easter vacation week when the group would not be meeting. Although the mood of the group was sad, the patients engaged in their highest level of closeness—doing deep breathing and giving each other back rubs.

The ninth and tenth sessions marked the termination of "dissolution" phase. Many members refused to come to the ninth session. A plastic sheet became "quicksand," which was unsafe to cross, as one could be "lost forever." The last session was chaotic, becoming organized only around the coffee and cake served at the end.

With prolonged contact with a caring therapist in a stable milieu, severely disturbed patients interrelate; functioning is stabilized and atrophy stopped. These groups must be regarded as long-term support systems, rather than as short-term intervention that will resolve problems (Sandel & Johnson, 1983).

Johanna Climenko (personal communication, 2002) documented work with seriously and persistently mentally ill women in a group that focused on self-esteem. She finds that using dance movement therapy along with more traditional social group work and verbalization helps patients to express themselves more fully. She emphasizes the importance of flexibility of movement styles and modulation of emotions through movement. Her group sessions are divided into a dance movement part and a verbal part.

The women ranged in age from 41 to 67 and had diagnoses ranging from affective disorders to chronic schizophrenia. An ethnically and racially diverse group, their family experiences differed. Some women had never been married, while others were grandmothers; some women lived in their own apartments, while others resided on hospital grounds.

Climenko finds modulation of emotion and behavior to be one of the most serious challenges facing these patients. During discussion, many patients equated strong feeling or expression with loss of control. Some group members had only experienced strong feelings in association with psychiatric disturbance.

Patients talked about their fear that if they were overcome with feeling, that meant they were "out of control" or psychotic. The notion of modulation was repeatedly explored by Climenko and used in the movement portion of the sessions.

Many group members experienced difficulty in modulating their movement. Jean's movement expression reflected her difficulty with modulation and presaged her themes throughout the sessions. She moved energetically, with phrasing that was dynamically and spatially complex. As soon as the movement spread through her body, however, she stopped abruptly, saying she felt dizzy. During dance movement therapy, Climenko tried to help Jean find ways to tone the movement down so she would feel more in control but still express her feelings.

The continuum of assertion to rage is also a major theme in work with modulation. Anger was perceived as dangerous by many patients. Group members frequently saw anger as manifest only in dramatic ways, most commonly when they were psychotic. Jean came to the group in crisis. She had been upset by her roommate for several months and had failed to share her feelings with anyone. Only when she was at a crisis point did she share how upset she felt. During a session she said, "I should pop her, just punch her in the face. That's what she needs." The group gave her feedback about the consequences of that kind of behavior. "You'd get thrown out of the residence. They might send you to the hospital. You might even go to jail."

A theme in the discussion sessions with the group became negotiating between saying nothing and reacting violently. In movement, Climenko worked on starting with strong, free-flowing impulses, which the women then learned to bind, so that the intensity of feeling could be felt and expressed in safe ways.

Patients became less threatened by their feelings of pain and anger and learned to handle the physical expression of these feelings. The use of movement modulation was an important factor in helping patients to feel comfortable with their emotions and make healthier choices regarding self-expression. The verbal part of the group further helped to give safe vent to their emotions (personal communication, 2003).

Climenko's work emphasizes the importance of movement flexibility, modulation and the use of movement as a vehicle for verbalization. A strong theme for most dance therapists working with this population is the role that movement plays in enabling individuals to articulate emotions otherwise unavailable. Climenko has been dedicated to working with this population for over 30 years and has taught in the United States and abroad.

Summary

Dance therapists generally stress the importance of the therapist/patient relationship in fostering growth for hospitalized patients, particularly when working in individual sessions. In group work, the importance of experimenting with various types of group structures and therapist leadership styles has also been emphasized. Special attention has been given to the many emotional stresses that this population places on the dance therapist, particularly stemming from transference and countertransference feelings.

In general, dance therapy with hospitalized psychiatric patients focuses on promoting body image, interaction, verbalization, modulation and self-expression. These goals coincide with the physical, social and emotional goals described by the early pioneers of dance therapy.

Sandel (personal communication, 2003) notes that today, individuals with severe disturbances are benefiting from the new and advanced psychotropic medications and therefore are able to live in the community with outpatient support and maintain a fairly good quality of life. Long-term in-patient treatment is used much less frequently.

20 Victims of Physical, Sexual and Emotional Abuse and Dissociative Identity Disorder (or Multiple Personality)

The following is an overview of dance therapy with adult patients who have been abused. The material has been abstracted from *Dance and Other Expressive Art Therapies: When Words Are Not Enough* (Levy et al, 1995). The patient populations to be discussed are multiple personality disorder sufferers, abused adults and battered women. Fran Levy, Bonnie Bernstein, Meg Chang and Fern Leventhal worked with these populations.

Multiple Personality Disorder (now termed Dissociative Identity Disorder)

Fran Levy's (1995) work with Rachel is an example of working with the effects of protracted abuse on the personality. In Rachel's case the abuse was emotional in the form of parental manipulation, removal and the use of rage to control a child's behavior. Levy had been working with Rachel through various art modalities for 12 years when she wrote the chapter entitled "Nameless: A Case of Multiplicity" (p. 7).

When Rachel first started therapy she was in her mid-twenties and working as a lawyer in finance. Early in treatment, Rachel presented her therapist with an incredible challenge, the challenge of an inner infant self that had been "living inside" Rachel for as long as she could remember. Essentially, the infant feelings remained suppressed until Rachel found someone she trusted enough to let this part of herself out. Because the infant part had been tucked away for so long without receiving the nourishment it needed (as explained by Rachel) she had never matured and was in pain.

After drawing a picture of a young girl and calling this girl "Nameless" Rachel revealed and began to discuss in ever increasing detail her internal experience of her child self. It soon became clear to Levy that she was working with an unusual form of multiplicity or Multiple Personality Disorder (today called Dissociative Identity Disorder). What made Rachel fascinating was her gradual and finally complete, awareness of her inner child as a distinct identity and her ability to creatively, through imagery, heal this child and help her to mature. Rachel spoke of the child always in third person.

Because this infant had been locked inside for so long, never acknowledged or identified by herself or her family, Rachel came to call this self, Nameless. Rachel explained to her therapist that Nameless had never been seen, in the deepest sense of the word and eventually she said that she needed someone to love and mirror this little self. As Rachel got over her initial feelings of shame and fear of rejection, she became unusually articulate and assertive about her needs. After seeing Levy for approximately three months, Rachel decided she wanted to adopt Levy as her therapy mom.

The combined use of the arts is especially helpful when trying to reach individuals who have become immobilized or fixed in different developmental stages. Many individuals experience themselves as divided into parts and this division is based largely on developmental experiences and ambivalent feelings. Often it is one or more traumatic events that create a dissociation of part of the self from consciousness (Braun, 1986; S. Levy, personal communication, 2000, Kluft, 1983; Putnam, 1989). The expressive arts approach to treatment lends itself to the clarification of different developmental stages, often referred to as inner selves and permits the dissociated identity to express itself creatively and symbolically.[1] This was the case with Rachel.

---

[1] See also Chapter 17.

The following is an excerpt from Levy's book (1995), which describes early sessions with Rachel.

> Although Rachel's early figure and animal drawings pointed in the direction of multiplicity and even possible multiple personality disorder, Rachel did not present alternate personalities during the first 2 months of treatment. In retrospect, her anxious pacing may have been expressive of the childlike feelings that were struggling to be released but were yet unidentified.
>
> At first Rachel only described Nameless' feelings and needs in a general way: "Nameless is cranky" or "Nameless is tired, she needs you." Later she began to talk about Nameless in more concrete terms—what Nameless did at home, the hour Nameless went to bed, the clothing she wore and the activities she enjoyed. When I asked Rachel if she actually saw Nameless in the room with us, she said, "I see her in my mind."
>
> Nameless' existence in treatment was expressed primarily through Rachel. She was spoken of in the third person: "Nameless needs to nurse." "Nameless is lonely." "Nameless is wearing her cute pink overalls." Within 3 months after Nameless emerged, her needs had become central in our sessions. If Rachel wanted to talk about her problems at work, Nameless gave her only so much time before she became visibly uncomfortable and irritable. Nameless made it evident whenever she was tired of "grown up talk." (p. 16)

At this time, Rachel's infant self was crying out for a mother figure to mirror and love her. Levy was confronted immediately with a challenge. She asked herself whether she should meet these compelling needs or if she should simply analyze the parental transference. Levy wondered if she could do something between or if she could do both. She found the thought of meeting Rachel's intense needs frightening and overwhelming, but to simply analyze the transference, while safe, seemed cold and inhuman in the light of Rachel's raw request for love and her battle against the shame these needs produced.

The answers to these questions were found largely through Rachel's own burgeoning creativity. With the help of Rachel's ability to use imagery to heal old wounds and create new "positive memories," and after much soul searching, Levy and Rachel together started out on a tumultuous journey. Through creative imagery, symbolic realization (S. Levy, personal communication, 2000) and movement, Levy, without ever touching Rachel, provided her with the nurturing she craved. The following excerpts taken from "Nameless: A Case of Multiplicity" (Levy, 1995, pp. 16-19) are an example of how this method worked and Levy's personal reflections on the process.

> Rachel progressed in treatment from talking about what Nameless was doing, wearing and thinking, to making specific requests, always in the third person, "Can you hold Nameless?" "Can she sit on your lap?" "Can she nurse?"
>
> Knowing that Nameless was an infant, I attended closely to Rachel's requests and spent considerable time trying to determine how best to respond. I reasoned: if Nameless lived in the safety of Rachel's mind and Rachel was able to reach Nameless through imagery and symbolization, perhaps I could also reach Nameless in this way. Perhaps I could find a way to speak to Nameless with Rachel's help. With this in mind, the next time Rachel said Nameless wanted to be nursed, I responded by saying, "Nameless is nursing now." Then, in a voice that sounded like a very young child, Rachel asked, "Is she in your lap now?" and I said, "Yes, she's in my lap now." None of this was acted out physically. With the help of Rachel's imagination, our dialogue continued.
>
> "Can you hold Nameless?"
>
> "I'm holding Nameless now."
>
> "What are you doing with her?"
>
> "I'm rocking her and stroking her hair."
>
> "Can she look into your eyes?"
>
> "Yes."
>
> "What does she see in your eyes?"
>
> "There is lots of love in them for Nameless."
>
> As our dialogue continued, Rachel's body relaxed and silent tears rolled down her face. Following these nursing sessions, Rachel's speech was more audible and articulate. After many repetitions of such mo-

ments, Rachel one day suddenly moved from lying in a fetal position to sitting up. She then unwittingly touched her belly as if to express contentment. As I watched these changes it was clear that Nameless was making a transition from a hungry, needy infant to a more mature and contented stage of development.

In a particularly significant session, Rachel asked, "Would you really hold Nameless?" This was a difficult question for Rachel to ask, as she believed herself to be profoundly unlovable. It was also a question I had anticipated and about which I had thought carefully long before she asked. I knew that Rachel's ability to ask for her needs to be met was a positive sign; yet, long-term ramifications for therapy had to be considered. Would it be helpful if I crossed over the line that distinguishes symbolic realization, which takes place through shared imagery, from the actual acting out of fantasy? .... Would it give her what she needed to grow or might it keep her in infancy? Might it seduce her away from trying to manage the difficulties of her adult life?

Because all of these ideas had already been considered, when the question came I said, "I don't think it would be a good idea for me to hold you in my lap. If I actually hold you, it might keep you a baby and prevent you from growing. I want Nameless to feel loved but I'm also aware of the rest of you and all of your different needs, not just Nameless' needs." I went on to explain, "Touch is very powerful. It could unintentionally constrict you." Rachel listened carefully to my words and seemed to understand that she was safe in her therapist's office and that her therapist would not attempt to either dominate or infantilize her as her mother had (pp. 17-18).

Even though Rachel's needs were intense, she had an extraordinary intelligence about what was healthy and safe for her. She understood the dangers of being swallowed up by a parental figure and said she was relieved to know that I would nurture her only in a fashion that would be safe ...

From our first attempt, it was clear that symbolic communication provided nurturance that was helpful to Nameless. In time, Rachel stopped asking to nurse and began to substitute images of bottle-feeding for breast-feeding. In much the same way as with nursing, I talked Rachel through the images of this more grown up source of nourishment. In time, even the bottle became less important to her and was replaced by symbolic hugs thrown playfully through the air—an activity that made Nameless giggle with joy. As time went on, Nameless also came to enjoy our singing together. She was growing up, weaning herself and moving from infant to toddler.

Nameless became increasingly comfortable with all of the playful gestures, love sounds and songs that are typical of a young child's interaction with parents. How, I wondered, was she so receptive to this language of love if she had not received it herself? Had she, somewhere in her past, experienced this quality of attention, perhaps prior to the birth of her brothers and before she attempted to assert her independence, thereby coming into conflict with her parents? Or, did she observe this behavior and take it in while watching her parents with her younger siblings? These questions cannot be answered at this time, but it is clear that she thrived from the experience of reparenting and she knew exactly what she needed (pp. 18-19).

Levy (1995) makes the following observations about the importance of the arts and nonverbal expression when treating victims of abuse who experience a fragmentation of the personality with dissociative states:

If we accept as fact that we carry pieces of our childhood with us, it is easy to understand why a variety of expressive modalities can help to elicit and clarify nonverbal experiences. We know that children tell us many things through play, art, dance and music that they may not be able to say in words. It follows that adults [especially those who have been traumatized], carrying aspects of their childhood with them, can also benefit from creative symbolic action.

... In the case of Rachel, a combination of movement, drawing, writing, music and symbolic realization gave expression to both the child and the infant Rachel had within. To keep Rachel solely in a verbal mode of expression would have limited her ability to experience and nurture the very young parts of herself ... In addition, because Rachel had not been allowed to express herself verbally as a child, she had stored many of her early feelings in art and symbol. In order for her to find these parts of herself, a number of expressive and symbolic activities were incorporated into her treatment. (p. 10)

In 2002, Levy continued to work with Rachel, but in a very different manner. Levy is in the process of completing a book on Rachel's growth written through excerpts from Rachel's diary intertwined with Levy's reflections.

For a thorough clinical discussion of the theory and methods that were used to support Rachel's early and most dramatic growth, the best source is *Dance and Other Expressive Art Therapies: When Words Are Not Enough*. In this book, work with Rachel is illuminated through an analysis of Rachel's drawings. Levy corroborated with psychologist Sidney Levy (no relation), a pioneer in projective drawing analysis, throughout her work with Rachel.

Finally, Levy explains, although it produced anxiety at first to take on the therapy mom role and stay aware of positive and negative transferences and counter-transferences, the work proved to be deeply satisfying and helpful. Today, Rachel functions as a highly successful and happy, integrated adult. Her therapy has taken many new directions including the building of an intimate relationship.

Edith Z. Baum

Another dance therapist who worked extensively with male and female adult victims of abuse who have Dissociative Identity Disorder is Edith Z. Baum. Baum worked in group dance therapy from 1985 into the late 1990s at the Institute of Pennsylvania Hospital in the Multiple Personality Disorder (MPD) unit. Baum collaborated with psychiatrist Richard Kluft (1983; 1991) who has specialized in the study and treatment of this disorder and who was also doing pioneering work at the Institute. MPD patients participated in dance therapy sessions for months to years.

The following excerpts from *Dance and Other Expressive Art Therapies: When Words Are Not Enough*, edited by F. Levy, et al. (1995, pp. 88-89) illustrates Baum's thoughts about the process of doing dance therapy in a group psychiatric setting with adult survivors of abuse who have a major dissociative disorder. Two case vignettes help to illustrate her work.

Eliciting Expressive Movement and Traumatic Material

> It is necessary that patients be encouraged to identify and express feelings without hurting themselves or others. Acting out needs to be contained. Once clear and supportive boundaries have been established and an environment for open feedback has been encouraged, patients can begin to learn new skills in managing the rages common to individuals with MPD.
>
> An example of eliciting expressive movement occurred when Randy, a relative newcomer to the group, fell to the floor in reaction to another group member's powerful expression of anger. Randy told the group that as a child she had never been allowed to express her feelings. At the next session she began to move gently and rhythmically and then began to stamp her feet. Next, she bent her knees and leaned backward and switched to another personality, a male [figure]. She brought her arm close to her side and quickly thrust it outward and lunged forward. Her whole body began to tremble and she retreated to a chair. The therapist suggested that the angry male alter ego step back and that Randy come forward. After a moment, Randy returned but was aware of what had happened and stated that she would have to punish herself for getting angry. The individual who had abused Randy as a child had not allowed her any display of anger. This inhibition had prevented Randy from expressing herself for many years. Her expression of rage came about as a result of the therapist's support ("all parts of the mind are welcome here") and her observation of a peer taking similar risks. (Baum, 1995, pp. 88-89)

Baum discusses the use of movement reflection to help a patient get in touch with repressed, often traumatic events. Reflecting a patient's movements can cause a spontaneous abreaction. Abreaction is a catharsis that accompanies the recollection of a repressed experience. Baum explains:

> ... Maya arrived at the movement group looking extremely anxious. She had just returned from a session with her doctor. During the warm-up she appeared preoccupied and had difficulty following others' movements. It was not until a peer suddenly began to initiate strong punches that Maya became involved. She replicated the angry movements, something she had never done before. As she punched, her eyes filled with terror. She clutched her throat, gasping that she had asthma and couldn't breathe. Maya was suddenly experiencing a spontaneous abreaction. During this she recovered a memory of having been sexually abused. While Maya punched at the air, she relived the traumatic experience. Behavior and sensation suddenly reassociated with affect and knowledge. The behavior was punching, the affect was rage and terror, the sensation was loss of breath and the knowledge was the memory of the abuse. (Baum, 1995, pp. 89)

Baum uses the BASK model, an acronym that stands for behavior, affect, sensation and knowledge (Braun, 1988a; 1988b). These are parallel processes. Dissociation is the separation of an idea or thought from consciousness. This separation can be mild or severe. Dissociation can occur in any one or more of the BASK dimensions. The example of Maya illustrates the reintegration of the self (BASK) through group movement interaction.

... movement stimulates the sensory motor components of repressed memories (the sensation and behavior dimensions of BASK). At the same time, increasing awareness of one's moving body supports the mastery of overwhelming affect. Although the fluid nature of movement stimulates both fear of disorganization and loss of control, it also has the potential for integration of feeling, thought and action. Alters emerge, making themselves known by movement patterns that tell different pieces of their stories. The validation received from the group's replication of these patterns can empower the patient regardless of which alter is moving. Images that spontaneously emerge during the group join kinesthetic sensation and slowly become connected to memories. This connectedness promotes a sense of personal autonomy and a gradual sense of integration. As one patient remarked, "This group is helpful because as I am able to reexperience the feelings that have been buried, I am able to begin to feel whole, rather than fractured into many pieces." (Baum, 1995, p. 89)

Work with Sexually Abused Patients

Bonnie Bernstein was trained by Blanche Evan and uses the Evan approach to dance therapy in her work with sexually abused women. Bernstein works in private practice in Palo Alto, California, and has specialized in survivors of sexual abuse for approximately 30 years, beginning with her work in New York City. Her chapter in Levy's book (1995) is an important historical as well as clinical contribution in that there is little written that integrates Evan's work with contemporary dance therapy practices. Since Evan did little to document her work, the writing of her protégés is invaluable. Bernstein's chapter clearly depicts Evan's technique and theoretical framework as it relates to the unique needs of the sexually abused person. Bernstein works with survivors of sexual trauma both individually and in groups.

The following is a brief discussion of this work:

> When a young girl or woman is sexually violated, she often experiences a trauma to every aspect of her being. As her body has been invaded, all normal physical and emotional boundaries have been disregarded. The combined psychological and physical impact of her experience may leave her with scars that alter her relationship to her body and to her world forever. Because dance therapy emphasizes the complex interaction of the psyche and the body, it provides an invaluable form of treatment for such women. (Bernstein, 1995, p. 41)

> Effective verbal therapy for the survivor emphasizes improving self-concept and working through painful memories. Treatment frequently includes improving relationship skills and changing the dissatisfying life-styles that may have evolved (Gil, 1988). In addition, dance therapy emphasizes improving the survivor's relationship to her body. Through movement she is helped to recognize and change the ways she uses, abuses or inhibits her body. In dance therapy the body becomes at once the vehicle for change and the focus of change, so that the client can begin to reclaim her body as an ally in her struggle toward health. (Bernstein, 1995, p. 42)

In describing her work with sexual trauma survivors, Bernstein states:

> My work emphasizes the individual client's autonomy and at the same time introduces the therapeutic assets of group interaction. Expressive movement serves as a diagnostic window, uncovering the client's history and its impact on her self-image and behaviors. The choreography of a dance therapy session based on the Blanche Evan Method introduces the client to a wide range of empowering tools inherent in the expressive body. Evan writes, "... to know her own body's gamut of movement and to make it the instrument for expressing emotions" (Benov, 1991). The client is helped to broaden her dance vocabulary and regains confidence in her creativity. She is supported in developing avenues for in-depth exploration of feelings and insight-oriented improvisations. This multi-dimensional approach opens powerful resources for growth and change.

> Each client enters therapy with a unique constellation of issues, strengths and therapeutic needs. There are, however, repeating themes that commonly arise in therapy with this population. These themes include unresolved issues of guilt, shame, dissociation, sexual dysfunction, problematic interpersonal relationships, unresolved developmental issues and the need for trauma resolution. I guide the client through experiences that address each one of these issues from a psychophysical perspective." (Bernstein, personal communication, 2002)

Following, Bernstein gives a description of a dance therapy group in which she addresses the survivor client's unresolved issues of guilt. The following passage is excerpted from *Dance and Other Expressive Art Therapies* (Bernstein, 1995). As in all sections of this book, all names, situations and identifying content have been altered to protect the confidentiality of the clients.

The rape survivor may come to treatment with feelings of guilt and responsibility about having been attacked (Brownmiller, 1975). The incest survivor, plagued by the aftermath of chronic abuse may believe that the sexual invasion was brought on by her own actions (Blume, 1991). One woman said, "If only I had run away when he said he had the knife, I might have prevented my rape." Another said, "My stepfather called me a sexy slut and said it was the way I moved that provoked him." In both cases, a reexamination of false assumptions helped to relieve guilt and self-condemnation (Bernstein, 1995, p. 50).

Residues of guilt are tenaciously retained in the survivor's body and may contribute to sexual inhibition, promiscuity, tension, inability to experience pleasure and fear of risk taking. Guilt may also manifest in the survivor's inability to trust her own choices and in an urgent need to remain in control. One approach is to focus on specific experiences that led to the guilty feelings. Another, as in the following session, is to focus on the survivor's body and to develop dance experiences that free the survivor from the physical restrictions that represent the guilt (Bernstein, 1995, p. 50).

In the first phase of this particular session, group members talked about how they inhibited themselves in their lives. Over and over guilt was identified as the root of the self-restricting behaviors and of decreasing self-trust. The discussion of guilt led to a focus on "letting go" physically. We began with mobilization directives. A series of full-bodied swing progressions were used to release muscular tension, to feel the spontaneity associated with building momentum and to invigorate numbed body areas. Frequently the survivor of sexual abuse numbs and constricts feelings and actions within the body. These symptoms are often routed in unconscious associations and guilt. Although the group members showed new freedom of movement in their dances, a consistent lack of resiliency in their knees and legs restricted full hip and pelvic action. Functional Technique (see Chapter 2) exercises for the knees and legs were introduced to encourage both loosening and strengthening. Releasing physical restrictions enables the expression of qualities such as assertion and sensuality which guilt may have inhibited. The group ended with a dance to Middle Eastern music, which integrated resilient knee action with full hip and pelvic movement. These movements encouraged locomotion through space without inhibition (Bernstein, 1995, pp. 50-51).

In the next phase of this session, I offered a creative dance directive in which each survivor was encouraged to select an image from nature to stimulate a dance of release and "letting go." In doing so they increased their expressive freedom without having to confront the content of their inhibitions.

The next task was to bridge the group's creative dance experience to their psychophysical manifestations of guilt. Again the group improvised themes of "letting go" and resiliency. One person let go of "beating herself up" with guilt. Her initially inward focus turned outward into a dance of powerful rage. Another woman concentrated on the ways guilt related to her tendency to dissociate. She used the resilient and stabilizing knee-bending exercises from earlier in the session in an effort to prevent her tendency to "leave her body." A third woman, who danced to explore her sexuality, expressed the flurry of thoughts that distracted her from being emotionally present with her husband during love making. As she worked on releasing her spine and thigh muscles, she danced images of "letting go" sexually. In the closing portion of the session, I encouraged each group member to create a poem for her images. Each recitation was accompanied by flute music and followed by individual improvisations. (Bernstein, 1995, p. 51)

This session demonstrates the interplay of several dance therapy interventions. Mobilization and Functional Technique altered habitual and constricting movement patterns. Creative Dance stimulated expression and imagination while broadening dance skills. Improvisations helped explore how guilt restricted personal freedom. Change in movement itself can bring about a change in attitude that, in turn, can liberate the survivor. The primary focus of this session was on the body and the issue of "letting go," rather than on the origins or specific content of guilt. (Bernstein, 1995, pp. 50-52)

In conclusion Bernstein states:

When a survivor participates in the dance therapy process, hope and positive feelings about her body can be restored. She is able to bridge her thoughts and feelings with action and to reclaim her body as her own. She becomes more expressive, more creative and physically stronger in her own eyes as she develops feelings of control and power. From an improved relationship to her body she finds her way to create a more healthful and satisfying life. (Bernstein, 1995, p. 57)

Battered Women

The subject of dance therapy with battered women is also discussed in Levy's 1995 book. The authors of this chapter are dance therapists Meg Chang and Fern Leventhal (a co-editor of *Dance and Other Expressive Art Therapies*). While their chapter focuses on the female survivor of abuse in male/female relationships, the material and ideas they discuss can be applied to the male victim in an abusive relationship as well and in homosexual relationships. The material for Chang and Leventhal's chapter grew out of their work in a shelter for battered women in Brooklyn in the 1980s.

> Domestic violence ... continues to be widespread and is devastating to all involved. A "battered woman is a woman who is repeatedly subjected to any forceful physical or psychological behavior by a man in order to coerce her to do something he wants her to do without any concern for her rights" (Walker, 1979, p. xv). Victims of domestic violence must be able to take action if they are to remedy learned patterns of helplessness, ambivalence and inactivity. Dance and creative movement offer a paradigm for action that can help women in danger take the steps necessary to reorganize their lives. (Chang & Leventhal, 1995, p. 59).
>
> Pervasive apprehension and paralyzing terror become a battered woman's chronic response to threats of abuse and violence. During an attack the woman's physical sensation becomes blunted; she develops the ability to cut off all feeling (Walker, 1979). Because she is unable to control the violence or defend herself, she psychophysically detaches or dissociates herself from the experience. (Chang & Leventhal, 1995, p. 60)
>
> Dissociation allows the woman to isolate herself from her fear, rage and hopelessness. At times, she may only be conscious of her feelings of love for the abuser. Her intensely negative feelings may split off from her consciousness and be denied (Paley, 1988). This splitting of her awareness inhibits the battered woman's ability to respond appropriately to signs of danger. Moreover, uncomfortable emotions such as anger, sadness and loss may be projected onto the abuser (Gillman, 1980). By assigning her feelings to the abuser, she minimizes her experience and thereby the ability to protect herself.
>
> Over time, a battered woman accepts the abuser's view of "reality," seeing herself as he describes her—worthless, stupid, ugly or undesirable. As her self-esteem is undermined, the ability to make autonomous decisions declines and she begins to accept her partner as all-powerful and all-knowing. A woman involved with an abusive partner wants to believe he is deeply sorry, that he will change and that the "honeymoon" period following the abuse will prevail (Walker, 1979, p. 60)
>
> Ambivalence, a prevalent factor in the psychology of battered women, is expressed as indecision about whether to stay or leave the relationship (Rounsaville, Lipton and Bieber, 1979). This ambivalence is fueled partially by feelings of helplessness, lack of a strong self-identity and fear of change. Lowered self-esteem and embarrassment may prevent a woman from seeking assistance from friends, relatives or professionals (Chang and Leventhal, 1995, pp. 60-61).

Broadening Movement and Life Choices

> Broadening movement patterns is [a] way of introducing new behaviors. Movement increases the battered woman's range of action and interaction. Living in a constrained relationship can lead to rigid movement patterns as well as limited coping styles. It follows that expanding the individual's movement repertoire is directly linked to changes in self-concept and interpersonal dynamics (North, 1972). For example, in a session a battered woman may be surprised by her own strength when she is encouraged by a therapist to push against a partner. Finding her strength, she begins to accept the therapist's observation that she is not the "pushover" she thought herself to be. This affirmation enables her to interact more assertively with the important figures in her life and begin to perceive herself more positively. Similarly, a woman who feels weak and helpless can mobilize feelings of personal power and a desire to fight back when provided with simple everyday props, such as small hand weights or a tennis racket. When props are used during improvisational dance they tend to increase muscle activity and thereby expand the person's total commitment to her actions (F. Levy, personal communication, October 12th, 1994). Bartky (1980) states, "without the active use of weight, there is little hope that these women will ever be able to stand up for themselves" (p. 135). (Chang and Leventhal, 1995, pp. 62-63)
>
> The technique of mirroring an individual's movement can be used to establish trust and promote a therapeutic alliance. It may be contraindicated as a long-term intervention, however, as it can reinforce dependency on the leader. Like all individuals in treatment, battered women move through stages of growth. As their needs change and mature, the treatment approach must shift to meet the new demands (Huston, 1984). The importance of the battered woman's increased independence and autonomous functioning must be recognized and validated.
>
> Clients who have become conditioned to rigid or hierarchical modes of relating may react to movement directives with either compliance or rebellion. Incorporating an approach that encourages self-directed action not only defuses the issues surrounding control but also taps sources of individual choice and creativity (Chang and Leventhal, 1995, p. 63).

Choosing Movement Directives

Thoughtfully articulated movement directives are essential, as illustrated in the following vignette. After the warm-up, the therapist noticed that several women were kicking. In an attempt to reflect the group's feelings, the therapist suggested that the women "kick him away." The reaction of the group to the interpretation was to perform a few explosive movements that quickly diminished into unfocused, peripheral actions. The intensity of feeling that seemed to be developing prior to the movement directive dissipated and the movements came to a premature and unsatisfying closure. The therapist, after reflecting on what had happened to the group, came to the conclusion that her suggestion to "kick him away" overdefined and overdirected the action of the women. When the kicking resurfaced, the therapist supported the group's physical intentions by saying, "make noise with your feet and legs and use all of the space in the room." This simple movement directive resulted in an exuberant dance.

The less interpretive suggestion emphasized expanding the women's ability to express themselves fully without burdening their movements with an analysis or preconceived formulation. Premature interpretation of the client's nonverbal experience "is liable to foreclose individual process" (Mackay, 1989, p. 300) and rob abused women of the opportunity to make meaning out of their own symbolic expression. (Chang and Leventhal, 1995, p. 64)

Because of the intensity of the emotions and stories that battered women bring to treatment, countertransference is frequently, often suddenly, evoked. In addition, when the abused woman is unable to recognize her own feelings she may project them onto the therapist. Analyzing this phenomenon provides clues to treatment and thus becomes an extremely important tool in the therapist-client relationship. (Chang and Leventhal, 1995, p. 67)

Summary

The preceding excerpts from *Dance and Other Expressive Art Therapies* show how dance movement therapy can help clients who have suffered abuse. In working with these populations, integration of body and mind is crucial, enabling empowerment of clients. At the same time, while working with patients with MPD or battered women, the therapist must work carefully; all work is predicated on trust, which, in these populations, is often difficult to establish. Fran Levy states (1995):

As [dance therapists and] creative art therapists we have a unique set of tools, which, when used intelligently and empathically, help us to reach deeply into the complex web of the human personality. By the same token, used carelessly or without a genuine understanding and empathy for the multileveled needs of the individual, the same tools can create further fragmentation and chaos. (p.10)

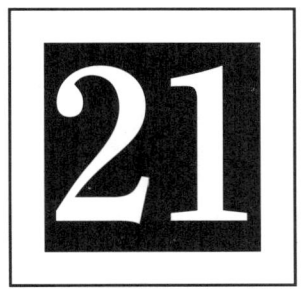

Women with Eating Disorders

Susan Kleinman and Terese Hall

Eating Disorders

A myriad of factors influence the development of an eating disorder. It is speculated that a complex interplay between biological, environmental and cultural factors contribute to this creative, tenacious and ultimately destructive force.

Women comprise at least 90 percent of diagnosed cases of both Anorexia Nervosa and Bulimia Nervosa. (American Psychiatric Association, 2000, pp. 583-595) In addition, a strong link exists between the development of eating disorders and the occurrence of emotional, physical and sexual abuse, although not all women with eating disorders have experienced abuse (Siegel, Brisman & Weinshel, 1988). The focus of this chapter is confined to the authors' experiences working almost exclusively with women.

Although a woman's height, weight and proportions are largely biologically determined, cultural standards of beauty have changed dramatically over the past 50 years. We are bombarded by images of increasingly thin women who bear little resemblance to reality. Since most women cannot conform to these rigid societal standards, feelings of pervasive inadequacy and insecurity often emerge. Regardless of age, race or socio-economic background, a woman may find herself withdrawing from experiences of living because she is unable to incorporate a healthy self-esteem, built on an acceptance of strengths and weaknesses that influence all areas of her life. Maureen Kelly addressed this issue in her book, *My Body, My Rules*, where she asserted that the women's movement of the 1960s gained momentum at the same time that the diet industry exploded. This, she believes, positioned women to feel pressured to achieve standards that were essentially unattainable (Kelly, 1996). The discord arising from this impossible dilemma sets the stage for the development of eating disorders, which have currently reached epidemic proportions (Davis, 2000, p. 1).

With regard to environmental forces, sometimes the avoidance of strong affect within a family system may contribute to the development of an eating disorder. For example, one member might "carry" the anger for the rest of the family and be very explosive. In this instance, the sufferer may fear that expressing her feelings will ignite a barrage of free floating rage, which could threaten to combust at any opportunity. Out of necessity, she may learn to censor her own spontaneous reactions, focusing instead on those around her for cues about how to behave.

Another sufferer may perceive her parents and extended family to be emotionally reactive to her feelings. Kim, a 16-year-old, described her mother's hysterical reaction when she told her about a problem she had with a friend. "She got so upset that I ended up having to calm her down. I didn't get the chance to have my own feelings." Kim needed to find a safer, less disruptive way to express her emotions and began to use her eating disorder behaviors as a vehicle to express her anger and sadness. Sometimes a daughter may feel pulled to live for others in her family and may engage in a never-ending succession of achievements, less for her own fulfillment than for others. She may be subtly discouraged from growing up and leaving home as a way to maintain a carefully constructed, albeit unconscious, homeostasis in her family. This sufferer may utilize her eating disorder to assert her independence.

An eating disorder is not merely an issue with food or weight, nor is it simply an issue of self-control. It is an attempt to cope with fearful, emotional conflicts that a woman acts out by binging, purging or starving, as well as acting on an endless variation of these themes. She, in essence, creates the illusion that she is in control by using eating disorder behavior to give her the courage to face her conflicts. For example, she may translate the concept "Am I good enough?" an abstract idea that cannot be concretely measured, to "Am I thin enough?" a notion that can be assessed. Her focus on food, body and weight becomes a way to escape from experiencing feelings and sensations, as well as to release the growing tension she feels. Her need to numb feelings grows progressively like any addictive process, becoming vicious and insatiable. Over time, she is forced to search for new ways to feel the relief that becomes increasingly elusive. Some ways include an accelerated devotion to an already known disordered pattern or "upping the ante" with some other kind of self-injurious behavior.

An eating disorder does not exist in a vacuum and always conveys a message that cannot be ignored. Sufferers generally heal more rapidly and profoundly when family and treatment professionals unite to decode the message that exists within the symptoms and behaviors. Patients can then become free to develop new methods of communication and interaction within their relationships, having to rely less on symptoms to express their needs.

Dance Movement Therapy in the Treatment of Eating Disorders

This chapter focuses on the use of dance movement therapy as a treatment method for women with eating disorders. Kleinman and Hall developed this particular method of dance movement therapy at The Renfrew Center in Philadelphia, Pennsylvania, and Coconut Creek, Florida. Based on the assumption that mind and body are connected, it serves as a powerful means for women with eating disorders to explore their relationship to their bodies and risk connecting to others. Because the experience of an eating disorder is such a bodily-focused experience, dance movement therapy is uniquely suited to helping women to address these issues directly. Dance movement therapy allows women to experience themselves more fully and to physically uncover connections between their eating disorders and the issues that underlie them.

Many women with eating disorders have difficulty expressing and articulating feelings and thoughts. Their tendency to cover deep feelings through intellectualization creates the need to access feelings and sensations directly, through the body. Dance movement therapy reconnects these women with their bodies so that they can identify and trust their sensations. Dance therapy also enables patients to explore what they communicate through body language. Discovering connections between how patients physically move through life and the problems they face enables them to process emerging feelings in movement experiences. This often leads to the development of insights and new coping skills and an understanding of the metaphoric meaning of their movements.

Confronting "Ed"

While desperate to present an outer appearance of perfection and control, the inner life of women struggling with eating disorders is filled with acute isolation, emptiness, pain, fear and a sense of disembodiment. As one patient explained, "I bury my feelings deep inside me and no one ever really sees what's wrong with me or how I really feel. Inside I am meshed with knots." Another explained, " I numb my body to keep from feeling. I can't stand being in my own skin and I isolate myself from others because I can't stand for anyone to come near me."

Focusing on food issues allows patients to detach from overwhelming anxiety and the emotional issues underlying their eating disorder. Patients often describe the ceaseless struggle they experience between their healthy self and their eating disordered self. Some even refer to their disordered self as "Ed," a mind shift that both personifies the eating disorder and helps them to gain distance from their illness.

The more therapists understand and convey their understanding of the patient's perspective, the more the patient will feel a sense of hope that a successful and lasting recovery is possible.

Fear of Change/Fear of Staying the Same

Although patients seen by Kleinman and Hall have willingly sought treatment, taking actual steps to accomplish change and recovery is usually terrifying. There is ambivalence and fear about giving up the eating disorder, which has paradoxically come to represent both "best friend" and "worst enemy." Convinced that the eating disorder provides a sense of control and well being, detachment from the physical self occurs in order to create and maintain the illusion. Simultaneously emanating from deep inside is a yearning to move toward health and freedom from the constricted parameters demanded by the eating disorder (Kleinman & Hall, 2001). Consequently, fear of change and of staying the same result in the patient's uncertainty about her ability to escape from this trap of her own creation.

Such was the case for Celine. At 55 years of age, she had been in outpatient treatment for many years. She entered residential treatment only because her outpatient team insisted that she needed more intensive therapy. Celine struggled with whether to stay in residential treatment or leave. The fears she had experienced in outpatient therapy resurfaced quickly. She had difficulty verbalizing her feelings, often became overwhelmed and was unable to comply with the eating regimen. She constantly tried to convince the staff that they expected her to eat too much. She liked the dance movement therapy group because she had the option to speak or remain silent and she felt more in charge and more successful in the dance movement therapy environment. Celine's primary therapist, a dance therapist, requested individual sessions, hoping that both the relationship with the therapist as well as the modality might spark a breakthrough. This is, in a sense, what happened, but not in the way her treatment team had envisioned. Celine identified her fears, needs and subsequent decision metaphorically through her first (and last) individual session. In this session, the therapist provided boundaries for Celine by giving her a pillow to use as a focal point. She purposely did not include other ideas regarding what the pillow might represent so that Celine could fill in her own details. Celine and the therapist then collaborated on creating an expressive movement phrase, subsequently exploring this movement in different ways.

Interpreting her experience, Celine said, "The pillow seemed like a goal to me. I think I started out very close to it. I was feeling burdened. I still wasn't moving toward it. I was moving laterally; just staying at the same level. I moved further and further away from my goal and again I felt burdened. I lunged forward trying to get back, closer, to the goal but then I discovered I couldn't do it. I couldn't reach the goal I wanted, so I lunged back." Celine made the decision to leave treatment the next day, recognizing that she was unable to commit to recovery and change at this time. The connection Celine made between her movement experience and her lack of readiness to change represented progress for someone so committed to avoiding her inner experience. Had Celine chosen to remain in treatment, the dance movement therapist may have been able to help her divide her goals into more manageable segments as well as identify obstacles to her recovery.

When the Facades Fade

Within the dance movement therapy session, facades fade and fears come to the foreground in many forms. A college student in treatment for anorexia explained, "Living in my body is the hardest thing I've ever had to deal with. It's maddening, scary, frustrating and suffocating."

Since exercise or stylized movement is more familiar and safe for these patients, who spend most of their time trying to detach from their bodies, it is often the place from which the movement experience begins. Patients learn to differentiate between moving to burn calories and moving to express feelings. Kleinman and Hall encourage patients to transform rote movements into feeling movements. Eventually, patients discover that they have the ability to cope with feelings and sensations if they can find it within themselves to take the risk.

Body Image

According to Adrienne Ressler, Renfrew Center Body Image Specialist, "Body-image is the picture in our mind's eye of how we look to ourselves. It reflects our beliefs about how we think others perceive us and captures how we experience the feeling of "living" in our bodies" (Kleinman, 2002; Ressler, manuscript in preparation.)

Body image distortions are a hallmark symptom of eating disorders. A patient's attitude to her body adheres itself so profoundly to her self-attitudes and self-esteem, that the two become indistinguishable from each other. She blames and attacks her body for whatever shortcoming she deems unacceptable. Her body becomes so littered with the refuse of such self-loathing that complete detachment is seen as the only way to survive (Hutchinson, 1985).

Lisa, who spent years of disowning her body and bodily felt experiences, discovered in one session that she could risk connecting with her body. During the session, she eloquently acknowledged, "Normally my body and mind are disconnected. I didn't try to use my mind [in the movement experience] to change my body, like I do with food. I am a body; it's not something I have. My mind is just another part of my body and my body is an extension of my mind. The whole 'thing' is one bodymind." Cognizant of the prominence of body image disturbances, Kleinman and Hall frequently weave in opportunities for patients to challenge the discrepancy between reality and perception. Tanya, a 27-year-old bulimic woman, found herself curled up in a corner of the movement room. When she risked stretching out toward the center of the room she later recalled feeling "like I took up the entire space." Peers reassured Tanya that she inhabited a small space in the room and, to her dismay, invited her to take up more space so that they might have an opportunity to interact with her more easily.

Body distortions often present themselves indirectly. For example, the need to please others as well as the ever-present fear of being imperfect may result in limited risk-taking. This fear can impact on the patient's self-esteem and perception of herself. Patients often need to be reminded that no mistakes are possible in dance movement therapy and that there is no wrong way to feel. Instead, they are encouraged to let themselves "be the way they are" and not to censor their needs or sacrifice their sense of authenticity. Support and connection with peers enables patients to take risks and expand their abilities, therefore challenging their distortions and self-imposed limitations.

Cognitive Markers

First developed by Kleinman (Kleinman, 1977; Stark & Lohn, 1993, pp. 130-131) Cognitive Markers serve as both a guide for the therapist to follow and a framework for patients to understand how their feelings and needs are reflected in their expressive behaviors. Cognitive Markers also give form to the therapeutic process and represent a frame of reference for what occurs in a session.

Cognitive Markers are used as follows: the therapist facilitates an experience that encourages the patient to *explore* herself inter- and intrapersonally and make discoveries regarding what she has explored. The *discovery* is then *acknowledged*; then the meaning of the discovery is *connected* with a familiar pattern or experience. Finally, the meaning of the discovery is *integrated* with the connection so that insights can develop and be further explored in the future. Integration provides a form of closure to end the experience (Kleinman & Hall, manuscript in preparation.)

The Cognitive Markers framework can be easily adapted by those who tend to over-intellectualize or by those dealing with alexithymia (difficulty putting feelings into words.) According to Zerbe (1995), "patients with eating disorders often struggle mightily to express their feelings in words. To develop their identity, they must learn to recognize and name these feeling states ... The first forays into naming feelings often come in other ways, such as through art, music or movement" (pp. 44-45).

In summary, the Cognitive Markers process is to: 1) explore, 2) discover, 3) acknowledge, 4) make connections and 5) integrate new information about the self.

Individual Dance Movement Therapy Using Cognitive Markers

Sara was diagnosed with anorexia nervosa while still a freshman in college. Away from home for the first time, she felt lonely and scared and soon found herself isolating from others and restricting her food. It had always been difficult for Sara to cope with change, but this time, the bottom seemed to fall out of her life. She felt depressed and her symptoms increased so much that others in her dorm began to notice. The resident assistant quickly arranged for Sara to see a therapist, who wasted no time in recommending more intensive treatment.

Sara was admitted to The Renfrew Center's Residential Treatment Program where she remained for approximately 10 weeks. She participated in biweekly group dance movement therapy sessions for the duration of her inpatient stay before being placed in a transitional level of care. Prior to discharge, Sara's primary therapist recommended an individual dance movement therapy session to help her identify issues related to a kind of physical rigidity or "wooden" state that Sara seemed to maintain.

The dance movement therapist asked Sara what she hoped to gain from this one session. Sara said that in the group sessions, she had been able to connect with feeling and would like this to happen again. "I have trouble actually feeling anything," she said and added, "I'd also like to know more about what my movements mean. Leaving is pretty scary and I want to learn as much as I can so that I can explain my needs to my new therapists. Maybe that will help me feel a little more secure." The therapist agreed with Sara that the goals she had identified could be invaluable for future work with her new treatment team and they explored some options for promoting these goals.

The therapist introduced the Cognitive Markers framework to guide Sara in connecting the meaning of her movements with her coping patterns. It was decided that the Cognitive Markers framework would be used throughout the session to help Sara identify and articulate an understanding of her nonverbal experiences.

The therapist suggested that Sara choreograph (marker 1—*explore*) a short movement sequence. Sara asked to use her favorite music, "Pure Moods," a moderately paced album of popular New Age music and quickly chose several simple movements to serve as the sequence to be explored. She moved like a precision dancer, stretching her arms upward, to each side and in an arc around the middle of her body. All her movements were punctuated with crispness. The therapist noted (markers 2 and 3—*discovered* and *acknowledged*) that Sara remained in one constricted area, never venturing into the broader expanse of space that the room offered. Aware of Sara's difficulty coping with life's transitions, it was clear that Sara might benefit from addressing this issue more directly.

With Sara's basic choreography complete, the next task was to fully experience the sequence. Together, the therapist and Sara repeated it many times. The therapist then stepped back and asked Sara to explore it with her eyes closed at moderate, slow and fast speeds and Sara soon discovered the pattern and this became the focus for the remainder of the session.

The pattern Sara discovered involved her tendency to move through life as if one task followed another with little regard for the "experience." Sara acknowledged that she repeated her movements in a rigid wooden manner, always, she said, "a step ahead of the present," never fully experiencing the moment and always worrying about getting to and completing the next task. The anticipation of the next task continually collided with the present experience. In *connecting* (marker 4) her discovery with her pattern of movement, she acknowledged, "I cut off the time I'm in and don't get the most out of it." In other words, each experience becomes a set of compartmentalized fragments that remain disconnected from one another.

The therapist pointed out the discovery she had noted earlier regarding a possible connection between Sara's difficulty coping with life's transitions and the pattern Sara had just acknowledged. It was as if a light bulb had flashed on in Sara's face and she acknowledged "Oh I get it! Because I'm so busy planning my next moves I don't experience what I'm doing ... I get so anxious when I'm faced with transitions...." Sara spoke further about several transitional junctures in her life and how paralyzed she had felt. Now that Sara had connected the meaning behind her movement patterns, it was time to explore strategies for dealing with this problem.

The therapist asked Sara how she thought she might like to explore this issue. Trusting that her body could provide further direction if she slowed down and listened to it, Sara decided to slow her pace, to invest more of herself in the present and to occupy more space. She discovered that she was using her movements in a different way. Not only did she transition from her largely perpendicular movements to a more horizontal focus, but she also began to expand her movements outwardly. Slowing down her movements and expanding them helped her to stay in the moment and not move ahead of herself or disconnect from her experience.

Further exploring her idiosyncratic movement patterns, Sara discovered and acknowledged more insightful connections. On repeating the movement sequence, she realized she tended to speed up in anticipation of the transition to the next movement. Transitions between movements did not flow smoothly.

Because of her difficulty conceptualizing the whole of her experience, the therapist suggested that Sara interject "flow" into her movements.

Sara integrated "flow" by focusing on only one movement and then slowly transitioning to the next. She automatically became less rigid and precise and the transitions between movements became smoother. With less investment in moving forward to the next task and more investment in experiencing the moment, i.e., moving from inner impulses rather than her head, Sara began to discover her expressive self. She acknowledged an awakening of emotional and kinesthetic experience. She felt more in charge.

Sara also realized that she could vary her movements, tilt her body, add a softer quality to her movements and allow a movement to extend and expand in space as long as she liked. She said, "The responsibility is on me! There aren't a lot of guidelines. It's different, like not having a specific plan to follow." Psychologically she made a significant connection.

Sara and the therapist reviewed the work they had just completed using the language of the Cognitive Markers. Since writing was a useful tool for Sara, the therapist gave her a Cognitive Marker Worksheet to use on a daily basis to help her process her experiences and to work toward *integrating* (marker 5) her expressive connections into her life experiences. She encouraged Sara to integrate her insights by building new coping patterns that could help her deal with change in a less fearful manner. The movement experience helped Sara to differentiate functional and rigid movement patterns from her "inner dance" that expressed her essence.

Conclusions

Although our actions give form to our feelings visually, experientially and cognitively, psychotherapeutic emphasis is more often placed on the exclusive use of cognitive thinking to process emotional experiences. Human beings communicate through their bodies long before they learn to talk. As we develop we add words to our communication, however, body language remains our most acute means of recognizing our needs and expressing ourselves (Chace & Dyrud, 1968). Communicating the depth of one's experiences through verbal dialogue alone may lead to an intellectual understanding without the added physical and emotional connection associated with sparking genuine and long-lasting change (Zerbe, 1995). Building on the basic foundation that experiential understanding begets cognitive understanding, rather then the reverse, dance movement therapy can help to transform idiosyncratic movement fragments into expressive behaviors. Subsequently, possibilities are created for disconnected experiences to ignite into meaningful expression that can contribute to insight and lasting change. Part of the material in this chapter will be published in W. N. Davis & S. Kleinman, (Ed). *Healing Within Relationships: The Renfrew Center Perspectives in Eating Disorders Recovery*, The Renfrew Center (manuscript in preparation).

Cognitive Marker Worksheet

Use these markers as a guide to process your experiences. Keep your descriptions simple. Remember that you cannot make a mistake because these are your feelings and thoughts. Imagine that you are a detective, collecting clues to solve a mystery—the mystery of your experiences (one at a time). Good luck!!

Exploration

Write about your experience by exploring and noting feelings, sensations and subsequent thoughts that are emerging from it.

Discovery

Write about your awareness of your feelings and sensations as well as any observations you've noticed regarding what you have just explored. What did you discover? Be as specific as possible.

Acknowledgment

Acknowledge that your discovery has meaning in your life or if not, why you think you made this discovery and it is not relevant in your life.

Connection

Recognize how the feelings, sensations and thoughts you've discovered and acknowledged are important in relation to your present experiences, fit into your life and parallel past similar experiences.

Integration

Sum up this experience noting any issues you think are important for further exploration, including questions or things that you think were interesting.

The Elderly

Dance therapy with the elderly began as early as 1942, when Marian Chace used her dance therapy techniques with older patients (S. Sandel et al., 1993). However, it was not until the 1970s that dance therapists began developing specific approaches to address the unique needs of a growing aging population.

Problems common to older adults, both those who live in the community as well as those who are institutionalized, include physical limitations, dependency on others, social isolation, loneliness, loss of self-esteem, death of peers and fear of death. As Stark (Samuels, 1973) points out, dance therapy can provide an outlet for relieving tension and building support systems to deal with later life stressors.

In accordance with the problems outlined above, the goals of dance therapy with the elderly generally focus on three major areas: social, physical and psychological. The social aspect emphasizes social interaction, sharing and support. The physical aspect attends to the aging individual's need for physical exercise and expression. Promoting personal integration, the expression of emotions and feelings of self-worth and well-being are the general goals in the psychological area.

Most dance therapists who work with older adults do so in a group setting. The group provides a safe and supportive atmosphere that fosters communication and sharing. Significant benefits are also derived from the effects of physical contact, especially touching. Sandel (1980) points out that "touching and being touched appear to have a rejuvenating effect on the participants which increases their alertness and responsiveness to others" (p. 2). In particular, physical contact helps to alleviate fears of loneliness and isolation and to allay the sensory deprivation that frequently befalls the elderly.

Some dance therapists stress the physical aspect of dance therapy with this population, believing that benefits in this area will give rise to parallel benefits on the social and psychological levels. This somatic approach is exemplified by the work of Irwin and Garnet (1974). Each describes the use of physical exercises to maintain and/or improve muscle tone, posture, flexibility, joint mobility and movement range. Relaxation techniques to release psychophysical tensions are also emphasized. These include calisthenics, Jacobson's progressive relaxation (used by Garnet) and techniques of yoga (used by Irwin). The re-establishment of coordination, spatial orientation, kinesthetic awareness and control are other physical goals.

Despite the physical limitations of many aging individuals, a wide range of movement sequences can be utilized. For example, Garnet uses swings, falls, suspensions, twists, stretches, bends and pushes and pulls, done in all directions. She finds that participants tend to discover the limitations of their own movement potential and do not go beyond them. Irwin notes that the "methods and techniques are innumerable, limited only by the training, experience and, above all, the imagination of the therapist" (1972, p. 169). She recommends that dance therapists who work with the elderly have strong medical backgrounds.

Although this approach focuses on physical goals, attention is also given to the social and psychological areas as well. Because the elderly are often restricted in their range of motion participating in even simple movements can give them a sense of achievement, vitality and self-esteem (Fisher, 1995). Pleasurable and recreational movement experiences, performed in a safe and nondemanding atmosphere, provide additional social and psychological benefits. Furthermore, movement often evokes memories of youthful feelings and carefree experiences.

The use of memory and past experiences, that is, reminiscence, can be a powerful tool in working with this population. Reminiscing may involve sharing memories of youthful experiences or acting out activities such as shopping, going out or working on a job or at home. The associations triggered by these memories and activities often work to give the person a stronger association with the present.

While those dance therapists who use a somatic approach often incorporate reminiscence into their work, other dance therapists use this technique as the basis of their approach. For these dance therapists, the social and psychological goals take precedence over the physical goals.

Sandel (1978b) conducted a study specifically on the use of reminiscence with the elderly. The study took place at a specialized center for long-term elderly patients and was conducted with five female residents, ages 78 to 98. The focus of her work was on the use of imagery and reminiscence, with the aim of fostering sharing among group members, increasing personal integration and releasing emotions, both positive and negative.

Based on the Chacian method, Sandel began sessions with a warm-up using music and structured exercise and elicited imagery by asking about the movement. She then guided the group through a progression from the sensory experience to a symbolic one and finally a verbal one, allowing a spontaneous unfolding or developing of thematic material. The atmosphere of sharing and support facilitated the expression of even the most painful, negative memories, which became less threatening and hurtful after being expressed.

Sandel's findings support the use of reminiscence as an effective means of achieving psychological and social goals.

In addition to the three major goals of dance therapy with the elderly, Fersh (1980) cites two other goals: cognitive and spiritual. The cognitive goal, Fersh notes, is to stimulate mental functioning and improve the patient's thinking ability. It can be achieved primarily through movement themes and improvisation. Sandel (1978a) has also observed that movement activities often stimulate short-term cognitive reorganization: "When people participate in movements that remind them of former competencies or pleasures, they often appear more alert, organized and competent" (p. 740).

The spiritual goal, according to Fersh, is to provide the possibility for a transcendent experience, which "offers the elderly the opportunity to connect with the ongoing energy force which supports the ... continuity of life" (Fersh, 1980, p. 36). This can help a patient deal with the fear of death. The focus here is on the individual's inner resources.

Caplow-Lindner, Harpaz and Samberg's book (1979) is devoted exclusively to dance therapy with older adults. It presents a comprehensive discussion on the sociological aspects of aging (especially in the United States) and the characteristics and special concerns of the elderly. It describes how to establish a geriatric dance movement program and gives a complete overview of a dance therapy session, including physical, expressive and creative activities. It also provides a list of musical accompaniment and equipment resources and includes a section on program evaluation.

The following quote from this resource summarizes the goals of dance therapy with this population:

> Therapeutic movement sessions are ideally offered to discover, prevent, arrest and reverse the damaging effects of aging. Opportunities to express emotions, both positive and negative and to release tensions through movement experiences are invaluable parts of the therapeutic session. The movement therapist also offers stimulation for constructive recall, reality contacts and social interaction. We are working to promote a freer relationship between body and mind by encouraging affirmative and meaningful gestures and movement. (Caplow-Lindner, Harpaz & Samberg, 1979, p. 38)

Sandel (1978b) offers dance and drama therapy approaches with institutionalized adults. In addition to group therapy techniques, there is detailed information about intergenerational arts programs. They demonstrate, using a systems theory framework, how creative experiences can transform nursing homes into healing communities:

> The healing community transforms passive receiving into mutual giving, inactivity into purposeful motion and waiting into creating.

Fisher (1995) offers creative activities for the body, mind and spirit for fit to frail older adults. This book includes sample lesson plans and suggested readings.

Sandel (personal communication, 2002) integrates dance movement and other creative modalities into her psychotherapeutic work with older adults in the community. Her approach, *Moving Into Meaning*™, facilitates self-expression, self-soothing and the search for meaning in later life. Playful interactions overcome resistance and promote the use of humor as a coping mechanism to deal with the stress of aging.

Dance movement therapy is an ideal medium in which older individuals can learn to cope with the unique problems and stresses of old age. It enables them, "... in the company of peers, [to experience] the sense of renewal, relaxation and purpose that comes from feeling one's body in motion, in harmony with others" (ADTA, n.d., p. 4).

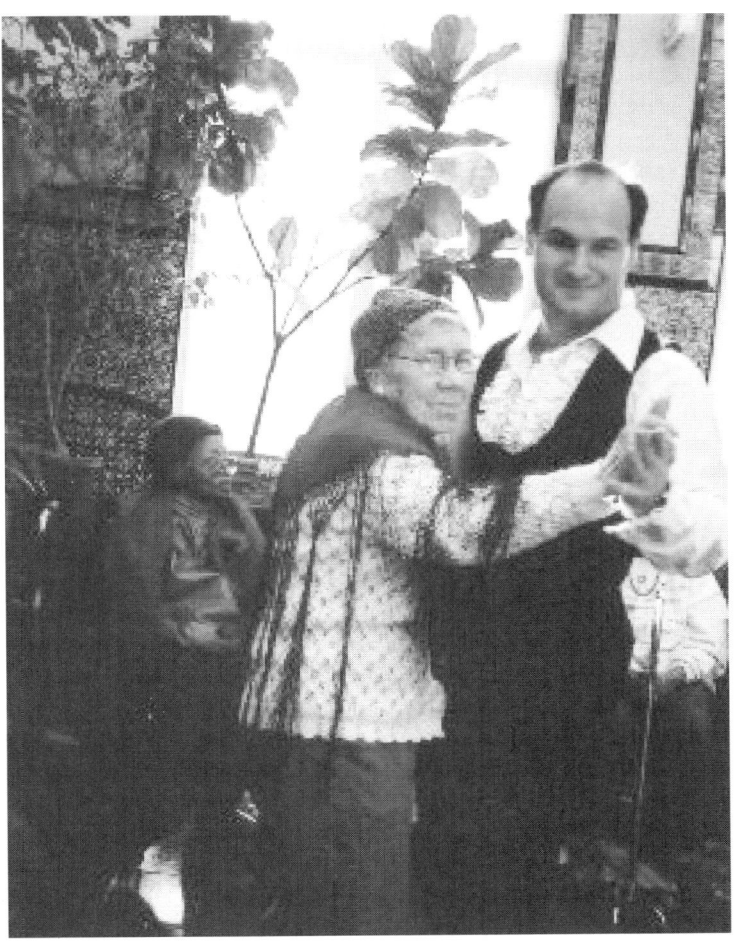

Professional dancer Peter Burroughs gently leads his senior partner (Photo courtesy Arts for the Aging, Inc. AFTA)

SECTION C

Work with Individuals with Varying Physical Disabilities

Rehabilitation

By Cathy Appel

The field of rehabilitation is diverse. It includes individuals recovering from illness or injury, as well as those who will not recover. It includes individuals born with a physical disability and those for whom the disability was acquired. Dance therapy is particularly well-suited for rehabilitation, because the goals of treatment so clearly encompass the need to integrate body, mind and spirit. With a physical disability as the entree to treatment, the dance therapist has an open and immediate invitation to connect with the patient in a dialogue, physically, as well as mentally and emotionally. The dance therapist's skills of attunement to the physicality of another are particularly useful and can readily facilitate an environment from which the patient can build self-awareness, awareness of others and of relationships, self-confidence and a sense of well-being, as well as increased perception and range of movement, and acceptance of and pleasure in the body.

The Early Work of Norma Canner

In the 1950s when the institutionalization of children with disabilities was under scrutiny, Norma Canner entered institutions that treated children, bringing dance, music and the spirit of play.[1] Because children are by definition more connected to their families and, because many parents of these disabled children were dissatisfied with their care, Canner was thrust early on into working with families and other service providers, helping her to develop her unique capacity to be inclusive and to contain many different elements. She believed in the family and in groups, and in reaching out to the service providers.

In the 1950s and 1960s, when the primary focus of dance movement therapy was on working with adults in psychiatric settings, Canner was developing approaches to, and applying concepts and principles of this modality, for children with physical and multiple disabilities. A pioneer in her early work with children in hospital, institutional and rehabilitative settings, Canner developed and employed a sensory-based approach. Rather than work on skills development only from a functional perspective as had traditionally been the case in many of these settings, Canner facilitated movement-based experiences that motivated children to be active through the medium of play. Gradually, her unique approach to working with these children found its way into the mainstream of early childhood, special education and public education settings.

Theater and dance were the two major influences on Canner's work. She had a background in the theater and the Stanislovsky method, and had studied with Barbara Mettler, a movement innovator and pupil of Wigman. From the former, she developed her empathic sense through the study of character, relationship and group interaction; from the latter, she learned a vocabulary of natural movement and improvisational structures.

Born in Boston in 1918, Canner worked as an actress in New York City from 1937-1942. Marcow-Speiser[2] has this to say of Canner's transition from performer to therapist:

---

[1] Institutionalization was being questioned by the parents of children with disabilities, some of whom founded United Cerebral Palsy/UCP in 1948 and the Muscular Dystrophy Association/MDA in 1950. As more children survived birth-related disability, more parents fought to keep them from being institutionalized.
[2] Vivien Marcow-Speiser, PhD, ADTR, LMHC, is currently a Core Professor in Dance Therapy and the Chair of The Institute of Body, Mind and Spirituality, both at Lesley University.

When her husband was drafted into the navy during WW II, she left the stage and returned to Boston where her children were born. While her children were young, Canner began studying dance with Barbara Mettler and this training taught Canner basic dance as well as a way of using dance to express herself and her inner life. She learned that everyone has the capacity to move and that dance has the capacity to heal. When she left Boston for Toledo, Ohio, Barbara Mettler encouraged Canner to continue to work with movement and told her that: "You will know more about the creative process and improvisation in this work than anybody from here to California." (Marcow, 1990)[3]

In Toledo, Canner began teaching creative movement for children and parents at the YMCA. Brownell[4] and Freeman[5] describe one of the first challenges she encountered teaching dance in the Midwest:

> Having said on a TV program that "anyone can dance," she was soon challenged in one of her classes by a little girl with braces on her legs who had cerebral palsy. Canner structured the class around this child, using movements which isolated separate body parts such as arms, legs, head, fingers, etc. Afterwards, she contacted the child's doctor for help and he invited her to accompany him on his rounds in the hospital. Thus began Canner's work with individuals with cerebral palsy and other medical conditions. (Brownell & Freeman, personal communication, 2001)

Typical of Canner's responsiveness to innovative ideas, according to Brownell and Freeman, she began working with persons with mental illness:

> A psychologist in one of Canner's classes with adults told her "you're doing group therapy." Canner had never heard of group therapy, but she accepted the psychologist's offer to work with chronic schizophrenics at Toledo State Hospital where she eventually initiated a movement and music program. Seeing the effectiveness of her work in engaging people and helping them to change their affect, doctors and teachers began to ask her if she could work with those who were deaf, blind, retarded, physically handicapped or mentally ill. She always replied, "I don't know, but I could try." In Toledo, she gave workshops for medical personnel, parents and teachers while working with children, adolescents and emotionally disturbed adults in clinics, housing projects and hospitals. (Brownell & Freeman, 2001)

Brownell and Freeman have this to say about Canner's relationship with Marian Chace:

> When Canner learned of the work of Marian Chace, she sought her out, corresponding with Marian between 1958 and 1961 and then taking a course with her in New York. Canner felt that Chace introduced her to a new kind of stimulation and awareness through her use of psychological insight. Chace also introduced Canner to the interpersonal theory of Harry Stack Sullivan which initiated her lifelong study of psychology, particularly the works of Jung, Perls and Reich. (Brownell & Freeman, personal communication 2001)

Canner returned to Boston in 1961 where psychologist Lewis Klebanoff hired her to work in the Clinical Community Nursery School Program. At that time, Massachusetts was unique in having a pre-school program for children with mental retardation, which hired teachers whose specialty was pre-school rather than retardation and who would look at these children as children rather than as patients. Brownell and Freeman explain:

> Canner was hired, not to instruct, but to help these children experience themselves and the world around them. Many doctors at that time believed that such children had short attention spans and therefore could not learn very much or develop social relationships. Canner challenged them by saying, "We don't know, no one has ever tried," and she then demonstrated that much of what was thought not possible was possible. She went on to establish a pilot program which grew to over one hundred schools and fourteen centers in Massachusetts where pre-school teachers and aides received training in the dance modality and which became a model for Early Childhood Intervention.

> Between 1967-1973, Canner taught at Boston University and at the Eliot Pearson School and the Occupational Therapy School at Tufts University. She also taught in Washington, D.C., at the National Child

---

[3] Marcow, V. "An Interview with Norma Canner." *American Journal of Dance Therapy*. (1990. 12(2) 83-93)
[4] Anne Brownell, MA, VDTR, LMHC co-created and co-produced with William C. Freeman, PhD, ADTR, the documentary film *A Time to Dance: The Life and Work of Norma Canner*. (1998)
[5] William C. Freeman, PhD, ADTR is the Director of Expressive Movement Project at Center on Disability and Community Inclusion at the University of Vermont and was the Executive Consultant on the film *A Time to Dance: The Life and Work of Norma Canner*. (1998)

Research Center under child specialist, B.J. Seabury; and in Massachusetts, Mississippi and Virginia for Operation Head Start, influencing a generation of teachers of children with special needs. Seabury said of Canner, "She concentrated on something different from their diagnosis: to move and be creative rather than focusing on their illness." For example, when confronted with a child with paralysis, Canner would put a drum in the crook of the arm that was paralyzed so that the child could hold the drum and then beat it with the other hand creating something in movement from a motivation rather than a prescribed exercise and using muscles never used by that child before. (Brownell & Freeman, personal communication, 2001)

Canner's methods with children are well-documented in the film, *A Time to Dance: The Life and Work of Norma Canner* (1998)[6], as pointed out by Brownell and Freeman:

> Canner engaged with children by meeting and supporting them at their levels of ability and by offering them opportunities to learn about themselves and interact with others within the context of movement groups. Canner used sound-making instruments, stretch band material, props and miscellaneous objects to encourage children to discover new movement patterns. This method increased sensory and kinesthetic awareness. With common found objects like wastebaskets and scarves, the children created their own movement patterns and uses making sounds, investigating textures and other kinesthetic properties, transforming "things" into meaningful objects which facilitated group interaction. Through this approach, Canner facilitated nonverbal and verbal interactive communication between children and their peers and adults.
>
> In this film, photographer and film producer Harriet Klebanoff describes Canner's early work with a particular child. The girl she describes is withdrawn and removed from the group and social interaction. Canner offers the girl a piece of cloth to touch, then returns to the group and periodically comes back to her, moving closer and touching her on the face and arms with the cloth. Over a fifteen-twenty-minute period, Canner encourages the girl's participation with verbal prompts, glances and use of the cloth, until eventually she joins the group by engaging with another girl. Klebanoff describes this as quite remarkable since no one had ever expected this child would ever do more than sit withdrawn into her own self and, maybe, watch. (Brownell & Freeman, personal communication, 2001)

Speiser, long-time colleague of Canner at Lesley College (now called Lesley University), credits Canner, saying:

> In the early seventies, Canner developed the Dance/Movement Therapy specialization within the Expressive Therapy Program at Lesley College. As an integral part of this unique cross-disciplinary multi-modal training program, Canner infused the program with movement, sound, rhythm and pulse and was instrumental in the development of dance therapy in the state of Massachusetts. (Marcow-Speiser, personal communication, 2001)

In 1973, Canner founded the Dance Therapy Core Group at the Institute for the Arts and Human Development at Lesley College, which she led for thirteen years. In 1974, she began a dance therapy program with her students at Perkins School for the Blind. From 1981-1994 she taught teachers, medical professionals and parents as consultant to the Arts with the Handicapped Program of the Kansas State Department of Education and to Accessible Arts, Inc. in Kansas.[7] She also traveled to Switzerland, Germany, Norway, Sweden and Israel to instruct therapists and teachers.

Brownell and Freeman emphasize that Canner's work with children informed her later work with adults. This is evidenced by her extensive commitment to providing over forty years of education to therapists, teachers, artists and parents, thirteen of which were spent developing and coordinating the pre-service education program for dance movement therapy at Lesley College. They observe that in working with educators:

> Canner engaged these adults in their own experience of dance/movement therapy, demonstrated this way of working with children in their classrooms and then discussed the theory, methods and applications of work with them. (Brownell & Freeman, personal communication, 2001)

Freeman, who has worked closely with Canner since 1979, emphasizes the far-reaching impact her work

---

[6] *A Time to Dance: The Life and Work of Norma Canner.* Feature-length 16 mm documentary film produced by Bushy Theater, Inc., Somerville, MA: 1998.
[7] Accessible Arts, Inc. is a not-for-profit organization, of which William C. Freeman, PhD, ADTR, was the Founding Director.

has had, not only on her clients, but also on other dance therapists, the field of dance therapy and the essential political and social issues of our time:

> Many have been profoundly affected by Norma and her belief in the power of dance and movement to be inclusive of all people and deeply touch the human experience. Many of us have witnessed her work with children, their teachers and parents, opening opportunities to explore and discover the rich resources that lie within themselves. Norma's innovative methodology illustrates her unique sensory based approach to integrating movement, dramatic action, sound and visual expression in facilitating growth for children, youth and adults. Norma's depth of feeling and compassion, reverence for our sacred and only home, planet earth and commitment to social and global consciousness to respond to those in need, is an inspiration for all of us to envision our opportunities to affect change. (Freeman, personal communication, 2001)

Perhaps these words by Canner herself provide the best insight into her underlying vision, which sparked a brilliant career, meeting the needs of children and adults for over fifty years in a range of settings:

> Dance Therapy, in my view, is really about spontaneous, creative movement and about experiencing oneself from a feeling place rather than an intellectual one. When we are moving spontaneously, we come closer to our primal selves and that is nurturing and healing. We use the language of movement to access deep emotions and early memories without censoring them. The focus is to go somewhere where you leave off your usual movements to find the ones that are just there. It's not to do more or less, it's just what happens— it's in your body, in your cells. This way of working brings you back to the time when you didn't have to think that you would have to learn to dance in order to move. Think of yourself as movement; you are the movement, the dance is in you and always has been. (Canner, personal communication, 2001)

Rehabilitation with Severe Head Injury Patients

Dance therapy with patients suffering from severe head injuries is a relatively new and rapidly growing field. Stephanie Katz has worked extensively with head-injury patients. She believes dance therapists are especially suited to work with this population because their training is both physically and somatically oriented. (Katz, personal communication, 1987)

Katz, along with Cynthia Berrol, two leaders in the field of dance therapy rehabilitation with traumatic brain injury (TBI) patients, have been extremely active in educating other dance therapists as to the special problems facing this population. Berrol is the Coordinator of the Special Graduate Major, Dance/Movement Therapy at California State University at Hayward. Katz is the former Program Director of Michigan Rehabilitation Center.

According to Berrol and Katz (1985):

> Every 16 seconds someone sustains a head injury; every 12 minutes someone dies of a head injury.... Approximately 700,000 individuals are admitted to hospitals each year as a result of severe cerebral insults. Of the survivors, upwards of 70,000 suffer marked, pervasive and long-term disruption of all domains of human function—physical, cognitive and psycho-social. Every facet of life is significantly altered.... Regardless of the level of recovery, a somewhat different person will emerge, a seeming stranger.... (p. 46)

TBI patients suffer emotionally, physically, socially and cognitively. Various degrees of paralysis and/or neurogenic movement disorders are common results of severe head injuries. Other physical problems that may occur are plasticity, ataxia, tremors, sensory impairments and perceptual-motor difficulties. In the cognitive realm, disorientation, lack of initiative and poor memory and attention are frequently seen.

Berrol and Katz explain that, even in cases of severe injury, the brain has some ability to repair itself. They describe several types of neuroplasticity; that is, the brain's capacity to dynamically reorganize its means of operating. For example, some brain functions are gradually restored after the swelling of brain tissue following trauma subsides. There is also a process called collateral sprouting, "...by which axons from intact regions of the brain send out axonal 'shoots' to the damaged zones to form new synaptic connections..." (p. 49). In addition, there are indications "...that axons and synaptic connections which are not normally responsible for a particular function may take over when the primary or dominant system is disrupted..." (p. 50). Berrol and Katz point out that other factors also have an influence on the degree of dynamic reorganization of the brain after trauma. These include age (being younger is an advantage), environmental factors (social interaction is an important part of rehabilitation) and drug treatment.

Frequently in their work with TBI patients, the authors divide their sessions into a warm-up, a theme development phase and a closure. The warm-up is designed for five purposes:

1. *To organize the group.*
2. *To organize the body.* They utilize "...a traditional warm-up of nonlocomotor type movement using body parts first in isolation and progressing to a coordinated use of the whole [body]..." (p. 54). Movement opposites range and dynamics are also explored. Specific movements are introduced depending on individual needs.
3. *To stimulate cognitive processes.* Using imagery stimulates the symbolic process. Asking questions, which encourage reflection on internal sensations, feelings, memories and images, helps to strengthen conceptualization and broaden the movement repertoire.
4. *To support group interaction and stimulate social awareness and a feeling of community.* When the group is ready, the leader relinquishes the role of movement provider and encourages the patients to take over. As group members alternate assuming this role, their independence, sense of initiative and leadership are promoted.
5. *To lay the groundwork for subsequent theme development.*

During the theme development phase of the group, issues of dependence versus independence are frequently dealt with. These are immediately relevant and potent issues. TBI patients find themselves suddenly thrust into a totally dependent situation in which they are continually being manipulated, pushed here and there, directed and controlled. Each patient reacts to this differently, some with extreme compliance and others with rage and aggression. For this reason leaders try to engage patients around these issues so that they can deal with them within the group.

Several group structures done in dyads are suggested by Berrol and Katz. One of these is called sculpting, a technique by which one patient sculpts another in space. The patient who was first instructed to be passive while being sculpted (i.e., physically placed into a specific shape or pose) is then told to resist being molded. Another movement dyad technique that encourages issues of personal strength and independence involves the use of large stretch bands, with the participants working to keep the band taut. A third dyad technique involves having one partner say "yes" while the other says "no," continuing until one gives in and says the other's word. These and other similar techniques evoke feelings and discussion among participants around issues of dependency, anger, fear and so on. Common problems and frustrations are aired; and group support and further movement development and reflection are facilitated. These structures also promote specific kinds of muscle activity awareness and coordination.

The closure of the group session promotes further benefits for this population. Closing techniques involving breathing and relaxation increase the individual's ability to attend to his or her internal sensations and in this way facilitate the development of a more intact body image. Recalling what happened in the session as a kind of summation fosters the ability to remember. "The importance of this sort of cognitive exercise, verbal and/or motoric repetition as a therapeutic technique with...this population cannot be overemphasized." (Berrol & Katz, p. 56)

Berrol and Katz provide two case studies in their article. At the Therapeutic Recovery Program in Southfield, Michigan, Katz conducted the case study of D., a 22-year-old man who suffered TBI in a car accident. D. was confined to a wheelchair. He could not feed himself, write or even go to the bathroom without help. He also suffered from partial facial paralysis, and impaired intellectual and proprioceptive functioning. His behavior revealed depression and impulsivity. Prior to his accident he had prided himself on his independence, prowess and reckless qualities.

Katz, seeing D.'s need for freedom and unconventional treatment techniques, provided him with the time and space he needed to explore movement in his own way.

> We developed a technique of D. sliding out of his wheel chair to the floor with my assistance so he could stretch out and feel the length of his body. Rolling across the room provided the freedom in space he so dearly missed. Pressing his lengthened body on the floor allowed for kinesthetic feedback as to more correct alignment of his spine and head. He was able to use... the mirrored wall...to make necessary

adaptations... D.'s true joy, however, was using the full space of my room, trying new movement activities.... (Berrol & Katz, p. 63)

The key to the success of Katz's work with D. was her ability to feel comfortable with D.'s needs for space, freedom and unconventional movement exploration. The traditional equipment used for rehabilitation was too confining for D. When Katz gave him the freedom he needed to feel in control of his body and space, he became an active participant in his own recovery and proud of his achievement.

Dance therapy with brain injured patients focuses on developing awareness, cognition, motivation, concentration, control and memory. Emotional issues are also important for this population. Dealing with feelings of anger, frustration, remorse and loss are all aspects of treatment, as well as dealing with pressing issues of dependency, sexuality, autonomy and others. Some of these goals and the methods used to achieve them, overlap with those of dance therapy with other populations. For example, work with the physically handicapped also focuses on issues of dependency and on "activating and motivating" patients—Bartenieff's main themes in her work with that population. In addition, the cognitive development stressed by Berrol and Katz is also a goal of dance therapists who work with learning disabled children, particularly those with organic brain disorder. However, Berrol and Katz are also charting new waters. As TBI research continues, a whole new body of knowledge and dance therapy technique is developing.

The dance therapist's work with TBI patients is complemented but not duplicated by the work of the occupational and the physical therapist. The latter, according to Katz (personal communication, 1987), is more task-oriented. The occupational therapist stresses development of dexterity in the upper body, fingertips to shoulder and activities. The physical therapist emphasizes development of the lower half of the body (gait training, adjustment to braces, etc.) and skill acquisition. In contrast, the dance therapist works with the whole person. Movement is the vehicle with which all aspects of the individual's life—emotional, cognitive, social and physical—can be dealt with. (Katz, personal communication, 1987)

In order to determine appropriate goals and objectives, a thorough knowledge of the pathological sequella of head injury is necessary. Problems due to neuropathology often require goals specifically compatible with the patient's neurological level of function. A therapist coming from a psychiatric background might initially make the false assumption that certain behaviors common to both populations have common etiologies. (Berrol, personal communication, 1993)

Group Dance Movement Therapy with TBI

Another important center for the rehabilitation of TBI and other traumatic injury and illness is the International Center for the Disabled in New York City. Cathy Appel started and runs the Creative and Movement Arts Psychotherapy Program in ICD's Mental Health Department. This urban outpatient facility has a Cognitive Rehabilitation Program, which helps people with TBI return to work and live with greater independence.

Appel leads a weekly TBI Movement Psychotherapy Group for this program. Members are all ambulatory but sustain in varying degrees cognitive, motor and visual impairment. While members like B., 40, a former psychotherapist who suffered a stroke two years ago and R., 55 and a former heroin addict who suffered several strokes in his late 30s, reconnect with their ability to move and experience sensations of pleasure, mastery and connectedness to others through dance, they also gain in physical strength, balance, coordination and self-awareness. Verbalization is an important part of this group; and, for many with TBI, talking while moving is no easy task.

The relaxed, supportive group environment facilitates spontaneous improvisation combined with clear, consistent structure and limit-setting. The dynamism of dance movement therapy makes it an excellent treatment modality for this population, to help them cope with painful losses while remaining hopeful and focused on abilities. Social interaction is emphasized and members are encouraged to integrate their experiences with dance in the group into their lives outside of treatment.

Members take turns leading and are encouraged to initiate movement opportunities in their homes and communities. For example, when R. attended a family wedding and was able to dance with his daughter, he thanked the group for its help in "getting me there." D., 22, blinded by a bullet at 18, has connected to his love of music and drumming through the group. His life of isolation and idleness is turning around since treatment. D. attributes his new drum set and the time he spends practicing at home and at his church directly to the group's support of his weekly efforts to play for them during the session. At first, D.'s drumming was started as an attempt to help him remain connected to the group during long movement improvisations with little conversation. Sightless, D. could only pick up on aural cues. Making sound kept him engaged and helped him feel a sense of control and accomplishment.

Dance Movement Therapy with the Chronically Ill and Dying

At ICD, Appel also does an Inner Movement Group for people seriously ill with cancer, multiple sclerosis, muscular dystrophy, Parkinson's disease, heart disease and diabetes. Here, the movement focus is on subtle aspects of breath and alignment, as the members are severely limited in their mobility and/or in pain. Group discussion is central, but members often limit the length of conversation "to be sure we get to move." Incorporated into the sessions are the practices of meditation, yoga and vocalization or chanting.

When the group lost one of its members, J., a former dancer and college dance teacher and breast cancer survivor, to heart disease at 58, they performed a ritual which consisted of placing a blooming plant J. had often admired in the center of their circle as they mourned the loss of J.'s vibrant presence and the sound of her theatrical voice during chanting. J. came to the group to prepare herself to die. She had abused her body through dance, alcoholism (although she was a recovering alcoholic) and neglect; finally to have it all catch up with her. In the group for two years, she opened to the nurturing aspects of movement through yoga and breath work. Even toward the end, when she was in constant pain and rarely able to attend, she would light up as the group did a simple alignment exercise.

J.'s bravery was astounding and a challenge. She would often talk about her life as a dancer and express the irony that she had come to this "inner" approach to movement only when she could barely move. Often J. would lament, "Why didn't I learn about this sooner?" and the group would give her support for "being able to learn it now with us." J. had no living relatives except a niece out of state and the group became her "family." In this family, unlike her own, J. was appreciated for her love of dance instead of being looked down on as she had been as a young woman in her family of origin and the dancer in J. was cherished and set free.

Others in the group will not live to normal life expectancy and frequently undergo risky surgeries or other medical crises, so it is especially important to honor the memory of those, like J., who are no longer in the group. The spiritual dimensions of group meditation and group movement experienced in an electromagnetic field, such as auras, transpersonal energy and the Eastern concepts prahna and chi, are sustaining themes. Periodically, one of those who remembers J. will suggest the blossoming plant be placed in the circle during meditation and will tell newer members about her.

Maintaining a vision of dance as a way of life is central to the approach of ongoing rehabilitation treatment in ICD's Creative and Movement Arts Psychotherapy Program. Daily, dance and movement receive support in the simplest and most fundamental ways, as with W., a woman from Trinidad with sickle cell anemia, who died at 36 after being at ICD for four years. Following a stroke at 27 due to a sickle cell-induced blood clot, W. was left with hemiparesis on the right side, cognitive deficits and severe aphasia. She was also in pain due to the sickle cell and endured frequent hospitalizations during exacerbations.

When W. first came to ICD for treatment, she sat in her wheelchair staring blankly at all who passed by. Her right arm was propped on a molded foam support along the armrest of her chair and her right leg was in a brace. She looked sad and isolated. She was also strikingly beautiful and well groomed. W. was referred to dance movement therapy by her doctor at ICD, who was concerned about her depression and complaints of loneliness. During the screening to determine her appropriateness for a twice-weekly dance therapy group for patients with limited mobility, despite W.'s difficulty with speech she eagerly communicated her love of dance and made known the important role dance had played in her life in Trinidad. W. expressed feelings of regret that she could no longer visit Trinidad, especially when her mother returned each year for Carnival without her.

In the beginning, W. was shy about attempting to speak and giggled, bringing her hand up to cover her mouth. She seemed childlike due to her cognitive deficits and had what appeared to be a waif-like helplessness. On her first day, W. sat and watched without moving as the group began a gentle warm-up. It wasn't until Carnival music was played that she began moving. It started in her torso, deep within her solar plexus and seemed easy, natural. In a matter of seconds, W. was transformed into an alert, cheerful, coordinated woman, connecting with the group through music with a wave-like ripple in her spine and a wide smile. When the music stopped, she resumed her collapsed posture and the life quickly faded from her face. Gradually, W. joined in the warm-ups and responded to all kinds of music.

Once, a group member brought a two-year-old to the group. The excitement level rose as the baby played with a small rubber ball and soon one member slipped onto the floor to play with the baby. Everyone followed. The session was held on the floor and, while for some the nature of their physical limitations became more apparent, W.'s disability seemed to disappear.

W. knew how to use the floor and moved with abandon, reaching and stretching in wide arcs. Without the threat of falling and the constraints of the wheelchair, she was radiant and the young girl who had studied dance in school was visible. The floor dancing demonstrated W.'s desire and ability to get out of her wheelchair. She always carried a three-pronged cane to transfer from her wheelchair when she used the restroom. Eventually, with encouragement from the group, she began transferring to a regular chair for the dance therapy session. It would take her a long time to accomplish this and then to return to her wheelchair at the end of group, but everyone waited patiently and the movement of W.'s labored determination was as riveting as her island reggae.

One day, W. sat forlorn and quiet in the group. When asked what the problem was, she began to cry. It took a long time and much coaxing for W. to explain she had seen a news report on sickle cell anemia the night before and had learned people with sickle cell only live to 35. As she cried, concerned group members blurted out, "How old are you?" W. used her fingers to communicate, "35." The group expressed their support and love. Horror at this illness, at W.'s having to hear such a thing on TV and at the group's denial and attachment to her, filled the room. It became evident the degree to which W. was mystified by her illness, her body and her losses.

An important group project for W. and others was the choreographing of individual dances for and by each member. This grew out of the success of several group dances made to express specific themes, such as survival, change or courage. Personal styles and individual movement qualities emerged more clearly and received recognition during these sessions. Eventually, each member selected her own music and worked on a solo. W. chose Aretha Franklin's "Natural Woman."

By this time W.'s movement range included reaching, twisting and stretching. At one point in her solo, she would reach for her three-pronged cane and stand up. The stretches grew more luxurious and expansive until she would finally let go of the cane altogether. The dance seemed to be saying, "I am free—look at me—I am free."

A year later, during a telephone conversation with W.'s mother, Appel learned of W.'s death. As she cried, W.'s mother talked of how happy W. had been at ICD and how much the dancing meant to her. She said, "I'm sitting here missing her so, looking at the photographs of her at ICD—she was so happy there—it's about now I'd hear her at the door—it's the time she'd be getting home." It was easy for Appel to envision W. arriving home with the same determination and regularity that she had exhibited in coming to dance therapy for years. W.'s participation in dance movement therapy until her death illuminates the importance of including one's culture in the healing process and of connecting to the unique life force in each patient.

Dance Movement Therapy in Pediatric Oncology and Hematology

Susan Cohen is the Supervisor of Child Life at Tomorrow's Children's Institute in New Jersey. In the treatment of seriously and terminally ill children using dance movement therapy she stresses the importance of being responsive to changes in pediatric care. Cohen observes that now these children are seen as having a chronic disease with an uncertain outcome, which means the stressors for the patients and their families have shifted from coping with the pending death of the child to:

> repeated invasive procedures, major side effects of treatments, radical changes in physical appearance, missing school, interactions with friends, financial burdens, trips to the hospital and missed work. Un-

certainty of outcome makes coping even more difficult because there is no specific recognizable endpoint or any guarantee that the disease will remit or be cured. (Cohen & Walco, 1999, p. 36)[8]

Cohen points to Kupst and Schulman's identification of a number of adaptive tasks for families, including 1) understanding the realities and implications of the disease, treatment and long-term survival, 2) management of emotional reactions and 3) developing the capacity to address medical issues, to deal with other responsibilities and activities and to use the available resources effectively.

In her work, Cohen integrates these findings in the context of normal development to provide a useful platform for the implementation of a dance movement therapy program in which specific content issues and modes of intervention are directly related to developmental stages. Of infants with cancer Cohen says:

> A central question is the degree to which these developmental processes are affected by chronic illness. On an ontogenetic level, development can be disrupted because of a restriction in motor activity, to invasive procedures that stimulate distress and pain and to the onslaught of multiple medical caregivers and treatments. Separations from parents, repeated hospitalizations, increased parental anxiety and disruptions in family functioning affect the infant's perceptions and reliance on a consistent environment with trusting relationships. (Cohen and Walco, 1999, p. 36)

School-Age Child Undergoing Stem Cell Transplant

The following case example, cited by Cohen (Cohen and Walco, 1999, p. 39), is about Greg who turned seven years old during a cord blood stem cell transplant, after extensive treatment for acute myelogenous leukemia (AML). For reasons not clearly defined, he developed hydrocephalus, with concomitant neuro-cognitive effects. This included excessive response latencies to various stimuli and a constriction and slowing of most motor and speech behaviors. Although Greg did not evidence overt awareness of these changes, he struggled with finding means of identifying and communicating his feelings and ideas.

Initially, a therapeutic relationship was established by mirroring Greg's postures, efforts, shapes, movement dynamics, spatial preferences, emotional tone and subtleties of breath. The dance movement therapist empathically adopted similar qualities, which facilitated opportunities for acceptance and rapport forming the building for subsequent therapeutic endeavors. Early on, Greg displayed a great deal of restriction and passivity in his movement and gestures, with only minimal changes in his body shape, breathing pattern and dynamics. Once eye contact and kinesthetic empathy were established, the therapist introduced slight changes to promote greater awareness and sense of self in the environment.

By suggesting that Greg gently touch various parts of his own body, he used sequencing to regain a sense of connection, as well as increased body awareness, boundaries and stimulation. The use of movement props helped Greg clarify unfocused thoughts and feelings resulting from limitations in his expressive and receptive range of communication.

Cohen points out that although children of this age lack the capacity to comprehend difficult issues on an abstract level, they are potentially adept at using analogous concrete representations or metaphor to resolve conflicts. She gives this example: A scarf represented a magic carpet and a stretch band became the reins of a horse in the service of bringing abstract themes to life in a more concrete manner. In this way, Greg was able to transcend his usual bland affect and withdrawal to relate to movement experiences that involved fantasy, spontaneity and interaction. Movement interventions were integrated with verbal associations to the context and were targeted to promote awareness and communication. (Cohen and Walco, 1999) Cohen concludes:

> At its very core, dance/movement therapy emphasizes the holism of mind and body, thereby providing a new avenue for exploring the complicated inter-relationship of factors involved in coping with cancer. (Cohen and Walco, 1999, p. 41)

Dance Movement Therapy in a Residential Group Home

Sandi Lieberman practices dance movement therapy in residential homes for severely disabled individuals

---
[8] Susan O. Cohen, MA, ADTR, CCLS and Gary A. Walco, PhD; *Dance/Movement Therapy for Children with Cancer*; "Cancer Practice," January/February 1999, vol. 7, No. 1, p. 36.

who also exhibit autistic features and/or psychotic processes. These clients are mostly nonverbal and sometimes engage in self-abusive behavior or aggressive acting out. Since "normalization" is the state mandate, group homes are required to provide the best therapeutic and home-like care possible. Lieberman says the difficulties in programming for this population, with its high degree of withdrawal and isolation, prompted her being hired to work specifically in the areas of communication development and relationship building.

Lieberman credits her training with Judith Kestenberg as the foundation of her work in these group homes. She says of Kestenberg:

> She was an extremely compassionate woman whose sensitivity and intuition fed her work constantly. In particular, I loved to watch her engage in her lively encounters with young children and infants. Time and time again she was able to empathize and relate to a child who was upset or sad or isolated or furious and more often than not, make it better for them. I wanted to learn this knack she had for relating so I watched her closely. I watched her use her hand to "visually attune" to a crying six month-old baby's leg kicking rhythm. The baby paused, gazed at her hand, cried again, paused, gazed, gazed, cried again until the crying ceased I also listened to her moan and wail in rhythmic synchrony to an 18 month old, until this back and forth "vocal attunement" gradually transformed from shrieking sounds to the pleasant toned singing of a soft melody that others joined. I watched her use "touch attunement" while holding a tantruming child modulating her rhythmic squeezes to match his thrusting impulses. Very soon, the child quieted. (Lieberman, personal communication, 2001)

Lieberman learned from Kestenberg that attunement in tension flow, visual, vocal and touch, are communications of empathy, which usually soothe and comfort because they instill a feeling of being responded to on a basic feeling level. She was also taught how to recognize and reproduce subtle shape flow changes in the body, in growing and shrinking movements. The adjustment of these responses interpersonally facilitates the development of trust. Watching Dr. Kestenberg, she observed first-hand the power of movement-based empathy and trust to connect deeply with another on a nonverbal level and prompt change and growth.

Examples of Dance Movement Therapy in a Residential Setting

It is apparent in Lieberman's description of her work how she employs KMP techniques:

> I walk into a quiet living room space; eight clients sit on couches, each in their own spot, all in their private worlds. There is some humming and idiosyncratic gesturing. Most of these will actively resist anything but the most superficial contact and mechanical handshake. Most staff are adept at creating structures for the clients, like putting chairs together in a circle, leading clients around, making them shake hands with one another in a mechanical way and giving behavioral commands. As a dance movement therapist, my approach is different and focuses on communicating empathic support and respect and inviting participation in a nonverbal dance of attunement and adjustment. I am in no rush to gather clients together and spend much time moving from one to the other.
>
> I approach Michael and match his low intensity in tension flow... in my whole body. I attune to his ... rhythm first by walking in place and later through touch on his arm. He "shortens up" in shape flow, gets up on his toes and begins flow adjustments in his hands. As we touch hands, I am sure to reflect back what I feel in his muscles, even when it is neutral flow. His eyes drift upward—there is a quality of being able to be blown away by the wind. I join him for a while—side-to-side—light on my toes, taking on the same qualities. Then I place my hand on his back attuning to his low intensity flow adjustments. A smile passes over his face for a moment like the sun poking out from a cloud—in recognition. I join him for an entire dance, adjusting my shape flow responses to match his, stepping forward and backward, fluttering touches—minimal eye contact. The song ends, I call his name softly and he leans over to lay his cheek gently on mine.
>
> I approach Valerie. She has a solemn face, her head is down and she gazes at her hands that are flexing in abrupt high intensity tension changes. She is humming loudly fragments of tunes I recognize. She moves with a high intensity bound pushing and release as she presses back into the couch and then rocks. I sit beside her looking straight ahead and lean against her side with a similar intensity and rhythm. I hold and release. After a time she pauses—then continues—she pauses again as if listening, waiting until I resume. She reaches over to grab my head and I set a limit. She grabs my hand. We do the same high intensity abrupt hand dance together for a long while. Then she starts wagging her head to the beat of "Sweet Honey in the Rock" with a big grin on her face. Her head is up, eyes roaming about the space with much more presence.

> I continue around the space, making connections to each as I can...I already receive anticipatory eye contact from clients in acknowledgment of my presence. Although it begins with a one-on-one attunement dance, I often will be relating to two or three clients at the same time. I may have my hand placed on Michael's back using touch to attune to his feathery flow adjustments while staring nose to nose in even bound tension flow with Dennis and swooping with my voice in high intensity free flow bursts to match Patty's singing. This attunement proves successful in catching clients' attention, in sparking their interest and curiosity in an "outside other" that is somehow mysteriously safe for them. By the end of the session signs of increased social interaction become obvious. One client approaches another and pulls a soft silk scarf over their head. Another presses foreheads with a staff member. Still another gives away their drum to the person who wants it.
>
> For many of the clients I work with, this attunement dance is the first step towards establishing some trust in relationship. Without it, our clients can maintain homeostasis in very regressed and isolated patterns for long periods, deteriorating in functioning.
>
> Again and again, it has been my experience that once a client can begin to take part in a relationship, their mastery on other levels follows. Doing by rote, the minimal behavioral expectations coerced by others, however well intentioned, does not compare with the leap in social functioning when a relationship with affect develops for the client. Now that we have worked together for some time, when I walk into the group home, the bells on my tambourine signal my coming. Staff report that heads look up, there are some smiles of recognition and anticipation. Some clients jump up and start their dance on the spot with no music. Two follow me around to the back room. The room is energizing, sounds build. I am reminded of the past when I longed to learn that knack of relationship building from my mentor, Dr. Kestenberg. And I am deeply grateful to her still, for this tool that I use constantly which so enriches the lives of my clients. (Lieberman, personal communication, 2001)

According to Lieberman, tension flow is not only important to use for increased relatedness, socialization and communication development, but, she points out, it is useful in crisis management situations. If a client is out of control, any connection to people and surroundings can help stabilize the situation. Attunement techniques, whether sound, visual or touch, communicate empathy and will often "take the edge off" a client's distress and lead to soothing and more adaptive behaviors. She cites this example:

> A client was becoming very self abusive, pounding her head with her fists rhythmically. In the process of restraining her, my arms were encircled about her. I was able to rhythmically press the client's arm with the same degree of intensity and rhythm. In a matter of minutes we gradually transformed the movement impulse into a softer more adaptive one. This touch attunement, the mediation of muscular responses without relying on the visual mode, is an especially important technique to use with visually impaired clients. (Lieberman, personal communication, 2001)

The growing emphasis in health care on inviting diverse and formerly isolated populations into community living has created opportunities for flexible, motivated professionals like Lieberman. These residential settings, which are smaller, more intimate and home-like, allow dance therapy to become a part of daily life.

Conclusion

As the field of rehabilitation has changed since Norma Canner first went into children's hospitals, so has the role of the dance movement therapist. Along with the legal and social empowerment of people with disabilities, the integration of the body, mind and spirit has become an accepted treatment goal. We have learned that the distinction between people with disabilities and the non-disabled or, more accurately, the temporarily able-bodied, is blurred. The dance movement therapist fosters inclusion and supports connection between all individuals and their bodies. Rehabilitation is an excellent setting for the power of dance movement therapy to create a sense of resilience and community.

SECTION D

Other Applications of Dance Movement Therapy

# The Developmentally Disabled

Generally speaking, dance therapists working with people who are developmentally disabled tend to work with the patients who are more severely limited individually and with patients with less severe limitations in group settings. The focus is generally on improving body image, coordination and motor skills, promoting socialization and communication and developing the individual's confidence and awareness through mastery and self-expression. All of these lead to increased intellectual capacity and growth.

The use of repetition is especially helpful for this population. Liljan Espenak (1975), one of the six major dance therapy pioneers, stressed repetition through the use of rhythmic exercises and music. The rhythmic beat, facilitated by music, provides a structure that helps to organize movement and thinking and leads to mastery of functional and recreational skills. These are important in fostering ego development, which, Espenak believed, is hampered in individuals with developmental disabilities because of the negative responses directed towards them from other segments of the population.

Espenak summarized her approach, called Psychomotor Therapy, with this population:

> The ... value of ... dance activity ... lies partly in the stimulating quality of rhythmic movement and activity, but partly also in the structuring properties of physical education.
>
> ... Psychomotor therapy's efforts for reaching and effectively changing the undeveloped self-image of the retarded has been of great help in removing some of their social barriers and in overcoming their fear of interpersonal contact by offering them a tool for communication and a physical-emotional program to help them grow as personalities. (1975, pp. 3-4)

Susan Moss and Stephen Anolik (1984) also emphasize the value of repetition in working with people with developmental disabilities. They believe that any clear structure of exercises, repeated for many weeks, builds body awareness and could be used to achieve other dance therapy goals with this population. They caution against the tendency to avoid teaching physical techniques that seem to be too complicated for these patients. In this connection, Moss and Anolik conducted a study to ascertain whether patients with developmental disabilities could be taught relaxation techniques and if learned, whether the relaxation response could be used to calm them when emotionally upset.

They taught Jacobson's (1929) progressive relaxation technique to five adults with moderate to severe limitations, in a group setting three times per week (6 sessions). Pre- and post-testing of skin temperature of the index finger were administered as physiological indicator that the relaxation response had occurred, since skin temperature rises in the hands and fingers when the muscles relax.

The authors found that the five clients of the pilot study were able to learn the relaxation response. The skin temperature tests of three of the patients showed significant differences between pre- and post-test; although the differences in the other two clients were not statistically significant, their mean temperatures did rise.

The authors attribute their success in teaching the technique to a high staff-to-patient ratio (2-5) and to repeated use of verbal and physical prompting during sessions. The verbal prompting focused on key words, such as "calm" and "feeling good." The physical prompting consisted of touching the body part to be tensed and relaxed. As the work progressed, fewer prompts (particularly physical prompts) were needed, indicating the patients were increasing their body awareness. In addition, they seemed to associate the room, the therapists and the skin temperature-testing machine with the relaxation technique. Contrary to the authors' initial concern about the effects of using the biofeedback equipment, the patients became progressively calmer when they entered the room, immediately and eagerly raising their finger for the skin temperature test.

As a follow-up project, two classroom teachers were trained in the relaxation technique. One used it on a regularly scheduled basis, three times per week. The other used it more informally when she felt her class was becoming restless. The first teacher got a positive response using the technique during crises; the second did not. Thus, it appears that "frequency of exposure and concentrated clinical attention are important factors in the client's ability to generalize the benefits of relaxation training" (Moss and Anolik, 1984, p. 55) and perhaps other forms of body movement training as well.

Because language may be poorly developed in patients with developmental disabilities, some dance therapists have concentrated on its development. The decision for emphasizing language development may rest on the extent of the client's retardation. With individuals who have more severe limitations, the focus is likely to be on developing remedial language skills, often as part of intensive one-on-one therapy. The individuals with less severe retardation, such as the trainable or educable patients, may already have developed basic language skills. Dance therapists who work with these patients, usually in group sessions, often stress further language development by encouraging conceptualization and verbal expression. This helps the patients organize their thinking and improve their communication with others.

Promoting verbal expression was one of the goals of a dance therapy program described and filmed by Weiner, Jungels and Jungels (1973). The dance therapy was part of a creative art therapy program, which also included art, music and drama therapy. It was held at a New York public school during 1970-71 for a small group of educable children with developmental disabilities. Its purpose was to determine whether ease and mastery in the creative arts would help improve the children's overall functioning in language, body image and coordination.

The dance therapy sessions included spatial exercises to "alter body-image disturbances, improve understanding of directionality and laterality and improve balance coordination" (p. 46). The authors stated, "no particular technique, style or steps were taught" (p. 46). Work was also done with fantasy, interaction and group and individual improvisations. Verbal reinforcement, music and various props were also used. By the end of the program, according to the authors, the children displayed increased self-confidence and greater control over their bodies and their movements were more aggressive and spontaneous.

Maureen Costonis' (1974) work with a nine-year-old with severe retardation and secondary emotional and behavioral problems concentrated on language development and on shaping the boy's self-destructive behaviors into expressive movement. She focused on developing the child's body image and body/environment awareness, using techniques that included mirroring his idiosyncratic mannerisms and free-flowing dance. Costonis believes that "... a client who engages in stereotyped gestures can transform them into dance movement and substantially expand his movement repertoire..." within a short period of time (p. 151). Costonis utilized her own notation system—the Movement Range Sampler (MRS)—to describe small changes in the boy's movement during the dance therapy sessions.

As a result of the dance therapy, the child's ritualistic behaviors decreased and ordinary behaviors (e.g., walking, running) became more normal. Also, the patient spoke more frequently during the dance therapy sessions. This increased frequency in language was attributed to the increased physical contact between therapist and patient.

Replacing the mannerisms of a child with developmental problems with "more appropriate social behavior" was also the focus of Elaine Siegel's work (1972). By encouraging free expression and the uninhibited acting out of fantasies, Siegel facilitated the intellectual and emotional development of a 10-year-old boy. The therapy sessions consisted of warm-up exercises, other physical exercises, games (rhymes, body image games), dance (polkas, made-up dances), specific movements (hops, jumps), spontaneous and fantasy movement and play-acting. In accordance with psychology theory, Siegel believed that the child's "bizarre behavior was not caused by his retardation but by an anal fixation, the reduction of which allowed for further growth" (p. 107). That is, by providing an outlet for the controlled acting out of the child's innermost fantasies, Siegel helped alleviate much of his anally compulsive behavior. Also, during the period of the therapy sessions, the child's IQ increased from 40 to 70, his social behavior improved and psychological tests revealed fewer emotional problems.

Summary

As with other populations, five major goals emerge for patients with developmental disabilities: cognition (which includes body image); physical and emotional mastery; self-expression; self-confidence; and socialization. However, with this population, there is less concern with transference phenomena and more stress on social participation, communication and interaction skills. The technique of repetition as a tool for refining and crystallizing new areas of growth and psychophysical education is also emphasized. In recent years, the term developmental disabilities frequently replaces the term retardation. The term retarded is no longer considered correct.

25 | Additional Applications of Dance Movement Therapy

Part A. Dance Movement Therapy in a Corporate Setting

Virginia Reed has been a consultant at J.P. Morgan Chase for five and a half years. Her title is Movement Therapist and her clientele consists of individuals from Chase who have been downsized and are in transition, looking for the same kind of job or considering new directions.

Reed was first asked to consult at Chase by an upper level employee familiar with her body-mind approach to healing and expertise in nonverbal communication. Reed works in individual and group formats. Her theatrical and practical approach is most influenced by Bartenieff and Laban. Movement, at once functional and expressive, is a cultural, social, psychological and physical event. Interventions are made in one or more areas (personal communication, 2002).

An individual complaining, for example, of carpal tunnel syndrome, may be reacting in body attitude and effort phrasing to a high-pressured office situation. Despite up-to-date ergonomics, the worker may tighten and constrict the muscles in her head, neck and shoulders, while bursting forward with quick advancing motions through her hands and fingers to type on the computer. Over time, with repetitive nonadaptive patterns, pain and dysfunction ensue (Reed, personal communication, 2002).

According to Reed, a systems analysis that includes a holistic view of the individual in the workplace, utilizing movement description can effectively facilitate new movement behavior. Reed has taught the rudiments of Laban analysis to employees at Chase and other corporations. She refers to a "stress model of behavior," and she teaches staff how tension has direction, texture and context. Awareness of the components of stress starts the healing process. Particularly helpful is Laban's concept of exertion-recuperation.

Reed leads one group that integrates Bartenieff Fundamentals, yoga and dance in the first half and hypnosis and guided imagery in the second half. Auditory, kinesthetic and visual cues are woven throughout the trance work, with language inspired by the participants. The work of Milton Erickson strongly influences her work (personal communication, 2002).

Another group utilizes improvisational theatre and dance therapy techniques to facilitate and rehearse new and daring responses in job interviews. "Pushing the envelope" and getting the edge are vital qualities in a competitive market. A third group educates clients in nonverbal communication within the job interview. An interactional model with Laban vocabulary is applied to interviews, team meetings and public speaking (Reed, personal communication, 2002).

Public Affairs and the Media

The skills of a dance therapist can be extremely diverse. Several dance therapists have worked as image consultants and body language experts in the public sphere. Martha Davis, whose Movement Psychodiagnostic assessment tools based on Laban's concepts informed the work of many dance therapists, has done evaluations of political leaders from the United States and other countries. Miriam Roskin Berger appeared on CNN in 1992 (personal communication, 2002), commenting on the behavior of Bush, Perot and Clinton. Virginia Reed is the body language specialist for Fox Cable News and has analyzed the movement patterns of George W. Bush, Jesse Jackson, Tom Daschle and others. Other dance therapists, such as Karen Bradley, have also used their dance therapy and Laban experience to analyze the movement patterns of political leaders. Their work has been presented in major media interviews.

Part B. Families

Dance therapy with families is relatively new, though a few dance therapists previously had some involvement with this patient group. In the 1960s, Bartenieff, Davis, Schmais and White were involved in analyzing the nonverbal communications observed in verbal family therapy sessions at Bronx State Hospital. Also at this time, Kestenberg was developing her correlations of psychoanalytic thought with effort/shape theory and applying this to her analyses of family interactions, specifically, of mother/child and mother/infant interactions. However, it was not until the 1970s that dance therapists began seriously discussing the possibility of using their observational and dance movement skills as tools for intervention for family systems.

Dianne Dulicai (1976) emphasizes the role of nonverbal communication in family interactions, referring to the work of Birdwhistell, Scheflin, Kestenberg, Davis, North and Hall. She also stresses the importance of considering "the family from which the patient comes, its culture and its place in the community" (1976, p. 4). She quotes Ackerman in his belief that it is necessary, when treating an emotionally disturbed child, to also evaluate and modify the disturbances or pathology, where possible, in the child's daily personal life.

Dulicai describes her work with a middle class family consisting of a domineering mother, a passive, dependent father who tries to fulfill his emotional needs through his son and a 17-year-old son who could not separate himself from the family. She illustrates through "family sculpting" (p. 7), the physical positions that characterize each family member's role in the family system. The family sculpture demonstrated the mother's central position, the father's dependence and the son's fear of his mother's seductiveness. Also revealed was an increase in the mother's anxiety level as the son moved farther from the family.

In this particular family, one of the major goals was in helping the son to leave the family and succeed in his adult life. Since both parents expressed an intellectual interest in this goal, Dulicai felt it was safe and feasible to expose the nonverbal "messages" around this issue, which were unconsciously encouraging him to stay home. Dulicai tried the following style of intervention. Her goal was to begin decoding nonverbal communications in a nonthreatening way.

> The father and the movement therapist stood in a circle and, with music accompanying, began a simple gesture that all were familiar with ... "thumbing." The [family's] association with this was, "someone is going somewhere." At this point, the mother directly asked her son where he wanted to go. The therapist asked the son to try and mimic the gesture of the mother, for it was clear that her gesture had changed radically to message "come here" rather than thumbing "go away." (Dulicai, 1976, p. 10)

The above is one technique that Dulicai used to expose the family to an awareness of their nonverbal communications, that is, "messaging." A second technique that utilizes "messaging" and effort/shape is described below:

> I would get a simple motion started choosing a simple rhythmic two phasic gesture and increase the intensity and decrease the strength of the gesture, then add directness so that the gesture was no longer directed to space but to another person. Observing the persons in the family and how they used strength and to whom, we would then reflect on what had happened. (Dulicai, 1976, p. 10)

The conceptual framework that Dulicai used in the 1970s is still being used today. Further studies building on this original work have been published and are available through Dulicai (Dianne.dulicai@cox.net) (personal communication, 2003).

This kind of intervention can lead to thoughtful discussion by the family on the role, thoughts and feelings of family members. In this case, the father discussed his role and how this role developed out of his past experiences.

In a movement sequence that involved the pelvis, it was noted that the mother directed herself toward her son. Because of the severity of the son's physical response, Dulicai believed it would be destructive to bring this into the family's conscious awareness at this time. She states this as one important aspect of family dance therapy, that is, knowing "what kinds of data need to be used ... and what kinds need to be defended against" (1976, p. 11). Dulicai also emphasizes the importance of interfering with destructive family messages and at times directing hostility that might otherwise go to the child toward the therapist. Over a period of 18 months, Dulicai helped the son differentiate himself from the rest of the family, partially by interfering with the nonverbal message he was receiving from his parents and by bolstering his efforts to break away. At the same time, she helped the parents deal with their son's breaking away by encouraging them to find ways to satisfy their needs other than through their child.

In another article, Dulicai (1977) describes her observation over an 18-month period of eight families with children ranging from three to seven years of age. This study combines elements from a number of theoretical approaches. It is designed to disclose family dynamics through observing interaction, which can take place in any setting (e.g., playroom, clinic, dance studio). She developed charts and an evaluation system for assessment of nonverbal factors and family interaction patterns. Her body movement assessment scale combines kinesic factors with emotional content. Based on the data assessed in this study, an instrument was developed to rate potential change within families.

Dulicai and Rogers discuss the use of Dulicai's scale, "Nonverbal Assessment of Family Systems," in a 1980 article. The authors conducted a four-month study of a mother/child dyad at the Developmental Center for Autistic Children in Philadelphia. The mother was reported to be chronically depressed and the child, seven years old, was functioning at the developmental level of a 2-1/2- to 3-year-old child.

Parent/child evaluations were made by rating videotapes of three sessions during the study period. The resulting data were discussed and treatment goals were based on these discussions. Further data were recorded on the basis of daily emotional growth and behavioral changes that resulted from movement therapy sessions. The goals of therapy were to promote a rapport within the family and to develop both physical and psychological dynamics that would facilitate the emotional growth of family members.

For purposes of observation and assessment, the early sessions were nondirective. The mother could play with her child in any way she wanted. The therapists encouraged her to respond to his initiation of play and try to reach him at his level, but they did not suggest any specific themes or tasks. During the first videotaped session, neither mother nor child exhibited a wide range of possibilities for a relationship. The mother seemed more concerned with her own needs than with her child's.

Based on this and continuing assessments, the individual sessions with the child concentrated on spatial clarity, phrasing and modulation. The mother/child session focused on movement interchange, particularly those aspects relating to sharing, relationship, accommodation and support. By the third and final videotaped session, considerable changes in movement and interaction were apparent. The mother was able to nurture her child for brief periods of time and could support him as he initiated and explored movement. The child was able to focus more fully, to complete movement phrases, to leave and return to projects and was more spontaneous in speech.

Judith Bell (1984) has integrated a number of movement therapy techniques into her work with families. She observes the family members' everyday movements, of which they are not aware, as well as "subtle shifts in breathing, skin tones and eye contact." (p. 194) She assigns structured and unstructured movement improvisations, which bring creative movement into conscious awareness. Also, she utilizes authentic movement, with stress on the ego's self-observation, to promote understanding of the feelings and motivation underlying behavior.

Bell describes movement processes at all levels of human experience—in the formation and expression of emotions, beliefs and values, as well as in physical action. Because she sees movement in all interactions, she finds it natural to communicate family behavior patterns as "Kinetic Translations" (p. 243). This is a nonverbal re-enactment of the behavior, which the family describes in the session.

For example, Sarah, a mother in her mid-thirties, complained that her boyfriend, Dave, was trying to "break up" her relationship with her 10-year-old daughter, Susie. The therapist asked Dave to communicate symbolically through movement how he was trying to relate to Sarah and Susie. He placed the two sitting next to each other on the floor. He then stood up in front of them and tried to drive between them, separating them with his hands and trying to squeeze his face between theirs. Sarah immediately screamed that that was exactly what she was talking about!

By stripping the behavior to its bare bones through nonverbal movement, the family members communicate clearly, dramatically and with full affective impact. Dave could not disown his behavior or deny its emotional effect. However, he stated that this first translation did not portray his true intention and that he wanted another chance. The therapist asked him to try a different approach. This time he gathered Sarah and Susie together in his arms in a big, tight bear hug. Sarah's reaction was to feel suffocated and angry.

The therapist then asked Sarah to advance beyond portraying the current reality in the family, to demonstrate the way she would like things to be. Sarah structured the scene with Susie standing and herself and Dave kneeling, so they would all be the same height. All three kept their hands at their sides. This not only gave Dave a clearer view of Sarah's feelings, but also gave the therapist rich material about additional themes, or "core processes," in the family's interaction, such as boundary issues between mother and daughter and power issues between mother and boyfriend. Bell stresses that the therapist should treat this movement information gained through improvisations as a "hunch," to be confirmed or discounted as the treatment progresses.

Bell has organized her thinking about family interaction by adapting William Schutz's Fundamental Interpersonal Relationship Orientation (FIRO). FIRO postulates three dimensions to categorize all interpersonal phenomena: inclusion, control and openness. Inclusion refers to "desires for belonging and togetherness, recognition of uniqueness, commitment to a relationship and desires for attention and prominence." Control is defined as the "desire to exert or relinquish authority." The third dimension, openness, revolves around the issue of vulnerability. It encompasses the "amount of transparency or privacy sought, ... the desire for personal and intimate or impersonal and distant relations" (Bell, 1984, p. 200).

Bell believes that the FIRO themes of interaction tend to proceed with the developmental stages of the treatment: inclusion in the initial phase, control in the middle phase and openness in the end phase (Bell, 1984, p. 233). Each theme and phase calls for a different behavior and role from the therapist. She summarizes this along with typical family behaviors, attitudes and goals for each stage, in two convenient tables.

Bell clearly uses the power of movement to effect change and turns to it as both a first and last resort. She then clarifies her thinking and systemizes her information through theoretical formulation and adaptation. Her work seems particularly useful to dance therapists interested in expanding their methodology and also for family therapists from other disciplines less familiar with nonverbal communication and the potential of body movement.

James Murphy (1979), a psychiatrist and dance therapist, has also experimented in the use of body movement as a therapeutic tool in his work with families. He describes his "experiential-educational approach," which "integrates dance and movement therapy with family therapy theories and techniques" (p. 61). Murphy's programs have been exclusively for families with infants less than one year old. Groups consist of four families each, with the infants present at each session. Sessions take place in a workshop setting. Murphy believes that it is possible, on a movement level, to observe, interpret and change the dynamics of family interactions. He makes the point that a therapist can work directly with an infant only on the nonverbal symbolic level.

For theoretical bases, Murphy refers to Klaus and Kennell (1976) who believe that patterns of family interaction and directions of infant development become established in the first days, weeks and months of a baby's life. He also refers to Speck (1964) who focuses on the use of space in particular rooms of the house as a nonverbal indicator of parent-child dynamics.

Murphy's techniques rely on specific movement interventions and behavior changes that will reduce tension-producing and conflicting behavior patterns, and will positively affect both the harmony and stability of communications between parent and child and the healthy development of the infant.

In conclusion, dance therapists working with families are particularly concerned with patterns of nonverbal communication and interaction, combining dance movement concepts (e.g., effort/shape) with family therapy concepts. Since both the dance therapist and the family therapist work with nonverbal communication and interaction, family therapy done through the medium of dance movement and verbalization seems quite natural.

Part C. Blind and Visually Impaired

Blind or visually impaired individuals often have tentative and restricted movement styles caused by fear of moving without sight. Joanne Weisbrod (1974) stresses the importance of having a safe place to work. A secure environment promotes a more complete use of the body and an atmosphere where more open and honest communication can take place. The therapist must pay careful attention to the patient's movements to insure safety and to help him or her dissipate anxiety. Allowing sufficient time for patients to become familiar with studio space is essential. Feeling secure in the working space facilitates the exploration of aggressive movement and space. Once the individual becomes secure in the space, he or she will feel freer to increase the range, scope and depth of psychomotor expression.

Weisbrod's overall goal is to provide the visually impaired with the means to "fully own, use and gain pleasure from their bodies" (1974, p. 50). Sessions are designed to provide this by increasing the participants' awareness of their movement strengths, weaknesses and potential, improving their body image and gross motor coordinations, reinforcing the positive aspects of their existing movement styles and increasing their range of responses and scope of movement. Activities include working with movement dynamics, energy flow, momentum, rhythm, space, multisensory experiences, relationship awareness and role-playing. Weisbrod emphasizes the need for auditory cues and uses musical instruments, clapping, finger snapping, recorded music and vocal instructions.

Martin writes of the blind person's inability to imitate the movement and to respond to the movement of others, as well as of the fear that impedes movement and results in poorly developed motor skills. Her main intervention style is the teaching of a wide variety of creative movements (not dance), which, she believes, can eventually help the blind individual to "participate in a larger share of life and come to move with more confidence, freedom and dignity (Martin, 1977, p. 62).

Martin believes it is important for the therapist to move with, narrate and reflect the patients' feelings by picking up on their actions and moods. She uses leaders to initiate exercise within the group. Though she sometimes suggests movement verbally, no orders are given and she makes it a point to use everyone's name during the sessions so each one feels special. Like Weisbrod, Martin also uses music.

For both Weisbrod and Martin the goal is the same: to help the blind and visually impaired increase their self-awareness and scope of expressive movement as a means of building self-confidence and the capacity for more meaningful relationships with others. As Canner (1980) points out, this is in marked contrast to the approach of past years, which saw as its goal teaching blind people those movement and behavior patterns that would make them more accepted by the sighted world.

Individuals who are blinded later in life through accident or illness often experience emotional problems stemming from a sense of loss and sudden dependence on others. Mary Frost (1984) describes her work with just such an individual, Richard, a 56-year-old man whose refusal to cope with his sudden blindness two years earlier had caused him to become obsessed with "calendar counting" (i.e., figuring out what day of the week a given day would have been x number of years ago).

The treatment was conducted in a partial hospitalization program two days a week for six hours each day. Clients participated in recreational therapy and received instruction in daily living skills. The object of the study, Richard was the only blind person in this program. Twice a week he participated in two hours of expressive therapy, which included 30-40 minutes of moving to music led by a dance therapist, followed by an hour of verbal psychotherapy that was co-led by the dance therapist and an art therapist. In three of the 26 sessions, art therapy was used to help Richard express feelings brought up by the dance therapy.

Frost's goal was to explore the relationship between the changes that occurred in Richard's movement repertoire and the changes that occurred in his psychological functioning during the course of the therapy. Frost described these changes from her clinical observations, then analyzed and charted them.

Richard's treatment goals were to reduce obsessive behavior (calendar counting) and, ultimately, to help Richard confront his situation and enter a school for the blind. The author used dance therapy to support these goals through focusing on his feelings, improving physical mobility and increasing social contact. In addition, verbal and nonverbal contexts were used to unearth the emotional conflicts that were fueling the calendar counting ritual.

The treatment assumed two stages. Initially, Frost worked to help Richard "shift from movements that were restricted and close to his body center to movements that flowed from the center to the periphery" (1984, p. 29). This expanding use of space and ease of movement began to break the grip of his obsession. In his first dance therapy session, Richard walked in a bent over posture with arms extended in front of him for protection and feet spread apart for stability. In the fourth dance therapy session, he learned to orient himself, using the sound of the therapist's hands clapping as "radar." After the sixth session (about three weeks in treatment), he could navigate by himself in the two rooms of the day hospital program. Later he took on the outside world, using a cane to walk down the street to visit a friend.

Interestingly, as soon as Richard began to make social contact with other group members, the link between his obsessive behavior and his loneliness became apparent; he did not calendar count on the days he attended the program. In addition, Richard's range of emotional expressions increased with his mobility. In the second stage of treatment, the dance therapist gave Richard ample opportunity to use symbolic movement to externalize his inner state. Over a period of weeks, Richard's psychomotor expressivity increased significantly. He began reaching into the center of the circle for, in his words, "good health"—when hopeful or "for nothing"—when despairing. He began trying to push away and symbolically throw off what he called, "his crazy head."

In session 13, he clapped his hands stiffly and pushed himself back strongly with his arms, stating that he was trying to push away what he believed to be "evil" (interpretation—his blindness). In sessions 14 through 16, these emotions climaxed as Richard accepted that his primary problem was blindness and expressed the intense anger he had felt at the restrictions and dependency this had imposed in his life. Using expressive symbolic movement, he angrily flicked with his hands and arms, pushed away and threw things down. In art, he drew a road with himself at the end of it, signifying that there was no hope. Outside the sessions, his calendar counting temporarily increased in intensity but could no longer cover his anger.

At this point, Richard used the verbal sessions to connect his angry feelings with frustrating events from his past: low paying jobs, social isolation and dependency on his family. His frustration and despair gave way to determination, as in movement session 20, he "punched forward on the diagonal and stomped his feet into the floor," while declaring that he was "burying calendar counting" and "was going to have a new life."

In session 25, Richard's last in the program (before going to a school for the blind), he enjoyed the support and strength of the group as all moved together in percussive stamping, arms interlocked around the circle. Richard received warm good-byes and good wishes and appeared on the verge of tears.

After one month at the school, Richard's calendar counting had totally stopped. One and a half years later, Richard had made friends, learned enough Braille to deal with everyday tasks and could maneuver around the city. He had married, was helping to raise his 13-year-old stepdaughter and worked 25-40 hours a week at the school.

Frost found an inverse relationship between the intensity of Richard's obsessive behavior (the calendar counting) and the expansiveness of his movement. In general, the more mobile Richard became, the less he calendar counted. Frost believes that more studies should be performed, correlating clients' emotional progress with movement changes, to statistically verify the patterns she observed in this case.

Part D. Deaf and Hearing Impaired

Peter Wisher (1974), a dance educator, is one of the few individuals to write about his work with the deaf and hearing impaired. He stresses that the dance experience (as in the case of blind people) reduces feelings of isolation and motivates social relationships and group feelings. This is particularly important for deaf and blind individuals, who frequently grow to be rigid in behavior and lacking in social consciousness. Wisher stresses group work for this reason and creates sequences that promote feelings of solidarity.

Because physical education is often unavailable to the deaf, they may lack neuromuscular skills. This is due to social deprivation, not to inherent physical weakness. Dance movement in conjunction with physical education can easily relieve deaf people of the stigma of appearing to have a muscular disability. Wisher also feels that deaf people are well-oriented toward movement, since sign language, the "language of the deaf," is communication based upon expressive gesture. He believes in total communication with his deaf students: a combination of signs and movement, manual alphabet, speech and lip reading. Through his methods, Wisher's students have experienced feelings of self-worth and confidence they previously lacked. These feelings come from within and extend toward others, both hearing and nonhearing.

Wisher's work with a group of deaf and some nonspeaking college students at Gallaudet College in Washington, DC, was the subject of a CBS News segment in 1987. Wisher described the students' training in dance improvisation based on exaggeration (i.e., expanding and broadening) of sign language symbols into abstract dance form. Because signing is essentially expressive nonverbal communication through body movement, Wisher believes that the hearing impaired have already highly developed the art of communicating emotions nonverbally.

While Wisher's work is not formally considered dance therapy, it is extremely therapeutic and could easily become psychotherapy; the joy, skill and expressivity displayed by these students as they danced in the CBS News segment were obvious. Wisher's work confirms that for deaf individuals, dance can be a major avenue for building movement skills, communication, self-expression, confidence and a feeling of community and belonging in the world.

UNIT IV

International Growth of Dance Movement Therapy

Introduction
By Miriam Roskin Berger

When the following chapter was written, the world had not yet experienced the trauma of Sept. 11th, 2001 and the ensuing war and threats of terrorism. It appears that now, more than ever, the nonverbal language of movement and dance is a crucial tool of communication and discovery throughout the globe and a critical channel through which to connect to others. Dance therapists from the United States have been to all parts of the world for many years. The first, in fact, was Marian Chace, who was invited to Israel in the sixties. It is also important to note that, even though dance therapy has grown most widely in the United States, several of the original dance therapy pioneers here were émigrés from Europe. There has always been cross-cultural interchange in our profession.

My own international journeys began in 1983, when I taught in Stockholm with Marcia Leventhal, who brought the New York University Master of Arts program to Sweden, where we had students from all the Scandinavian countries. Since 1990, I have worked most extensively in the Netherlands, Sweden and the Czech Republic and have led workshops in many other countries. In Sweden, I have taught at the University College of Dance, Umea University, the Royal College of Music, supervised dance therapists at Lowenstromska Psychiatric Hospital in a center that used the creative arts therapies as the only treatment, conducted research in this center and taught dance therapy in the Swedish Expressive Arts Therapy Program. In the Netherlands, I first taught many introductory courses at the Rotterdam Dance Academy and then set up a full curriculum there for dance therapy training. Judith Bunney was my co-teacher and, in

1998, we also began a training program in Prague initiated by Dr. Radana Sourkova and Corrinne Ott and taught summer courses in Poznan under the auspices of the Polish Dance Theatre.

In Germany, I have taught and lectured in Bonn organized by Sabine Trautmann-Voight and in Hamburg at the Psychotherapeutisches Institut für Tanztherapie directed by Anna Pohlmann. And, I had the honor, in 1994, to be one of the six keynote speakers (all of us Americans) at the First International Dance Therapy Congress organized by Maria-Luise Oberum in Berlin. Janet Adler, Joan Chodorow, Penny Lewis, Susan Loman and Elaine Siegel were the other American keynote speakers.

I have had a wide variety of experiences in many countries and have been impressed with some of the striking and touching similarities I have observed. There truly is a universal culture of dance therapy comprised of diverse people in all nations who understand and feel the meaning and the power and the potential of movement. The variety of students abroad seriously interested in our discipline is astonishing—among them dancers, artists, actors, social workers, journalists, psychiatrists and other physicians, cinema directors, politicians, psychologists, rehabilitation counselors and clergy. Many of them are already respected professionals in their own fields. And, somehow, I have not found either the tension or the disrespect toward dance that one sometimes encounters in the United States.

Dance is an accepted part of the intellectual and artistic world in other nations and, in several cultures, still part of the religious arena. Its use as therapy, therefore, seems organic and logical. The students are all extremely disciplined and intelligent, as well as creative. In groups of diverse nationalities, the language of movement binds them together. Their interest and passion is energizing. In Russia, a two-hour workshop lasted five hours, as the students did not want to stop and, during the summer floods of 2002 in Prague, not one workshop was cancelled and all students diligently attended. A dance therapist teaching in a foreign country has a special advantage, of course, in learning and adapting to a new culture. The universality of movement, along with our conscious and unconscious understanding of it, provides an immediate attunement to nonverbal subtleties of communication. We all learn the language of movement more quickly than the spoken language wherever we go. One tunes in very quickly to the patterns of the society and of the individuals we teach and, as we know, this creates a deep sense of mutual trust.

I have always felt at home whatever my destination. And I have learned so very much in my travels from the students and the pioneers in each country. In addition to knowledge of a new culture, I have learned much about dedication, commitment, the endurance of hardship and tragedy, humor, discipline and, of course, unbelievably fresh and creative perspectives on the possibilities of dance therapy. I have also found that the dance forms in each country reflect the principles of dance therapy in their own unique manner.

It is not the intention in the following chapter to describe dance therapy developments in every corner of the world but rather to illuminate the activities of Americans in their travels. Information about some who have worked abroad did not arrive in time for inclusion: Patricia Capello taught in London and Taiwan; Amber Gray works with war trauma survivors in Europe. And the work of Elaine Siegel in Switzerland and Germany and Dianne Dulicai in Great Britain and Mexico, of course, has been extremely important. So, what follows is a representative history of what American dance therapists have accomplished in their international journeys and an inspiring and insightful overview of their personal reflections. The issue of diversity is rampant in our precarious world and the personal reflections that follow and about which Cathy Appel has so skillfully written help to clarify these delicate multicultural issues. It is my hope that our dance therapy journeys will continue to strengthen cross-cultural trust and the diverse global growth of our unique profession.

26. International Growth of Dance Movement Therapy

By Cathy Appel

Industrial, nuclear, bacterial and viral threats to the environment and world safety are universally compelling issues which invite unity and cooperation among members of the healing professions, especially among dance movement therapists whose earliest roots stem from sacred rituals employed in the service of untenable forces.

Dance is a universal language and, as with the development of modern dance internationally, the growth of dance movement therapy around the world has been inevitable. By the 1980s and 1990s, the pioneer spirit so deeply embedded in the practice of dance movement therapy led many professionals to accept, or even seek, opportunities to work abroad. Unifying trends such as the development of the European Union, the globalization of commerce and the creation of common currencies like the Euro point not only to increasing interaction abroad but to growing similarities in the treatment issues presented to the dance movement therapist.

Increasingly, healthcare providers and their communities—regardless of nationality—are challenged by multiple problems. Immigration, epidemiological crises and expanding populations of the elderly and chronically ill, along with the deinstitutionalization of people due to greater access to psychotropic medications, the growing acceptance of difference and the inability of countries to meet the high cost of residential care, are now global issues. In addition, growing numbers of women are in the workplace, creating a shift away from the nuclear family toward after-school childcare programs and community centers, and new demands on these institutions.

With the start of a new millennium, it is useful to assess the impact of globalization on dance movement therapy. This chapter offers a glimpse of the quickly evolving international reach of dance movement therapy through the work of several members of the ADTA abroad. As with the codification of standards by the ADTA in 1966, continued attention is being paid by dance movement therapists around the world to training, credentialing and the integration of methods and standards of practice.

In 1995, at the ADTA's Annual Conference in Rye, New York, then president **Miriam Roskin Berger** instituted the first International Panel of Dance Movement Therapists. The Panel is now a highlight of the Annual Conference. In 1998, in conjunction with the ADTA's decision to affiliate with the NBCC (National Board of Certified Counselors), Sally Totenbier was appointed the leader for the International Hub of Task Force II, to consider the implications of this affiliation internationally and to maintain communication regarding this process. In 1999, after the completion of Task Force II's mission, Totenbier was asked to serve as the first chairperson of the Global Membership Services Subcommittee.

Sally Totenbier, who has lived in the United Kingdom for periods of time, became involved in the Association for Dance Movement Therapy (ADMT), which was started in 1982, by editing their newsletter. She says of the ADMT that its outreach includes lobbying with labor unions for affiliation and representation and working with the educational system to create job descriptions for dance movement therapy.

The following are Totenbier's observations on dance movement therapy in the UK:

> One feature of dance movement therapy work that is unique in the UK is that it often occurs within the context of "community dance." This most typically is via government programs housed in what would be community centers or recreational centers in the USA, but offering various health and mental health services. Community dance programs aim to be inclusive, offering persons with special needs the opportunity to participate in mainstream dance classes and performances. Community dance has a longer

history than dance movement therapy, but its presence has opened the doors for focused dance movement therapy practice and offerings for those with emotional or physical challenges. Many dance movement therapists operate within the school system as well. These foci are undoubtedly part of the legacy of Laban's work, which was part of the school curriculum in the UK for many years and still plays an important role in many UK physical education classes.

Dance movement therapy provides a service to the community at large and to children with special needs within the school system, as well as its more traditional role in the mental health services. The UK also is serving as the hub for European dance movement therapy information exchange, having the oldest of the European dance movement therapy associations. The UK has hosted many expressive arts conferences and symposiums that have attracted practitioners from throughout Europe; efforts are being made to standardize education and practice throughout Europe to meet the needs emerging with the Common Market. Many persons from other countries visit or live in the UK for the purposes of studying dance movement therapy, which contributes to both the economy and the cosmopolitan nature of this country. (I personally have known people from Brazil, Portugal, Hungary, Holland, Israel, Japan, Canada and the USA who traveled to the UK for this purpose.) (personal communication, 1999)

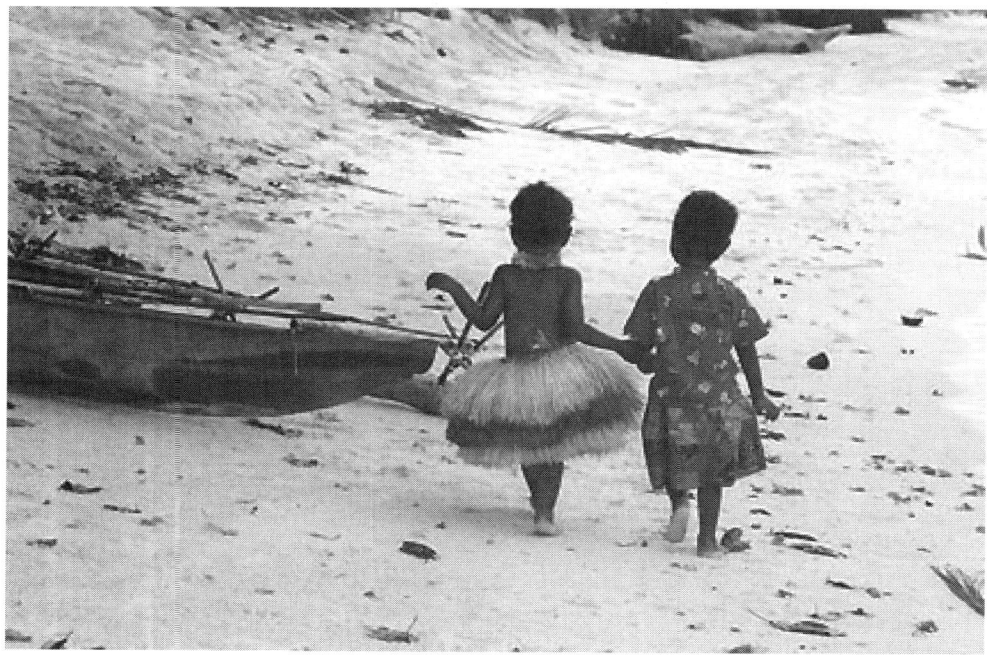

The nonverbal language of movement is a crucial tool of discovery throughout the globe (Photo courtesy Leonard Forrest)

Totenbier was present for most of the deliberation, which led to the creation of the UK registry. The ADMT followed the American decision to incorporate multiple tiers from the onset, but they also created a system unique to their heritage. Totenbier says, as there is now reciprocity between the ADMT and ADTA registry, the differences in requirements will not impact the work opportunities for herself or for future American dance movement therapists in the UK.

Sharon Chaiklin first worked in Israel in 1976 and 1977 doing workshops and individual work. Subsequently, in 1980-1981, the late Mara Capy initiated a year-long course at the University of Haifa in conjunction with Antioch New England, for the purpose of bringing together those who were already working in an isolated manner and to offer them common terms and ways of communicating with one another. During that year, Chaiklin was involved in teaching and supervising students. The Israelis now have their own organization, an annual conference and several programs. Yael Barkai, a member of the ADTA, is the director of the dance therapy program at Seminar Kibbutzim outside Tel Aviv, which recently affiliated with Hahnemann so that it can offer a Master's degree. Chaiklin observes:

> What makes dance therapy a fertile profession in Israel is that people are familiar with and supportive of dance and social services, and are used to absorbing many different people with myriad problems. There are many government-supported agencies. While funds are limited and the bureaucracy is difficult, nonetheless there is general understanding of the purpose and value of dance therapy. Many professionals make use of complementary therapies for themselves and their clients.
>
> The patient populations treated are within the total range of human problems. There are many problems in a country that is surrounded by hostile nations and has had several wars and is made up of immigrants from many cultures and varied languages. There is a high stress level as a result. Children are offered many services through not only mental health agencies but also through the department of education. There are hospitalized patients and the full range of family and social services.(personal communication, 1999)

Chaiklin also has experience in Japan. She first went to Japan in 1985 to visit a family member. While in Japan, Chaiklin contacted a psychiatric hospital to observe Japanese methods of treatment. The professionals there were interested in dance therapy and asked her to do a workshop for the professional community and speak to the staff. Her offer to do a session with their patients was accepted and the session was videotaped. This tape was seen by others; so when Chaiklin returned to Japan in 1990, people were already familiar with her work. As a result, she was invited to participate in a two-day workshop and subsequently in their annual conferences.

Chaiklin has maintained contact with those involved in developing dance therapy in Japan, like Shoichi Machida. The Japanese now have their own organization, a newsletter, an annual conference and a journal. Machida, who is the executive director of the Japanese Dance Therapy Association, attends the ADTA conferences and has compiled a booklet on international information for the ADTA that is available in their Maryland office.

Chaiklin has the following observations about dance movement therapy in Japan:

> Japan is open to the use of the body through such things as martial arts and an understanding of the body through meditation and other Buddhist influences. There are many rituals and ways of doing things and no one wants to be embarrassed in having "lost face," but these are choices that people make. In Japan, the body has not been repressed, i.e., public baths being quite common and until fairly recently, used by both men and women together.
>
> The Japanese did not have the "puritan" perspective that we inherited from the Puritans about the body being a source of sin. It is rather a source of pleasure and accomplishment, i.e., martial arts, noh, kabuki. For the Japanese, there are factors other than repression that have to be overcome in relation to feelings about using social services and mental health agencies, but this is slowly evolving in a positive direction.
>
> There are services for the elderly developing as a result of fewer extended families living together, also services for children and the developmentally delayed and other social services. The level of stress for families is high as work hours are long, and there are new stresses as the economy is fluctuating and westernization increases.
>
> I totally enjoy working within the country as people are gracious and kind and want to learn. The main obstacles of course are my own inability to speak the Japanese language and subtle forms of cultural differences that are difficult to pick up ... particularly without use of the language. However, the nonverbal still rules. (personal communication, 1999)

Nana Koch, who has had a long-standing interest in Japanese culture, had the opportunity to travel to Japan through a former Japanese Hunter College Dance Therapy student, Kyoko Jingu. After returning to Japan, Jingu invited Koch, in the spring of 1998, to teach the work of Liljan Espenak. Jingu served as the translator of the workshops of Koch as well as Chaiklin. She also practices dance therapy in a psychiatric hospital in Gunma, Japan, and runs ongoing dance therapy study groups for people in Japan who have some dance therapy training and want to increase their theoretical understanding. Koch also mentions Yoh Yahata, of Tokyo, who is an author and licensed counselor affiliated with the Holistic Health Society of Tokyo and a strong supporter of dance therapy in Japan. Koch offers this observation:

> In Japan, as is true of eastern thought, the mind and body are seen as one. This idea, distinctly different from what has been perceived as a split between mind and body in the west, gives the Japanese a particular openness to using dance as therapy. (personal communication, 1999)

Amy Wapner's connection with Japan happened early in her career. Due to her pioneering use of videotape and e-mail for long distance supervision, her initial contact evolved into an integrated clinical program through which dance movement therapy is offered on several inpatient units as well as in a daycare setting at independent psychiatric Hasegawa Hospital, in the outskirts of Tokyo, Japan. An American dance movement therapist, Wapner lives and is able to maintain a private practice in New York, while continuing to be an integral part of the institute-style approach she developed at Hasegawa.

Wapner started her career as a dance movement therapist at a state hospital in New York. She was part of a family therapy team there, when, unbeknownst to her, a routine exchange with a new staff psychologist from Japan planted the seed for a dramatic career shift which has had the most profound effect on her life. Wapner's openness to people and belief in dance movement therapy made it easy for her to meet Dr. Yasuichiro Yusa's inquiries about dance movement therapy with a challenge: she invited him to attend a dance movement therapy session. Their collaboration in the early 1980s made such an impression on him that in 1988, after returning to Japan, he, along with Dr. Tsunehito Hasegawa and Dr. Mikiko Hasegawa, invited Wapner to provide an introductory two-week workshop to the progressive Hasegawa Hospital.

The two-week seminar evolved into a 14-year comprehensive process that has produced a focused, integrated clinical program. An institute-style approach has been utilized successfully for training staff at Hasegawa Hospital. In addition to an annual intensive two-week seminar, the team maintains a monthly supervision dialogue with Wapner via videotape and e-mail. An interdisciplinary group of staff are periodically screened and added to the existing core group that comprise the dance movement therapy team. Several talented individuals from various backgrounds work together and provide a strong clinical dance movement therapy program which functions in concert with all other treatment approaches at Hasewgawa Hospital.

Current members of the team are: Miyuki Kaji (clinical psychologist, dance movement therapist ADTR), Tadashi Miyagi (clinical psychologist, dance movement therapist), Chiyoko Komori (nurse, dance movement therapist), Yokoko Matsuda (clinical psychologist, dance movement therapist), Toshiko Matsuo (occupational therapist, dance movement therapy assistant), Kumiko Horiuchi (occupational therapist, day care administrator, dance movement therapist), Makiko Khoda (occupational therapist, dance movement therapy assistant, team coordinator), Kunitoshi Iwai (occupational therapist, dance movement therapist), and Asuka Itou (clinical psychologist, dance movement therapy assistant). Miyuki Kaji and Tadashi Miyagi are collaborating to provide training to others in Japan through the dance movement therapy seminar based at and sponsored by Hasegawa Hospital. At present, they offer level one and level two short-term courses, and are actively working with many other dance movement therapists in Japan. They present their work in many venues, including those provided by the Japan Dance Therapy Association, the Japan Art Therapy Association, and other world congress settings.

Wapner expresses gratitude for her ongoing, long-term work in Japan and emphasizes her process and the importance of her learning Japanese:

> My work in Japan continues to emerge as a rich and powerful experience in my life. With strong support from director, Dr. Mikiko, Dr. Yasuichiro Yusa, administrative, clinical, business staff, and my frequent translator, Elli Uchida, access to the inner mechanism of a hospital, to individual patients, and to many aspects of Japanese culture, has been provided. So many have embraced the program and have collaborated closely with me, making this an exciting, often challenging, and fulfilling process.
>
> In the beginning, despite months of study and anticipation, my struggle to understand the culture forced me to slow down and to listen attentively to what was said, and what was *not* said. Even though I was often baffled and in error, my renewed discovery and awe of the healing dance, which is at the root of our practice with people, encouraged me to persist. It became apparent, in fact, imperative, for me to learn the basics of the Japanese language. I realized that without understanding the language, it would be difficult for me to teach, assist, support, and treat the Japanese people.
>
> In learning the language, I began to understand why, even with translation, I had been confused, or confusing to them. It took a long time for me to grasp that context within language is often implied or left unnamed, that pronouns, tenses, and other definitive terms are often not used in interpersonal dialogues. I realized that with Japanese culture, so much is understood, not stated, inferred, but not heard. I felt as if I had to make a full body shift from within, to rely on my kinesthetic and visual senses to hear. For instance, the gesture of bowing was initially just that, a gesture for me to practice while in Japan. Over time, somehow, the bow has become ingrained in me. At the beginning and ending of each session with patients, regardless of diagnosis or severity of pathology, the bow just happens ... initially with the greeting, finally with great thanks to all. It is filled with honor and respect for others. The bow

is part of the language and it starts somewhere in my toes and rises up through me, allowing me to be natural and authentic in speaking with the patients. In teaching verbal intervention, it was important to realize the necessity of "please" and "thank you," of stating imagery and discovery within the format of questions, softly. (personal communication, 2001)

Wapner has gleaned many keen insights from Japanese culture and dance movement therapy during her 14 years of close work in Japan. She comments on a few elements of Japanese culture and how they informed her work, as well as assisted her personal growth:

> In fourteen years of close work in Japan, not only at Hasegawa Hospital, but in school, university, and city hall venues, a few important elements of Japanese culture shine for me. Paramount to the culture are the inherent right to personal privacy and the emotional right to feeling ambivalent. Despite the common tendency for formality and privacy, many of my colleagues there have been drawn through the experience of dance and the movement, and through the experience of an intimate, safe setting, to open their hearts, to explore deeply private issues, to discover and tell their personal stories. Perhaps our work together helped them to release and grow.
>
> A second element that is prominent for me involves what I have learned from the Japanese regarding ambivalence. In really listening to them, in paying close attention, I have been taught to let go of the need for definitive answers in most circumstances, Western style. They have shown me that ambivalence is not necessarily a sign of weakness or a lack of clarity; rather, feeling two conflicting emotions about one issue at the same time is merely human and real, and perhaps, a strength. I remember the concept, which grabbed my attention in undergraduate school. In *Art and the Creative Unconscious*, Erich Neumann speaks of things that are "numinous," that are simultaneously compelling and threatening. It was this concept, which had first spurred my interest in therapy years ago, and here it was again.
>
> The third element, which strikes me profoundly in Japan, is the inherent ability for people to empathize with others. A profound and touching sensitivity to other people's struggles, growth and passages, has inspired and reinforced my adamancy about empathy as a tool in therapy.
>
> I feel enriched and forever changed by my opportunity to know and love a small part of Japan. Witnessing authentic self-exploration and development, valuing my own ambivalence, and perhaps most importantly being keenly aware of and emulating the sensitivity to and empathy for others by which so many Japanese people live, and feeling the instinct to bow, are only some of the treasured gifts I have received. (personal communication, 2001)

Marcia Leventhal's work worldwide is unique. With multiple visits and intensive work in several countries, Leventhal has been instrumental in the start of many dance movement therapy programs. She was an invited speaker in Sweden for DACI (Dance and the Child International) and the International Dance Council. Leventhal says there was a real ground swell of interest to do professional dance therapy training out of which began the Master's program in the early 1980s. Students spent two intensive summers studying in Sweden with either Leventhal or other New York University (NYU) faculty including Miriam Roskin Berger, the former Director of Education at NYU. The students then came to the United States to complete their internships and last year of study. Leventhal reports the dance therapy community in Sweden is very strong, with many individuals having earned advanced degrees and working throughout Scandinavia.

Leventhal has been presenting workshops and training, and developing graduate studies internationally since 1976. One of her first invitations was to Skyros, Greece, where she did intensive training in Athens and on Tinos. Leventhal says of the graduates in Greece, "Besides a deep understanding and experience of dance and body movement, their ability to grasp quite deep and sophisticated concepts from psychology, creativity, quantum physics, etc., is remarkable, but understandable when one realizes how much the word concepts developed from Greek language roots."

Leventhal was first invited to Australia in 1987 as the keynote speaker for the first dance therapy conference there. At present, she is the Director of Education and Training for the International Dance Therapy Institute of Australia. The Dance Therapy Association of Australia Inc. (DTAA), founded in 1994, supports and promotes dance therapy practitioners, practice and education throughout Australia. Leventhal observes:

> The dance movement therapists in Australia work with absolutely every population with great care and skill. They remind me of the kind of vision my teachers had (Mary Whitehouse, Blanche Evan, Alma Hawkins, Valerie Hunt), and which appears to be getting harder to discover in the United States as our practitioners align with other disciplines and seem to be separating themselves from their powerful dance roots. (personal communication, 1999)

Marcia Leventhal feels re-inspired by her opportunities to work internationally and says the only obstacles she's had have been the same ones encountered early in our profession—the creation of a professional identity and the development of jobs.

Penny Lewis[1] has been teaching in Germany. Her book, *Creative Transformation: The Healing Power of the Arts*, was translated into German. Lewis sees the Germans' "natural analytic minds, the intensity of their expressive connection, and their appreciation of learning" as strengths in their practice of dance movement therapy. Lewis observes:

> Germans have been known for their interest and involvement in philosophy. Existentialism was fostered in this country. Jungian dance therapy with its focus on individuation and higher consciousness can meet the needs of a highly sophisticated population.

> The populations often treated by DMTs in Germany are private practice populations focusing on recovery from early childhood abuse, post traumatic stress disorder as well as classical psychiatric conditions. (personal communication, 1999)

Of challenges she found in Germany, Lewis says, "Chace always told us to *meet the other where they are*. I believe this is as true for a client-therapist as it is for a student-teacher relationship." Like the majority of dance therapists who have worked internationally, Lewis expresses gratitude for the opportunity to expand her own repertoire.

Beth Kalish-Weiss, whose articles were translated into German, is another dance/movement therapist who has taught in Bonn and Munich, Germany. She was impressed with the educational advantages German students have. In Germany, education is free through graduate school and this gives students ample opportunities to learn and become highly skilled in a field of interest. Kalish-Weiss observes:

> It was my impression that DMT is filling a particular need in certain parts of Germany in which the medical model has dominated for years ... These professionals are looking for fresh, innovative ways to work ... This was particularly clear to me in many discussions with Sabine Trautmann-Voigt who directed the training group in Bonn. She and her husband, a psychoanalyst, are fine examples of how the pendulum seems to be moving there towards the creative arts therapies interwoven with those who have been trained traditionally as psychoanalysts. Still, the restrictions of licensure to practice are there, so it is necessary to have the proper credentials for practice. (personal communication, 1999)

Susan Loman started going annually to work in Germany beginning in 1993. The majority of her focus has been on teaching Kestenberg Movement Profile (KMP) notation. There was an International Dance/Movement Therapy conference in Berlin in 1994 and Loman, along with several dance movement therapists from the United States, was invited to give a keynote speech. Loman presented the application of the KMP as a tool for dance movement therapy. She believes the successful interaction among people from several countries led to networking and increased opportunities to teach. Loman observes:

> Germany has had a history of emphasizing physical education programs even for very young children. There is a value placed on keeping the body fit through hiking and mountain climbing. Today Germany offers several graduate-level education programs in body work such as Psychomotor Therapy and funds research projects in nonverbal methodology.

> More recently, I understand there have been difficulties about who is allowed to practice psychotherapy and this affects those specializing in dance/movement therapy.

> There are a wide variety of populations served. One clinic was entirely for skin disorders. They had a staff including dance/movement therapy and music therapy. Also, psychiatric hospitals hire dance/movement therapists. Other dance therapists work privately with children, adolescents and families. (personal communication, 1999)

Loman found it challenging at times not to be able to rely as much on humor, since what is humorous cannot always come through in another culture. She is also sensitive to the differences in movement styles between cultures and notes responses to certain experiential exercises will vary according to culture, based on the assumptions each country has with particular movement qualities. For instance, Loman reports she assumed flow-adjustment would elicit playfulness, but instead she found in Germany abruptness supported playfulness.

---

[1]Penny Lewis died October 10, 2003, subsequent to the writing of this chapter.

Loman was also invited to Bologna by Rosa Maria Govini to teach Kestenberg Movement Profile concepts at Art Therapy Italiana.

Marcia Plevin, an American modern dancer and longtime resident of Italy, has worked in Rome for many years. In 1986, Plevin left the position of dance chairperson at Southern Methodist University in Dallas, Texas, and moved back to Rome to join her Italian husband. She says, "I was very fortunate! Just two years before, Arthur Robbins and Debra McCall of Pratt University had set up Art Therapy Italiana in Bologna along with Rosa Maria Govini." Plevin's fortunate timing continued:

> As I left Dallas I knew that DMT was where I was headed and two weeks after I returned to Rome I connected with a workshop that Debra McCall was giving in Rome. That workshop put me on the road I am on today. The National Italian DMT professional association was formed in 1988. We are a conglomerate of about five different dance therapy schools. Still very much in the pioneer stage, but with didactic, ethics and registry committees and an annual meeting. I am on the didactic committee. Art Therapy Italiana (ATI) now has 14 DMTs who have graduated from the four-year program. It usually takes around six years to complete. (personal communication, 1999)

Of working as a dance movement therapist in Italy, Plevin observes:

> It is an uphill fight here. Although now we are practicing in psychiatric institutes, in state hospitals, in therapeutic communities and privately, the strength must come from us to help educate the mainstream "psychology-psychiatric" model. Therefore it has been very important to establish a National Association that can help with visibility, etc. However, the various regions in Italy respond differently. For example, in Lombardia (Milan) there are state hospitals that have established ongoing dance therapy treatment programs, whereas in Rome this has been more difficult. As it is everywhere, one needs the sympathetic head of some department who is willing to start the ball rolling.

> The populations served are psychiatric (children/adults), mentally disabled (children/adults), eating disorders, adolescents and in private work the range of neurotic disorders.

> There are political problems that belong in the category of state qualifications; i.e., in some cases one must be a psychologist before one can work as a DMT. If we do not have the psychologist or psychotherapy qualification we cannot advertise that we are doing psychotherapy. For example, this year I sat for and passed the Italian State exam in psychology so that I can call myself a psychologist even though that is not the work I do. (personal communication, 1999)

Plevin has a private practice in Rome where she does individual work. She also runs a Creative Movement training program with Teresa Escobar, a DMT teacher for Art Therapy Italiana. Plevin and Escobar's training is for counselors, educators and therapists in other disciplines who do not want to use movement as dance therapists but do want to understand the creative process in movement.

Joanabbey Sack says dance movement therapy was introduced in Quebec in the early 1980s. At this time, returning with an MA in Dance Movement Therapy from New York University, Sack met a visiting DMT from California who was giving sessions at a major hospital's psychiatric unit (Jewish General Hospital). Sack continued these sessions until she offered a pilot program to the Montreal Children's Hospital. This three-hour-a-week introduction became ten hours within the next six months and 40 hours within the next several years. This full-time position that began in psychiatry grew to encompass oncology, internal medicine and head injury. Sack was part of a team that developed a multi-disciplinary eating disorders team and adolescent treatment program. Both of these programs have welcomed dance movement therapy interns and continue to incorporate and, at times, highlight the creative arts therapies.

Sack feels that the experience of training in the United States has been a strong theme in Quebec:

> Those interested take workshops and intensives...those passionate leave to train in the United States (or France); some return, some move and practice elsewhere.

> DMTs in Quebec continue to work in hospitals, in private clinics, in a center for the Arts in Human Development and as consultants to education and public service institutions. Most continue to teach and several are busy producing the next generation. (personal communication, 1999)

Sack believes it is imperative that a Quebec organization (as well as a Canadian one) be formed and sustained by local training in Canada. She reports the development of dance movement therapy in Quebec is challenged by political and economic issues. However, it is the language issue that has the most immediate impact on the future of the field. The majority of the Quebec population is French speaking while the majority of the DMTs in Quebec are English speaking. A few French Canadians have studied dance therapy in the United States, yet Sack says it is not realistic to expect that many others would follow. Given the difficulty of training in a second language, the cost of higher education in the United States, and the low value of the Canadian dollar, studying in the United States is prohibitive for most Canadians.

Sack mentions some master's-level course work in dance therapy available in English where French-speaking students can submit their written work in French, and says bilingual dance therapists are available for supervision, thus making it possible for a French-speaking student to fulfill the professional requirements of the ADTA Alternate Route. She remains hopeful that efforts to start new programs and create an official dance movement therapy association in Canada will succeed.

Laura Peralta, an Argentinian psychologist and dance movement therapist, emphasizes the social and political factors in her country:

> Identity is important in Argentina. We are a mixture of mainly Spanish and Italian, among other European cultures. Europe and the United States model and are cultural references for Argentina.
>
> Decades of economic and political instability—not knowing what to expect—reinforces individualism. We pass on our fears and uncertainties, our children grow up with an outstanding sense of the present grief, resentment from the past and uncertainty for the future. It is both a strength and a weakness that we are adapting day by day with a high tolerance for frustration and a great deal of anxiety.
>
> Inherited from the Italians and Spanish, we have a strong sense of family unity. People have many children with large extended families where hugs, kisses and a lap to find refuge allow for the free expression of feelings and physical contact. (personal communication, 1999)

Peralta cites the dominant trend in Argentina until the 1980s as being psychoanalysis. She says the intellectualism, rationalism and dissociation from the body associated with psychoanalysis were extremely popular at a time when people had the time and money to spend on themselves. Things changed radically in Argentina economically in the 1980s and 1990s making the fees for four sessions per week impossible. Peralta observes:

> The hospitals were full of patients and the traditional approach didn't promise results in short-term therapies. Furthermore, in the 1970s, Argentina went through one of the most remembered internal conflicts. A great part of the population was involved and both sides suffered losses, grief, anger and desperation on a daily basis.
>
> A great need emerged. Loneliness, anguish, pain and rage were stored in the body creating emotional blocks which restrained movement, and caused insomnia, eating disorders, aching muscles, allergies, ulcers and strokes in response to the emotional stress and daily harassment. Our bodies were fragmented, distorted, injured.
>
> Slowly and firmly a new trend is opening. Body and alternative therapies are being accepted more each day and are responsive to the need for recovery, providing a "holding" space in which to integrate body-mind-emotions behavior. (personal communication, 1999)

An invitation by Diana Fischman, psychoanalyst, body psychotherapist and bioenergeticist, to Mariano Perez de Villa, group therapist, body psychotherapist and bioenergeticist, and Peralta, led to the formation of the first formal training program for dance movement therapists in Argentina in 1996. Directed by co-founder Fischman, this program is hosted by Brecha, a private institute founded by Fischman. The word Brecha means *gap* as when something *leaks* or can *get through* and there is the possibility of change. Subsequently, three 20-hour International Workshops a year were held. The following ADTRs were instructors: Marcia Leventhal, Fran Levy, Sharon Chaiklin, Jane Ganet Sigel, Joan Chodorow, Maralia Reca and Susan Loman. Levy and Chaiklin were the main consultants and supervisors. Weekly staff meetings and group supervision were the main tools used to accommodate and include changes while teaching, consulting, training and screening their own personal processes.

The institute, under the leadership of Fischman, continues to grow and now offers its services to the health care plans. Annual symposiums are held and opened to the public and DMT is being presented at conferences and seminars. Fischman and Peralta say one of the main goals of Argentinian dance movement therapists is to become part of the universities and be accepted in the hospitals. Through joint efforts with Brecha staff and others, the Asociación Argentina de Danzaterapia was formed. Fischman notes that she receives e-mail from Spain, Costa Rica, Colombia, Peru and the United States with questions and interest in the program.

The need for training programs, as well as the need to obtain academic and professional acceptance, are common themes no matter what the country. An example of this is the Netherlands, where Miriam Roskin Berger has taught at the Rotterdam Dance Academy since 1992 and, in 1995, helped start a formal training program, according to the ADTA alternate route guidelines. Several American ADTRs have taught in this program, such as Judith Bunney, Robyn Flaum Cruz and Johanna Climenko.

Robyn Flaum Cruz, a researcher of note, says the research and consulting she has done in Europe have been concentrated on individuals in England and Germany, but adds she also gets e-mail requests from individuals in South America, Australia, Spain, Italy, etc. In Rotterdam, she taught research methods and dance movement therapy for special populations (children). Cruz finds the Netherlands extremely welcoming to dance therapy and says Dutch DMTs work with similar mental health populations as well as with social issues such as child sexual abuse, domestic violence, etc., and function similarly to DMTs in the United States. Cruz says that her students all speak excellent English, but notes most have to use reference materials written in English and that is sometimes difficult for them. Hopefully, in time, reference materials will be translated and new materials written in many languages by dance therapists around the world.

Johanna Climenko has had extensive work experience in the Netherlands. She worked and taught for one year in Holland in 1971 and says of that year, it was one of the most profoundly transforming of her life and set the backdrop for Holland being her "second home" in which to teach and consult on an ongoing basis.

Climenko worked at Veleweland, a residential treatment center for neurotics that was created by visionary Willem Arendsen-Hein and is located in a manor house in the Dutch countryside. She comments:

> Holland is clearly a country of rugged individualists and in general the Dutch are practical, grounded and very clear thinking. There is a level of tolerance and values around caring for one another that sets a tone of real safety. There are many approaches to dance therapy in Holland, and in many respects these differences have been focused on rather than commonalities in trying to develop a professional organization. (personal communication, 1999)

Climenko speculates that this passionate individualism also impedes the development of a unified professional organization in the Netherlands. Climenko points to differences in the Dutch educational system as a challenge to the field of dance therapy. She observes:

> Although the work of foreigners is frequently embraced, developing understanding and acceptance of a new profession is even more challenging in a country where professional hierarchies are even more fixed than in the United States. For instance, the level of schooling a child will attain—i.e., University or Trade School—is determined when she is in elementary school. This is quite different from the American premise that anything is possible with enough self-application.

> Despite these challenges the field has developed in the Netherlands. DMT is practiced in many of the same contexts in Holland that it is in the United States, such as in psychiatric daycare centers and clinics. In some situations—as seen in the work of Annemieke Plouvier in Rotterdam and Frank Polak in Alkmaar—DMT is used [more] with healthier populations than it is generally used in the U.S., such as regional clinics for people with "regular life" problems rather than focusing primarily on the SPMI (seriously and persistently mentally ill) populations that are most frequently served in the U.S.

> There are also some other areas where the Dutch have made major inroads in DMT applications. There is a setting in Amsterdam to treat Holocaust survivors where Ruth Meier, one of the original Dutch dance therapists—and former Graham dancer—has practiced since the late 60s. Zweike Frank, one of my former students who is both Dutch and Israeli, has developed a specialty working with survivors of sexual abuse. He works with both women and men in groups and individually. In the past several years he has done extensive work with male abuse survivors. Not only has his work received a great deal of attention from the media, his facility has created a dance therapy studio according to his specifications and supports his work on all levels.

> Thanks to the indefatigable work of Sima Van Dullemen, the grande dame of Dutch dance therapy, there is a regular newsletter that reports events and news and profiles people's work. In short, it is the most unifying influence in Dutch DMT. (personal communication, 1999)

There is a continual exchange of dance movement therapists venturing out to new locations bridging cultures and sharing styles and techniques of dance movement therapy. An example is Meg Chang, who taught a workshop in Korea through Boon Soon Ryu, a pioneer dance therapist in Seoul. Ryu is the president of a private organization called the Korea Dance Therapy Association. Following this workshop, Chang, who has a longstanding interest in Korean literature and culture, was able to return to Korea for four months. Chang finds the Korean dance tradition to be rich and respected, and found shamanic healing practices primarily done by women and a Buddhist monk's dance, of particular interest. She notes that there is a great love of music and dance in Korea, as well as a tradition of linking dance with emotional expression.

According to Radana Sourkova and Corinne Ott, the first DMT training program in the Czech Republic began in July 1997 in conjunction with the Duncan Centre Modern Dance Conservatory in Prague. Miriam Roskin Berger and Judith Bunney are the principal instructors in dance therapy and Janet Kaylo, from the Laban Centre in London, is the guest instructor in movement analysis. This program follows the ADTA alternate route guidelines and their goal is to be a recognized training institute in the Czech Republic.

Conclusion

It is a challenge to keep up with all that is happening around the world. Due to the limits of time and space this chapter represents only a portion of the work being done. The dance movement therapists who have traveled, taught, practiced and supervised internationally are pioneers in their own right. They have surmounted barriers in language, culture, movement style and regulatory procedure to support the practice of dance movement therapy around the world. In the process, they have encountered numerous pioneers wherever they have traveled, as well as devoted students eager to learn. Every therapist represented in this chapter testifies to the enhancement of her own life and practice of DMT through her international experience. These leaders have deepened and broadened their understanding of DMT and have refined skills and perspectives that will help carry DMT forward into the 21st century.

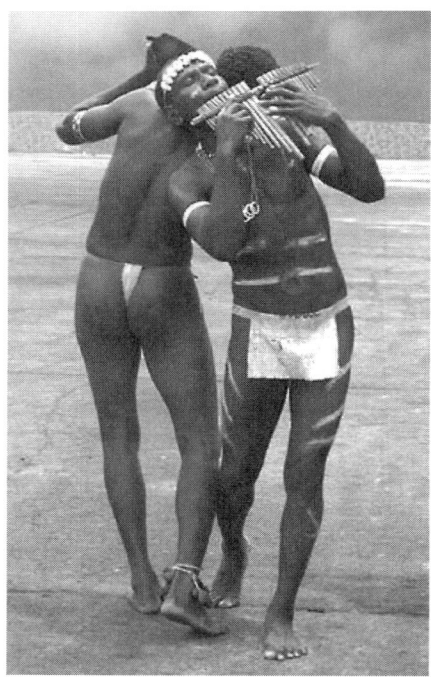

Music and dance may both be considered international languages. Noumea Dancers, in the capital of New Caledonia, South Pacific (Photo courtesy Leonard Forrest)

UNIT V

Dance Movement Therapy Research: Survey Results and the Heritage Trees

Today, the field of dance movement therapy is fortunate to have a group of dedicated researchers (discussed below) who are trying to inspire dance therapists to engage in research. Up until now research has been limited. Researching the effectiveness of dance therapy is difficult, as is researching other areas of psychotherapy. Standards for assessment have to be created and change needs to be evaluated. Movement and feeling are fleeting and recording what one sees in a patients' movement is subjective in art, difficult to evaluate and quantify. Moreover, there is the question of what sort of language to use in describing and quantifying movement change. Over the years, dance therapists have drawn up evaluation charts and have tried to evaluate as best as possible a patient's progress. Lenore Wadsworth Hervey, an innovative thinker, addresses these issues in Section A, Chapter 27. Hervey's book, entitled *Artistic Inquiry in Dance Movement Therapy* (2000) outlines creative movement-orientated evaluation methods.

In the future, further work assessing the effectiveness of movement in therapy should become available, including the work of Dianne Dulicai, William Freeman and Elise Billock Tropea, who have designed a framework to assess the movement of children. Also, Ilene Serlin and Susan Sandel, independently and with uniquely different perspectives, have been working in the area of dance therapy research for breast cancer patients (Sandel, personal communication, 2003).

Section B is an abridged version of the original dance movement therapy survey published in the first (1988) and second (1992) editions of this book. It was designed to discover the roots and development of dance movement therapy pioneers on subsequent generations of dance movement therapists. The data for the updated trees was collected by Anne Mitcheltree.

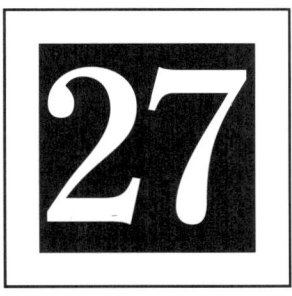

Contemporary Thought on Research

By Lenore Wadsworth Hervey

Historically, much of the published literature of dance movement therapy has taken the form of a story of an individual case or group told by the clinician, complete with the interventions he or she used that were successful and the theoretical rationale that supported them. These are valuable teaching stories and they serve to pass emerging and innovative clinical methods on to colleagues and students. Stories like these help build a profession by defining what dance movement therapists do and who they are, as distinct from other mental health practitioners. Reading these stories continues to be an essential part of learning to be a dance movement therapist.

It has become clear over time, however, that research in the field needs to diversify, increase in quantity and improve in quality to meet the needs of a growing and changing profession in a demanding mental health market. There is an ongoing concern that research is needed to validate the clinical work of dance movement therapists, to support legislation regarding state licensure and to endorse inclusion in health insurance plans. The intensity of this much-vocalized need seems to be matched only by the oft-recognized difficulty within the profession to meet it (Chaiklin, 1968, 1997; Ritter & Low, 1996; Cruz & Hervey, 2001).

The Research Subcommittee of the American Dance Therapy Association was formed with the primary mission of supporting research in the field. Three of its members, Cynthia Berrol, Robyn Flaum Cruz and Lenore Hervey, contributed in this effort through a variety of strategic efforts.

The founding chair of the subcommittee, Cynthia Berrol, with colleagues Wee Lok Ooi and Stephanie Katz, published the first large-scale experimental research project funded by the Chace Foundation in (1997). (The financial support of the Chace Foundation has been instrumental in the production of research and research-supportive projects.) Berrol later published a definitive educational article on the diversity of research methods available to dance movement therapists (2000).

Robyn Flaum Cruz used her expertise in quantitative research and statistical methods to support increasing complexity and accuracy of statistical analysis in traditional quantitative research. She worked for years to establish a tradition of annual research poster sessions at the ADTA conferences. As editor first of the *American Journal of Dance Therapy* and later of *The Arts in Psychotherapy*, Cruz supported and stimulated quality research in dance movement therapy and facilitated its delivery to the creative arts therapy community.

With the publication of *Artistic Inquiry in Dance Movement Therapy* (2000), Lenore Hervey encouraged the profession to move beyond the restrictive vision and methods of traditional scientific research. Many years of teaching research protocol in a graduate dance movement therapy program led her to believe that a new approach was needed that would more accurately reflect the interests, aptitudes and values of her students. Building on expressive arts therapist Sean McNiff's art-based research (1998), Hervey identified three unique characteristics of artistic inquiry:

1. Artistic inquiry uses artistic methods of gathering data, analyzing data and/or presenting data.
2. Artistic inquiry engages in and acknowledges a creative process.
3. Artistic inquiry is motivated and determined by the aesthetic values of the researcher(s). (2000, p.7)

Hervey argued that if dance movement therapists wanted validation of their work, they needed to use their most highly developed abilities as their primary research tools, not methods borrowed from other fields with which they might have only minimal familiarity. She identified DMT skills that could be extremely useful in artistic methods of research, such as:

1. Facilitating expression through dance as a method of gathering data in response to a research question.
2. Understanding the meaning of movement by experiencing it in one's own body as a method of data analysis.
3. Observing and recreating movement as a way to present research findings.
4. Creating dances that convey powerful affect and meaning as a way to communicate research conclusions.

Hervey also argued that if dance movement therapists wanted to create research that was meaningful and rewarding, they needed to see their fellow dance movement therapists, not outside authorities, as the primary audience for that research. She frequently worked with groups of dance movement therapists as co-researchers to examine questions such as: "How do you feel about doing research?" Through artistic inquiry, they would create short movement phrases representing their responses to the question. She might also ask them to draw small pictures outlining the shape and direction of the movement. The co-researchers would then view their creations all together and form small self-selected groups with the other creators of phrases or drawings having similar aesthetic qualities. The small groups of co-researchers would then examine their collective movements and drawings in greater depth, looking for common themes and patterns. These themes were then translated into a single group art form, such as a poem or a dance that was used to share their research findings with the larger research group.

Whether using traditional or alternative methods, dance movement therapists need to perceive themselves as researchers as well as clinicians. The research product needs to be relevant to practice, accessible and of high quality. The research process needs to be understood as rigorous, yet manageable, meaningful and congruent with the values and practices of dance movement therapy.

Review of Survey Findings—Past, Present and Future Trends

This survey explored changing trends in the theory and practice of dance therapists and aimed to understand the foundations on which dance therapy was built. One hundred and one dance therapists took part in the study in 1985. The results are summarized below, providing a baseline for further studies on developments in the field. We are aware that this study would show different results if repeated today, however, interestingly, many of the themes cited seem to reflect current issues and concerns. To our knowledge, no recent surveys of this type have been carried out. Charts have been omitted from this revised version of the book.

Respondents were asked to list significant influences on their work in the areas of dance, psychology and dance therapy. An assessment of the relative overall importance of certain areas was requested and compared. These areas were dance, LMA training, dance therapy training, psychological theory, one's own experiences as a participant in dance therapy and one's own experience as a participant in verbal therapy.[1] Respondents were asked to differentiate between influences that were most important in the early part of their careers and influences that are now important. Finally, respondents were asked to briefly state any significant changes that have taken place in their theoretical and/or practical orientation. The following is a summary and discussion of the results.

Dance Influences

Since dance therapy arose out of the modern dance movement, with all pioneers having started their careers as performers, choreographers and/or dance teachers, one part of the survey focused on the particular dance influences affecting the respondents' work. The respondents were asked to name the most influential styles of dance and/or dance teachers and could list as many as they wanted.

Modern dance is the most influential dance style on dance therapists (72 therapists cited it as the most important), followed by improvisation, then by ballet, folk, African, jazz, multicultural and creative dance. Mime/pantomime was thought to be important by only six respondents. This is not surprising since modern dance was propelled by the need for intense emotional and intellectual expression and psychological probing. It is surprising, however, that only 11 respondents cited creative dance as an influence in their work. Many of the dance therapy pioneers—notably Evan, Espenak, Polk, Boas, Hawkins and Whitehouse—had extensive training in creative dance and believed strongly in its power as a medium for self-expression. One explanation could be that creative dance was frequently integrated into modern dance classes, but was not always labeled as such.

Twenty-four respondents cited Martha Graham as the most influential dance teacher, followed by José Limón and Merce Cunningham. Respondents also mentioned Alwin Nikolais, Rudolf Laban, Hanya Holm, Mary Wigman, Isadora Duncan, Margaret H'Doubler and Doris Humphrey. The breakdown of influential dance teachers confirms the continuing and widespread influence of modern dance on today's dance therapists. All of the dance teachers cited at least six times by respondents were from either the European or the

---

[1] It is well known that a psychotherapist's own therapy is an important part of his or her training and often considered a prerequisite for any kind of advanced clinical training. A similar sentiment exists in the dance therapy field. For this reason we thought it especially important to find out what kind of therapy experiences dance therapists sought and what they found most helpful.

American school of modern dance. The only possible exception is Isadora Duncan, who was cited as important by seven respondents. Duncan's work cannot be easily categorized. While many consider Duncan to be an original pioneer of modern dance, others refer to her work as experimental or interpretive.

Although the Denishawn School was never cited, Denishawn descendents Martha Graham and Doris Humphrey were. This might be explained by the fact that both Graham and Humphrey branched out from Denishawn to make their own unique contributions and as a result, they and their descendents are not frequently associated with the Denishawn School. Moreover, Graham, who was cited more frequently than any of the other dance teachers, is considered by many to be the original pioneer of modern dance. Innovators St. Denis and Shawn, however, were from a much earlier period.

To obtain a more complete picture of the role of dance in dance therapy, the dance influence must be viewed in relation to other influences. In this context, respondents were asked to rate the degree of influence, both in the past and present, that each of the following factors had on their work: dance, Laban Movement Analysis, dance therapy training, psychological theory, being a client in dance therapy and being a client in verbal therapy.

In order to explore the possibility that areas of influence may have shifted for the younger generation of dance therapists, the results were grouped into two categories of respondents: dance therapists in the field for 15 or more years (the 15 + group) and those in the field for 13 or fewer years (the 13- group).[2]

Survey results indicate that the strongest influences in the past and present have been dance, dance therapy training and psychological theory, though to different degrees with both the 15+ and 13- groups and with changes over time. For example, members of the 15+ group were highly influenced by dance early in their careers (82%), but 64 percent rated dance as an influence on their current practice. For both groups, the influences of dance and dance therapy training have decreased, while the influence of psychological theory has increased.

While the importance of dance has declined for both groups, it was and still is a stronger influence on the 15+ group. One possible explanation may lie in the fact that the process of professionalizing the field of dance therapy began only 20 years ago. Therefore, many of the older generation had strong backgrounds in professional dance before becoming dance therapists, some moving into dance therapy at a midpoint in their dance careers and a few in the latter part of their careers as performers, choreographers and/or dance teachers. One can see how dance would be the major influence for this group, especially early in their dance therapy careers.

In contrast, the advent of formal academic programs in dance therapy and recognized career paths meant that the younger generation was more likely to be informed of this option early in their dance training and general education. This would have enabled them to gear their interests toward a career in dance therapy rather than in professional dance and accounts for the overall lower influence of dance for this group.

The survey indicated that the average number of years of dance training for the respondents was 20+ years. Generally, a solid dance education is very much a part of the lives of dance therapists and many respondents noted that their dance education continues today. Nevertheless, it can be speculated that the difference in professional dance experience is a contributing factor to the different stress that each group places on dance. It may also be a contributing factor to the difference in the influence of Laban Movement Analysis.

The LMA influence was not rated highly by a large percentage of the respondents in either group; however, it increased in importance for the 13- group while remaining the same for the 15 + group. It is possible that many of the older generation, because of their rich and diversified dance backgrounds, had already internalized the concepts of LMA inherent in a thorough modern dance education, while the younger generation may be making up for deficits through LMA training.

Psychological Theory and Its Relationship to the Dance Influence

The most significant factor affecting the decreasing influence of dance is the increasing influence of psychological theory. Theory has become the most important influence on the current work of both the 15+ and 13- groups.

---

[2]This breakdown resulted in two groups of equal size, with 45 respondents in each category. The six respondents who fell between the two groups were eliminated from these analyses, but are included in the data from the total field.

Dance therapists are for the most part eclectic. A large majority of the respondents have been influenced by three or more psychological theories. Psychoanalytic theory was by far the most influential for both the 13- and the 15+ groups, with 64 respondents citing it as the most influential. In addition, respondents as a whole have been influenced by a wide variety of other theories. These include: ego psychology, object relations, Gestalt theory and developmental psychology. A few respondents mentioned behavioral, bioenergetics, psychodrama, transpersonal and other theories.

According to the findings, the majority of dance therapists see the value in understanding their movement work in theoretical terms. This has often led them to investigate established theories and relate them to their clinical experiences. The dance therapists' ability to integrate established psychological theory into their work serves the purpose of linking dance therapy more directly to other psychotherapies, thus aiding communication among the various mental health disciplines. In addition, it can at times help dance therapists to broaden and clarify their observations and insights into the amorphous and often confusing nonverbal aspects of dance therapy. This is undoubtedly the role that theory plays for all psychotherapies.

Another factor contributing to the increasing influence of psychological theory is the tacit pressure exerted on dance therapists, from both outside and within the discipline, to bring dance therapy more in line with traditional and established forms of psychotherapy. Dance therapists too often speak a language unfamiliar to the broader community of mental health. Thus, they are in a position of trying to prove their worth to those who view dance therapy as esoteric, ancillary and/or recreational rather than as a legitimate, in-depth treatment approach. This has put pressure on dance therapists to explain their work publicly on more complex levels than previously required. This could account for the greater influence of psychological theory in recent years. As a result, dance therapy is becoming assimilated into the larger mental health community.

Assimilation always has its positive and negative features. Gaining more acceptance within the field of mental health is a positive result of this process, as are the many contributions of dance therapists in integrating personality and development theory into the theory and practice of dance therapy. On the negative side, however, it can be argued that dance therapy is losing its uniqueness, as reflected in the decreasing influence of dance on dance therapy practitioners. The importance of the purely nonverbal experience may be losing its power in the eyes of some dance therapists and those outside the field trying to understand dance therapy. This is unfortunate.

In light of economic pressures and pressures to conform and enter the mainstream of the mental health profession, one can see how it would take great strength and a deep commitment to the values of dance to maintain an emphasis on this aspect of dance therapy. It is not surprising that some dance therapists are beginning to feel that the dance aspects of their work are being threatened.

This conflict was elaborated further when respondents were asked to describe any noteworthy shifts in either the theory or practice of their work. The two shifts reported most frequently were: 1) a shift toward a greater emphasis on and/or a reaffirmation of the importance of dance in dance therapy; and 2) a shift toward in-depth psychological training as the theoretical foundation of dance therapy.

As for the respondents who indicated a move toward dance, some respondents said dance was the most important aspect of their work; some said they had moved from an emphasis on psychological theory to an emphasis on dance; others noted that they have moved from a Chacian approach to a Whitehousian or authentic movement approach to dance therapy; and finally, a few indicated their concern that the profession was losing the dance in dance therapy by becoming too theoretical and thus removed from the essence of dance.

Among the respondents who noted a shift toward psychological training, some noted that they had moved from a pure movement orientation to the incorporation of a particular psychological framework as the basis for their work; others said they have shifted from one psychological framework to another. The theoretical area cited most frequently by these respondents was psychoanalytic. It is important to note that of all the individuals who indicated this shift, only a few said they were moving away from dance. One respondent stated she had shifted toward a "developmental perspective, i.e., psychology of self, ego psychology, etc., while continuing to develop the art of the dance in the process."

While the trend toward an increasing influence of psychological theory remains strong, there are indications that the accompanying trend toward a decreasing influence of dance may be slowing down and, perhaps, even beginning to reverse. One may speculate that dance therapists are coming to realize that there need not be a conflict between these two aspects of their work and that, in fact, they can support and strengthen each other. These changes in the field are part of the maturation process any discipline needs to experience if it is to challenge itself and grow.

Dance Therapy Training and Dance Therapy Influences

Survey findings indicated that the influence of dance therapy training has dropped in recent years for both groups of respondents. Nevertheless, it still remains relatively important overall, ranking second for the 13- group and third for the 15+ group. The younger generation is significantly more eclectic in their dance therapy training, a large majority having had three or more dance therapy trainers.

Being a client in dance therapy has remained relatively stable over time as an influence for both groups. However, compared with the other influences it has generally not been important overall.

Verbal Therapy and Verbalization

Verbal therapy (specifically, personal psychoanalysis) is frequently a prerequisite for becoming a psychoanalyst and in recent years has become more common among dance therapists. Consequently, being a client in verbal therapy has had an increasing influence on the work of both groups of respondents. This raises a question as to why dance therapists, in seeking continued personal and professional growth, seem more likely to turn to verbal therapists than to their fellow dance therapists.

One hypothesis, relevant especially for the 15 + group but also to a certain degree for the 13- group, is that they tend to seek those outside the field for reasons of confidentiality, since their fellow dance therapists are often peers, friends and colleagues. More importantly, the healing aspects of dance for both groups have perhaps already become an integrated part of their lives, whereas the verbal idiom as an expressive and exploratory modality may need development. Finally, until the 1970s, there were very few dance therapists providing in-depth individual treatment.

Since dance therapists frequently go to verbally oriented psychotherapists, one might ask if they are increasing their use of verbalization in their work. If so, is this contributing to a decrease in the use of dance movement? Although the survey did not specifically ask respondents about their use of verbalization, in response to the question concerning shifts in dance therapy theory or practice, several respondents did note that they are including more verbalization in their current work. These respondents on the whole did not indicate whether the dance movement aspects of their work have become any more or less important as a result of this shift. We can only speculate that the use of verbalization may be replacing some aspects of dance movement for some dance therapists, while for others it may have the effect of simultaneously deepening and broadening movement expression. One respondent stated, "I used to view myself as a dance movement therapist who could talk; I now see myself as a psychotherapist who knows how to use movement."

At the extreme ends of the spectrum, some individuals need an almost purely verbal form of expression, while others may require an almost purely physical mode of expression. However, more often than not, different individuals at different times require varying combinations of psychic and somatic work. The expressive and exploratory needs of most patients are bound to change many times in the course of dance therapy treatment, especially in the case of long-term work, demanding verbal and dance movement approaches. Thus, dance therapists will by necessity alternate between movement, verbalization and other idioms as well.

The shift toward more verbalization goes hand in hand with another shift, that is, the shift toward dance therapy as a primary therapy, also noted by respondents.

Other Shifts

Other shifts were reported. One was a shift toward systems theory, particularly family systems. Some respondents indicated that they work with families, while others noted they use the systems theory as a framework for their work with various populations.

The other shift was toward the incorporation of the spiritual into dance therapy. Several respondents indicated a shift toward one or more of the following: spirituality, Jungian thought, ritual movement and/or transpersonal and transformational experiences.

This move toward spirituality is not surprising in light of the history and meaning of dance. Throughout the literature on dance, be it folk or primitive, ballet or modern, there is reference to various forms of faith and spirituality. Dance has often been attributed with magical and transformational powers. It has served as a form of prayer and meditation and as a way to reach the collective unconscious. In addition, some of the major dance mentors, including Wigman, Holm and Boas, spoke often of the spiritual aspects of dance.

In current times, there appears to be a resurgence of faith and spirituality expressed in many different forms throughout society as a whole and since this element always has been present in dance, it is not surprising to find this same resurgence among dance therapists. It is possible that this trend toward spirituality is one contributing factor in the trend toward a reaffirmation of the dance aspects of dance therapy.

Summary

The survey findings indicate that the discipline of dance therapy continues to grow and expand, and within that growth and expansion dance therapists struggle to sort out their professional identities. The question of how to view oneself professionally is not unique to dance therapists. With the proliferation of contemporary psychotherapies, all mental health professionals have to carefully consider and choose their treatment styles. The question, which is pressing for today's dance therapists, is how to incorporate complementary theory and practice borrowed from the more traditional verbal psychotherapies, while still remaining true to their belief in the healing powers of the dance. Financial and political pressures confronting today's dance therapists further complicates this issue.

29 Dance Therapy Heritage Trees—The Spread of Influence of the Major Pioneers

The following Heritage Trees represent the spread of dance therapy influence on dance therapists who carry the ADTR status. Individual trees were constructed for the six major dance therapy pioneers discussed in Section One, as well as for Rudolf Laban and Irmgard Bartenieff. Trees were constructed for these pioneers because they, according to the original 1984 survey, either directly or indirectly influenced the largest number of respondents. The tree for Laban was added to the book in 1992. It is important to clarify that Laban was not included as a pioneering dance therapist. He was not a dance therapist but, according to the survey results, he influenced such a large number of practitioners and teachers in the field, including Bartenieff, that, from a historical point of view, it was important to add him.

Original pioneers for whom trees were made grew out of the 1985 survey (Chapter 28) and so reflect research results that cannot be altered. All dance therapy pioneers began teaching in the fifties, sixties and early seventies and are deceased today.

In 1992 and again in 2001, these trees were updated. In 1992, notices were placed in the ADTA Newsletter requesting dance therapists (ADTRs only) to clarify who, of the pioneers listed in *Dance Movement Therapy: A Healing Art* (Levy, 1988), influenced their work. Approximately 75 letters were received in 1992 and 115 in 2001. One reason for the increased response in 2001 was thanks to the hard work and dedication of Anne Mitcheltree, ADTR, who facilitated sending letters to all ADTR's with a form to fill out requesting information about who their teachers were. In response to Mitcheltree's efforts, the trees are now affectionately referred to as the "Mitchel Trees."

It is important to note that there are other pioneering leaders and contributors who also made and/or continue to make significant contributions to the field. The individuals listed below were cited on the survey for pioneering their own approach to dance therapy or for their unique integration of several approaches. The Heritage Trees, as they are now organized, only track the influence of some of these leaders. This is because not all ADTR's answered the questionnaire and Registered Dance Therapists were not included. Hence, the following list is not inclusive of all the leaders in the field but is a reflection of survey results.

J.Bell, M.R. Berger, N. Canner, D. Dulicai, M. Dyer-Bennett, E. Dosamantes-Beaudry, L.Deihl, B. Kalish-Weiss, F.J. Levy, P.P. Lewis, M.B. Leventhal, S. Lovell, M.North, F. Paulay, E. Polk, C. Simcha Ruben, M. Schade, E. Siegel, J. Ganet Sigel, S. Silberstein and R. Winter-Russell.

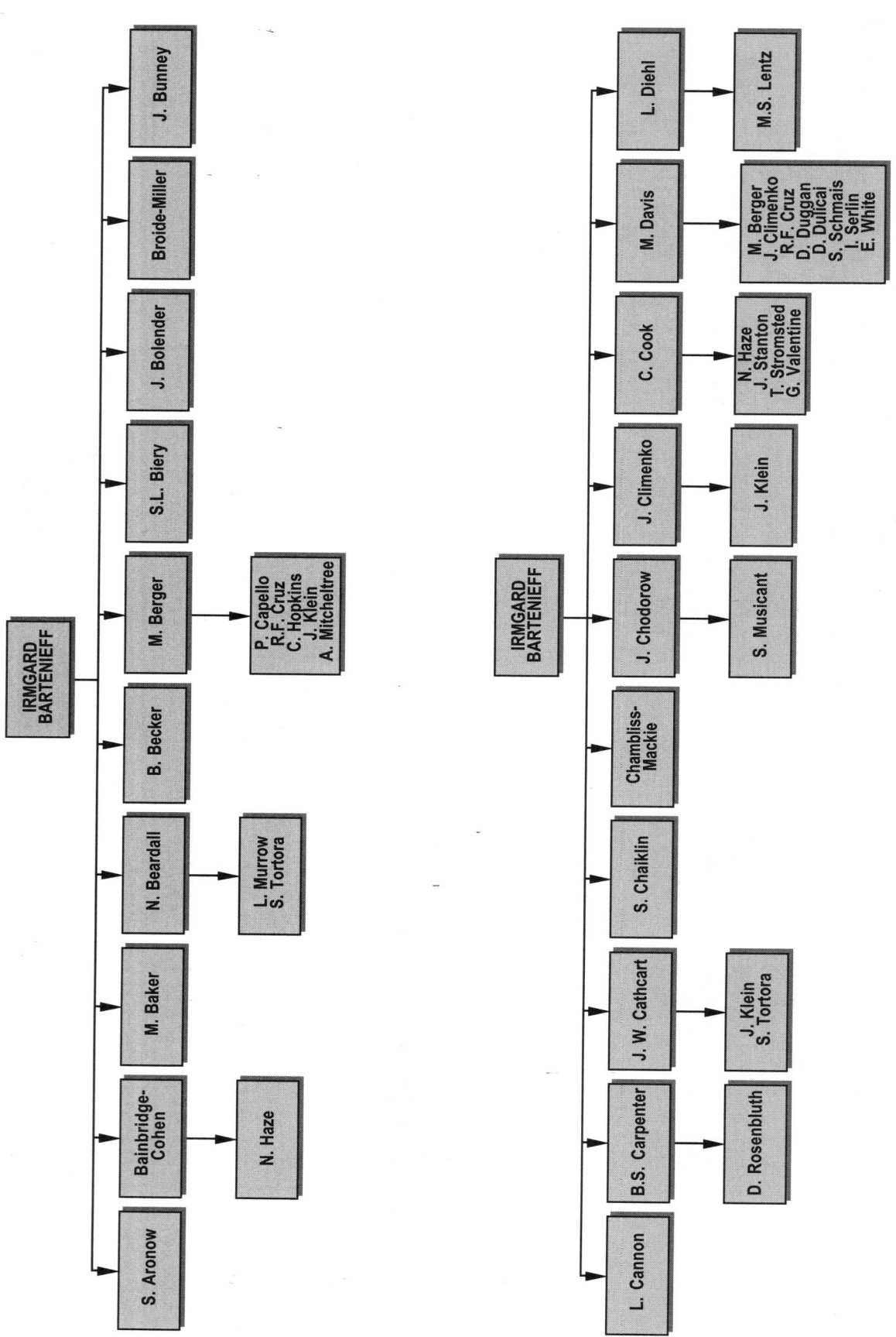

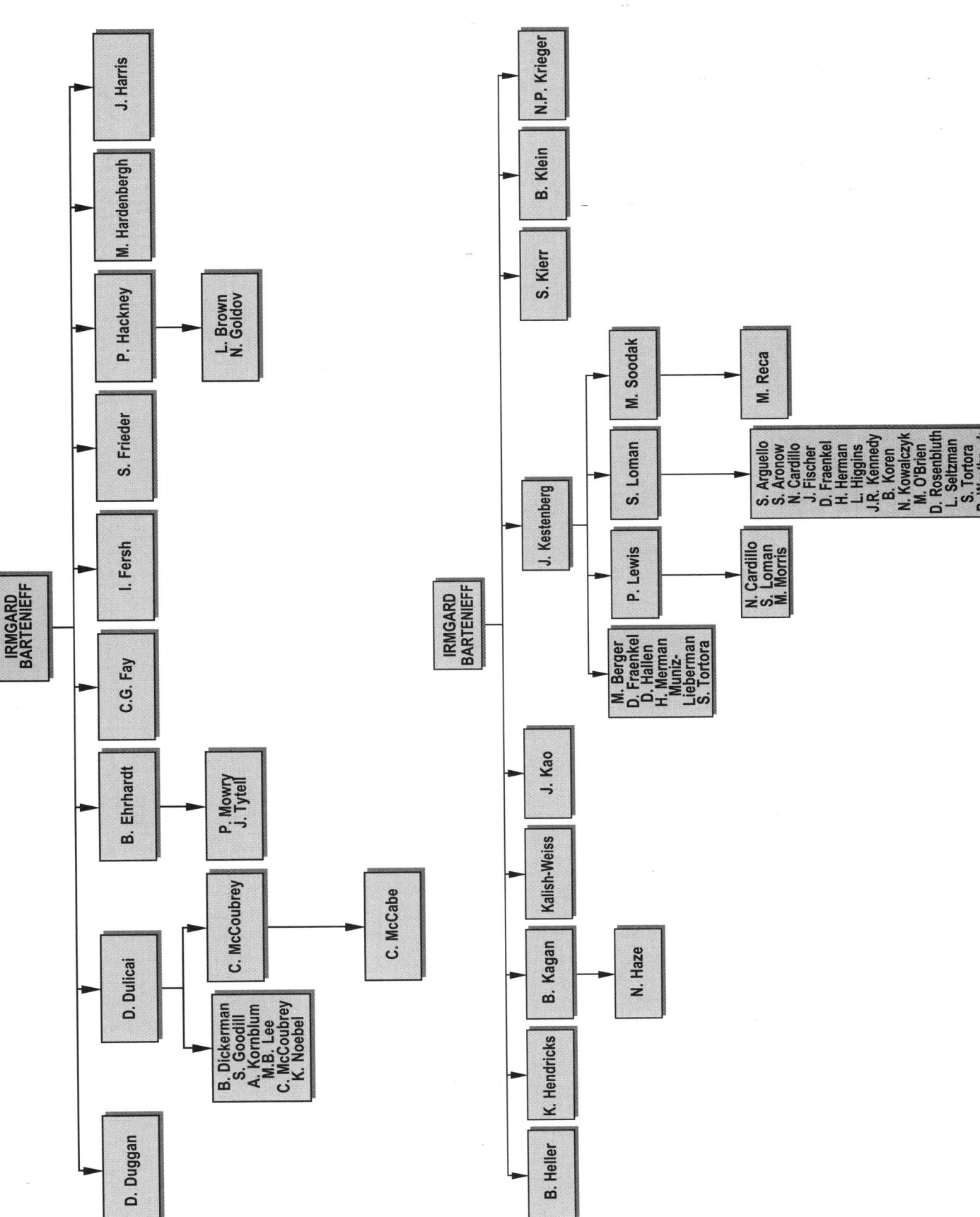

Dance Therapy Heritage Trees—The Spread of Influence of the Major Pioneers

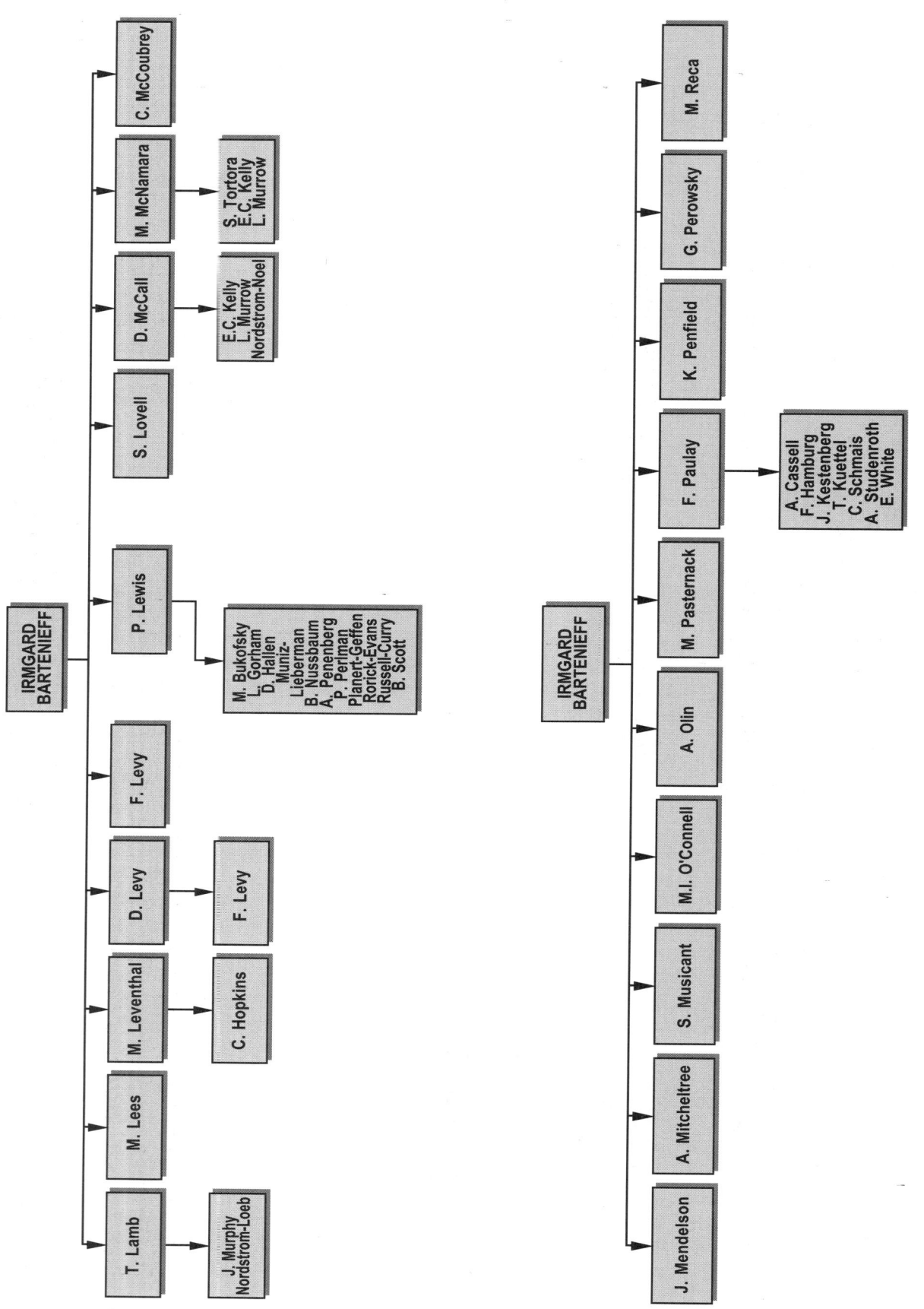

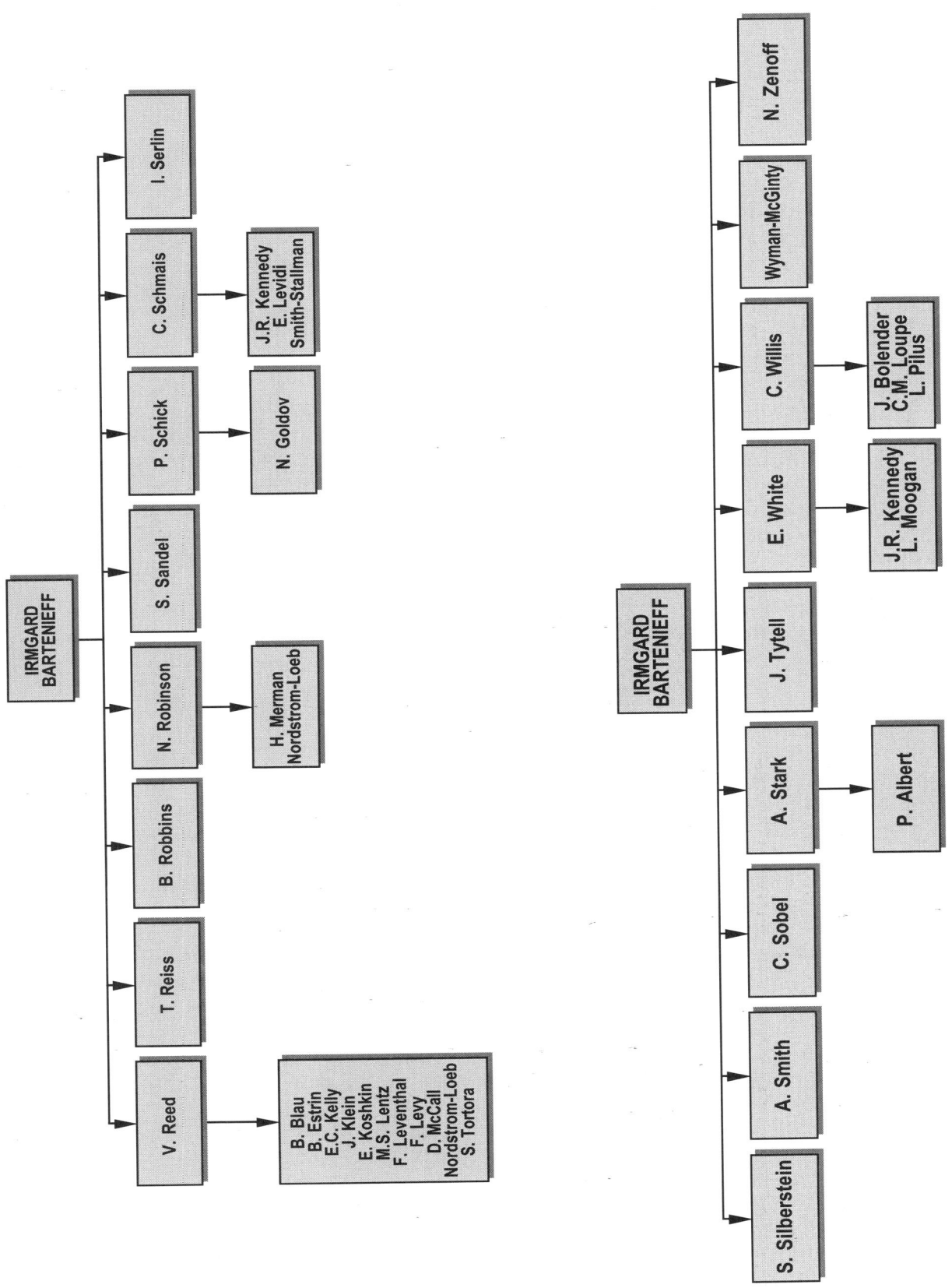

Dance Therapy Heritage Trees—The Spread of Influence of the Major Pioneers 287

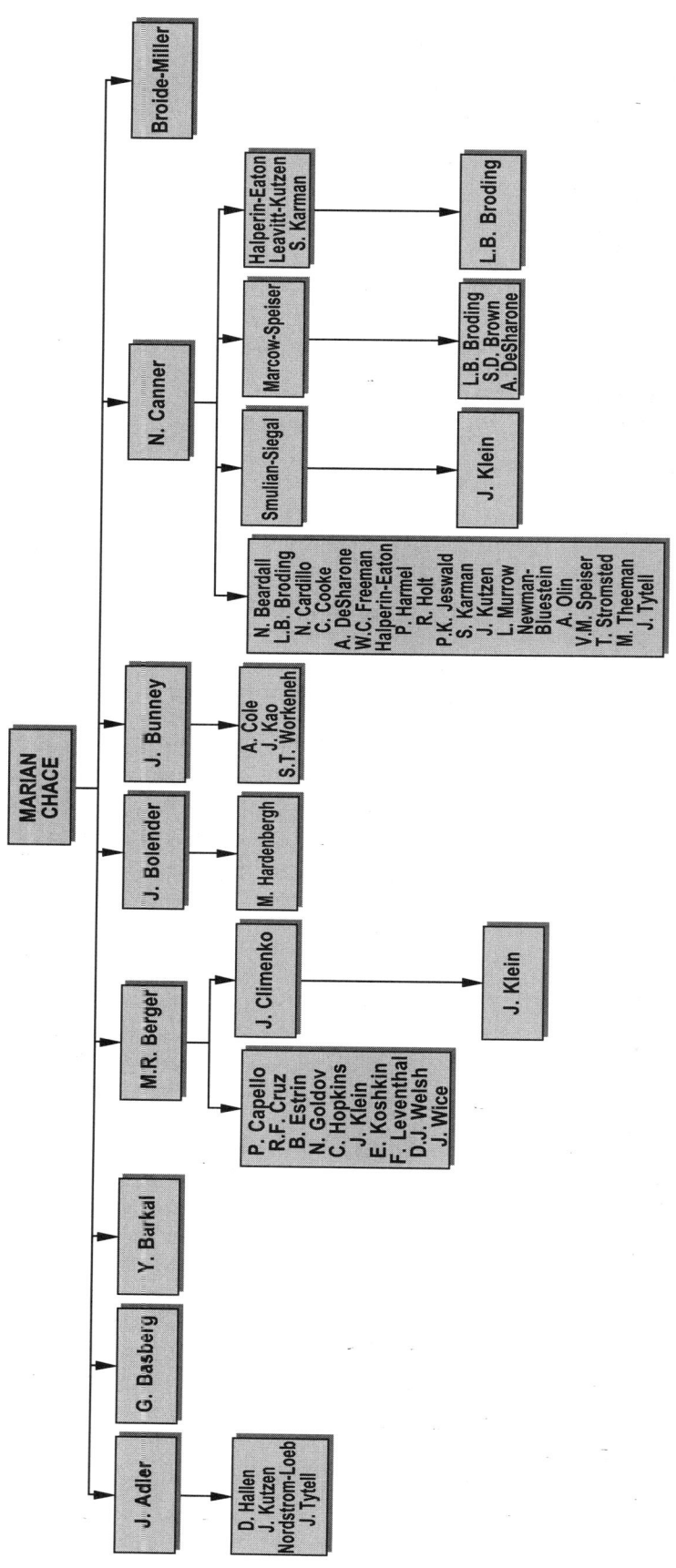

288 Dance Movement Therapy

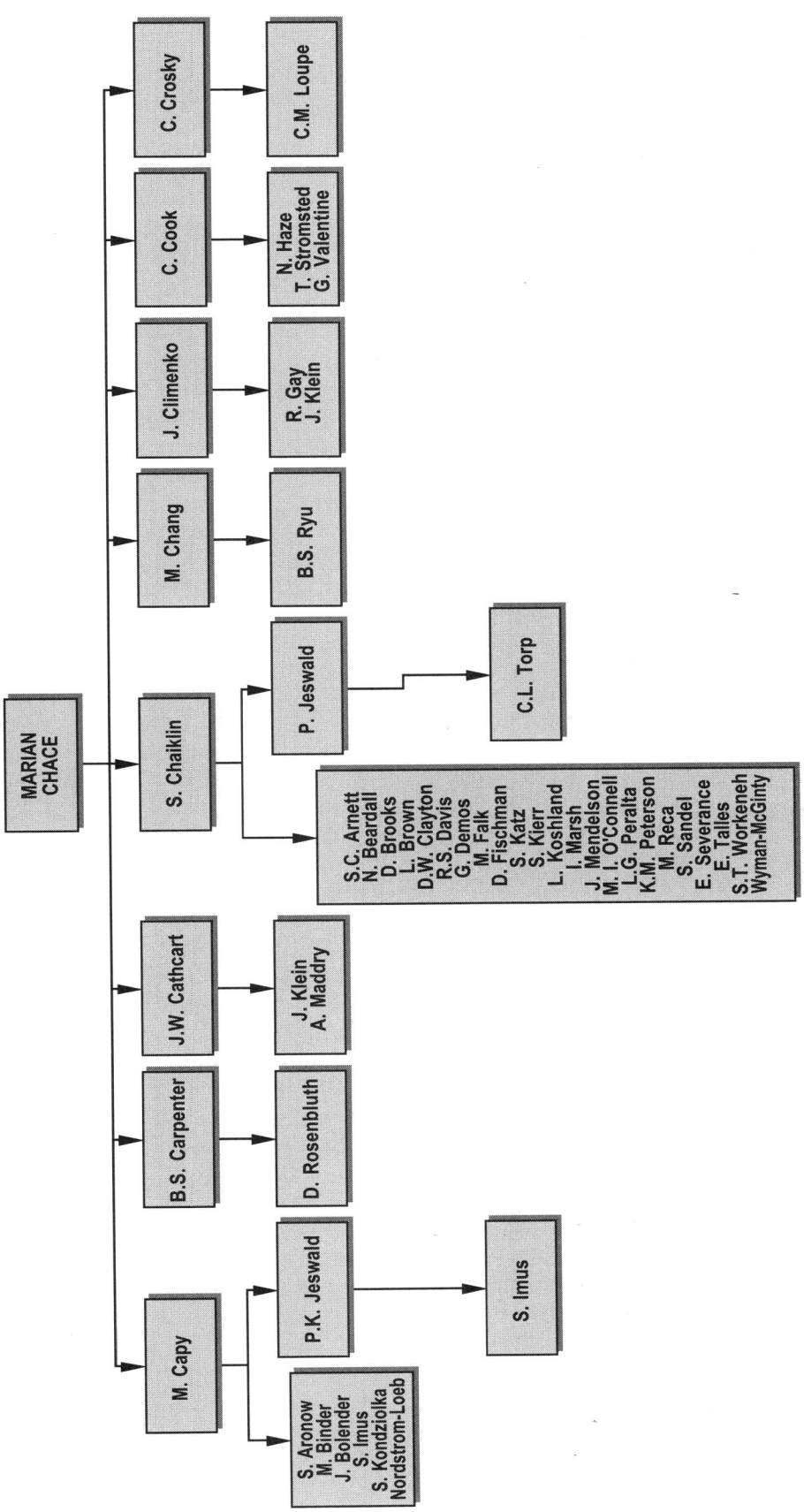

Dance Therapy Heritage Trees—The Spread of Influence of the Major Pioneers 289

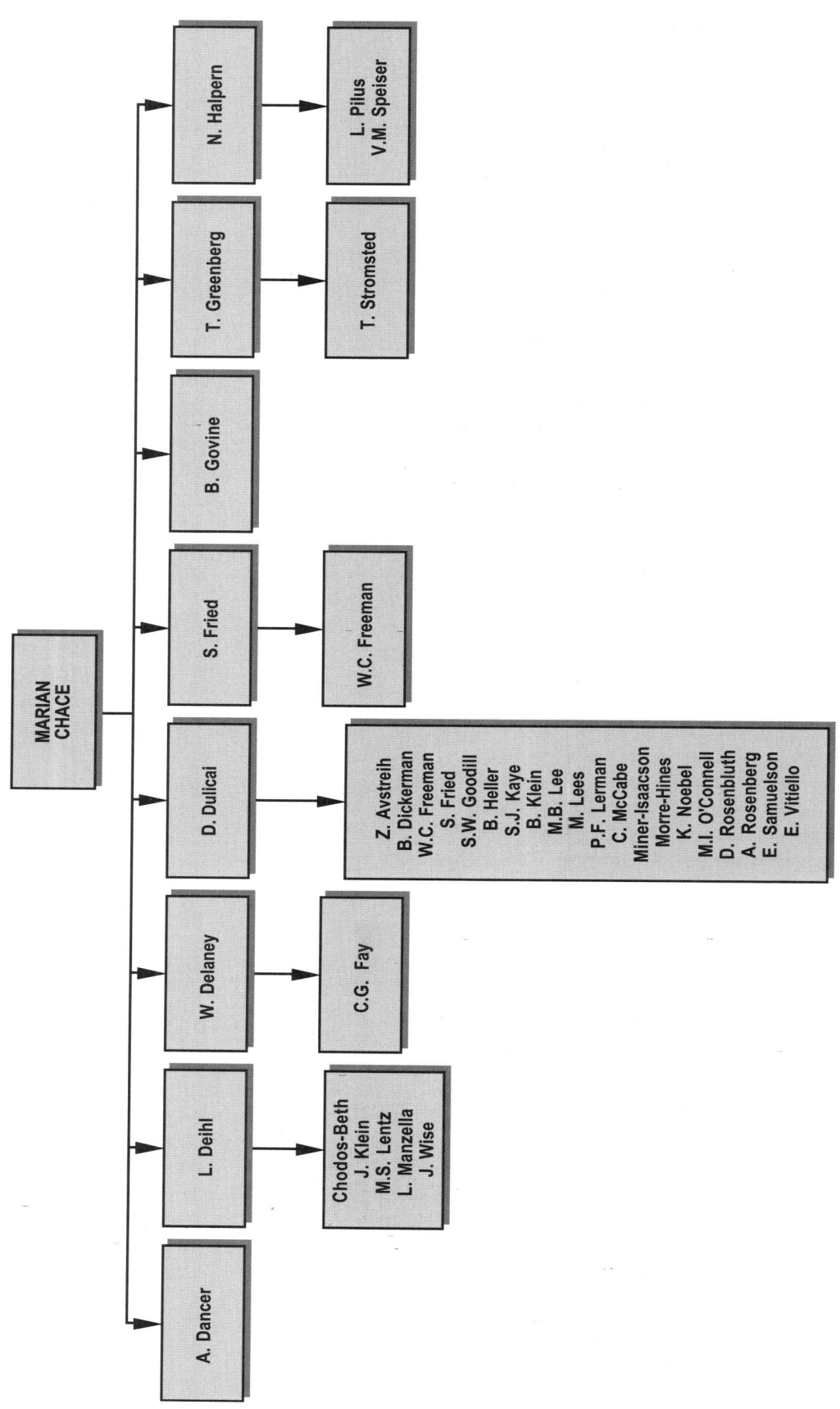

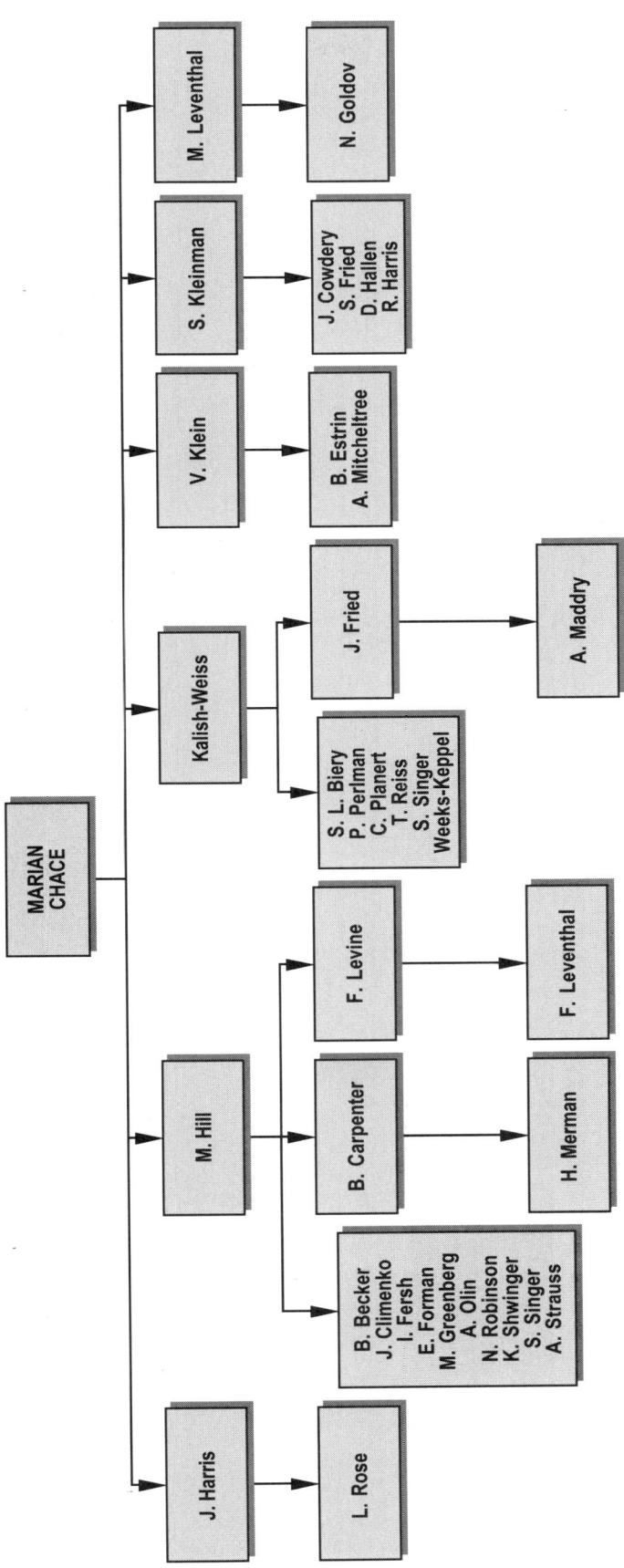

Dance Therapy Heritage Trees—The Spread of Influence of the Major Pioneers 291

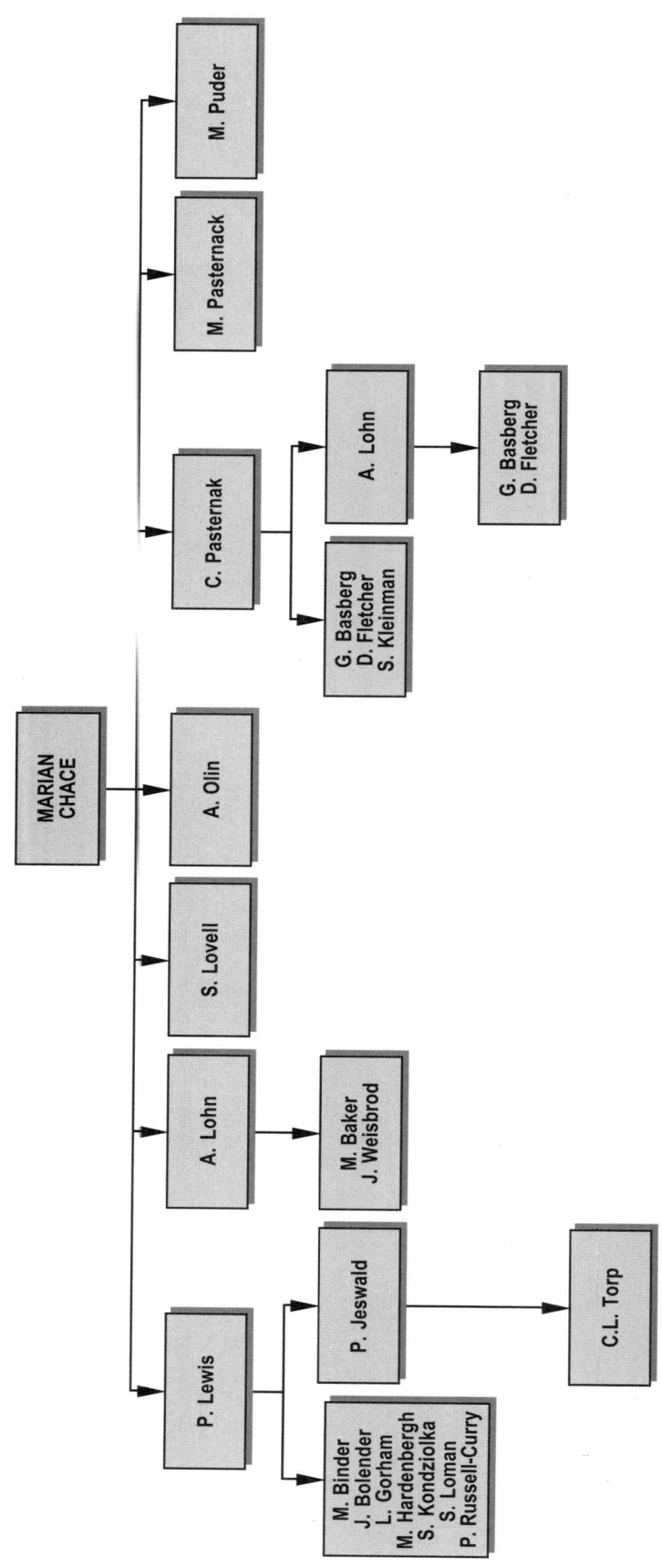

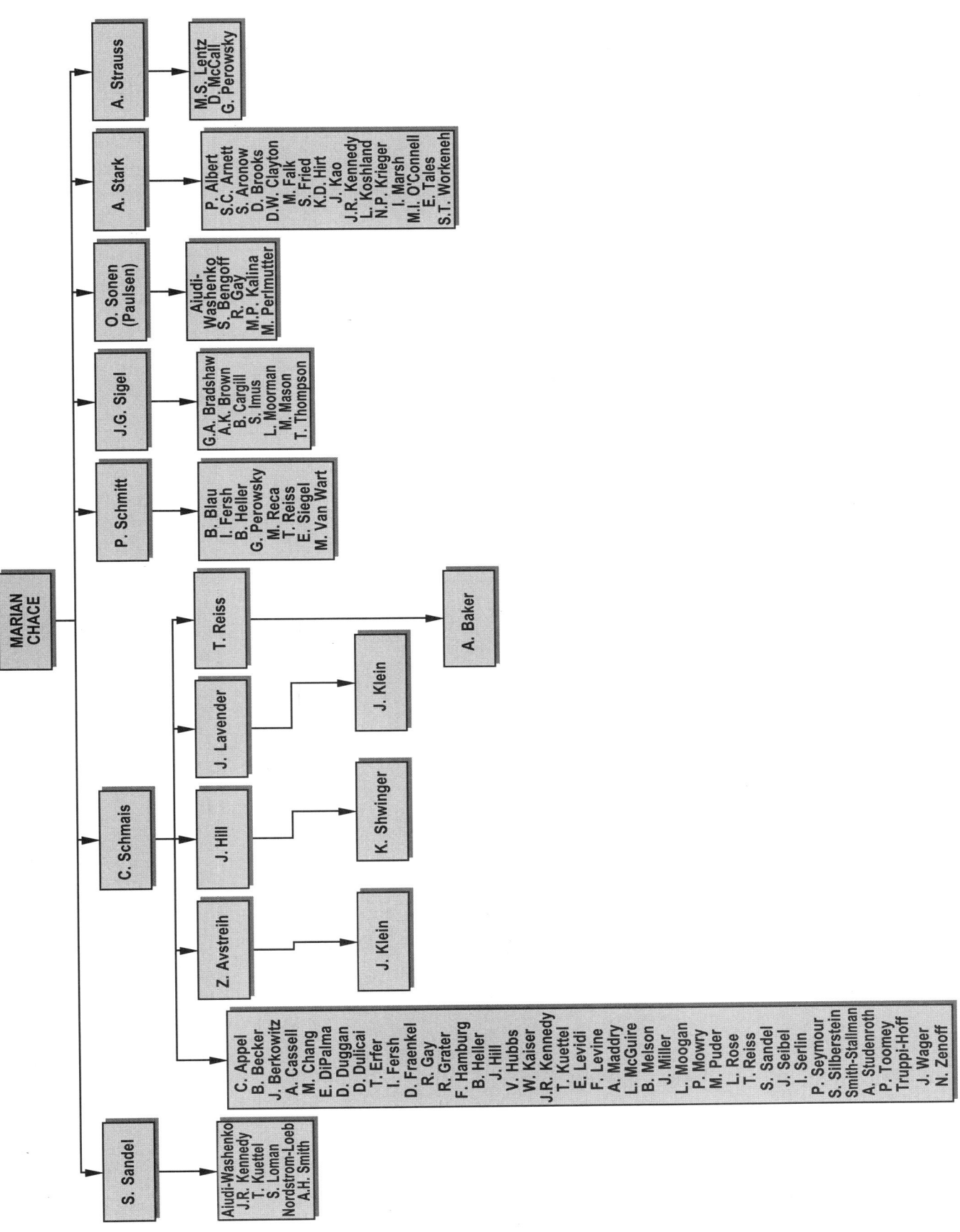
Dance Therapy Heritage Trees—The Spread of Influence of the Major Pioneers

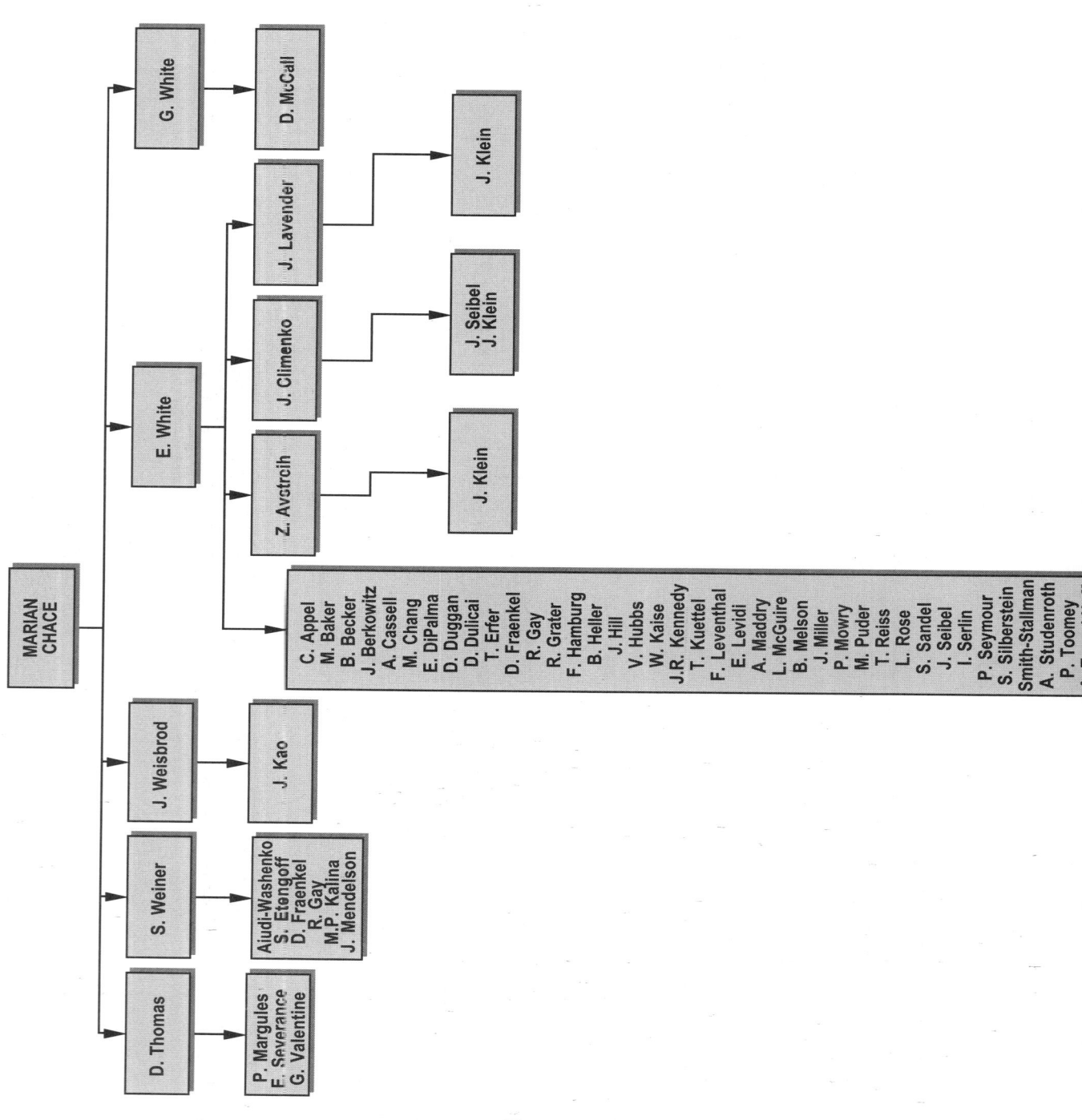

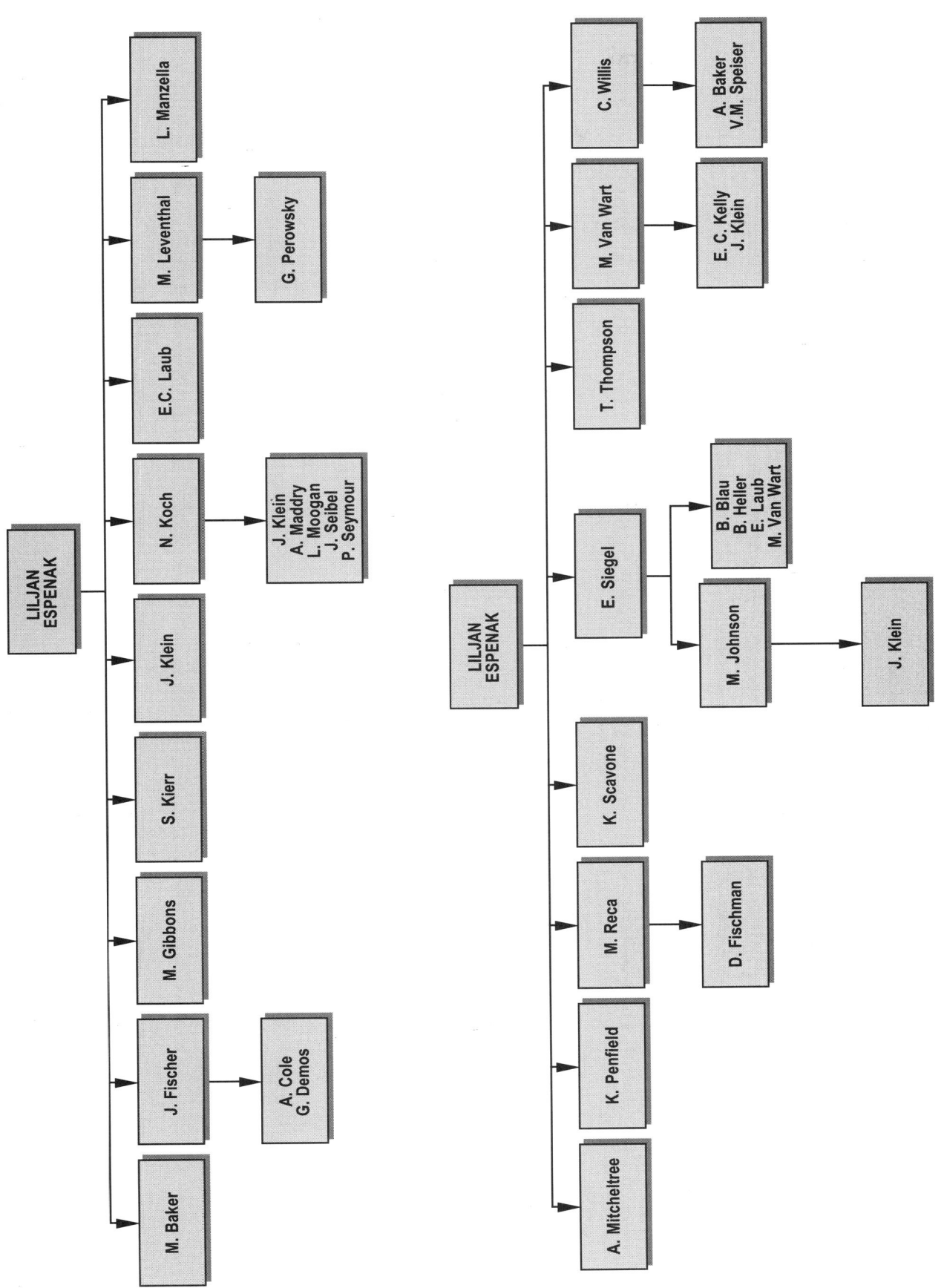

Dance Therapy Heritage Trees—The Spread of Influence of the Major Pioneers

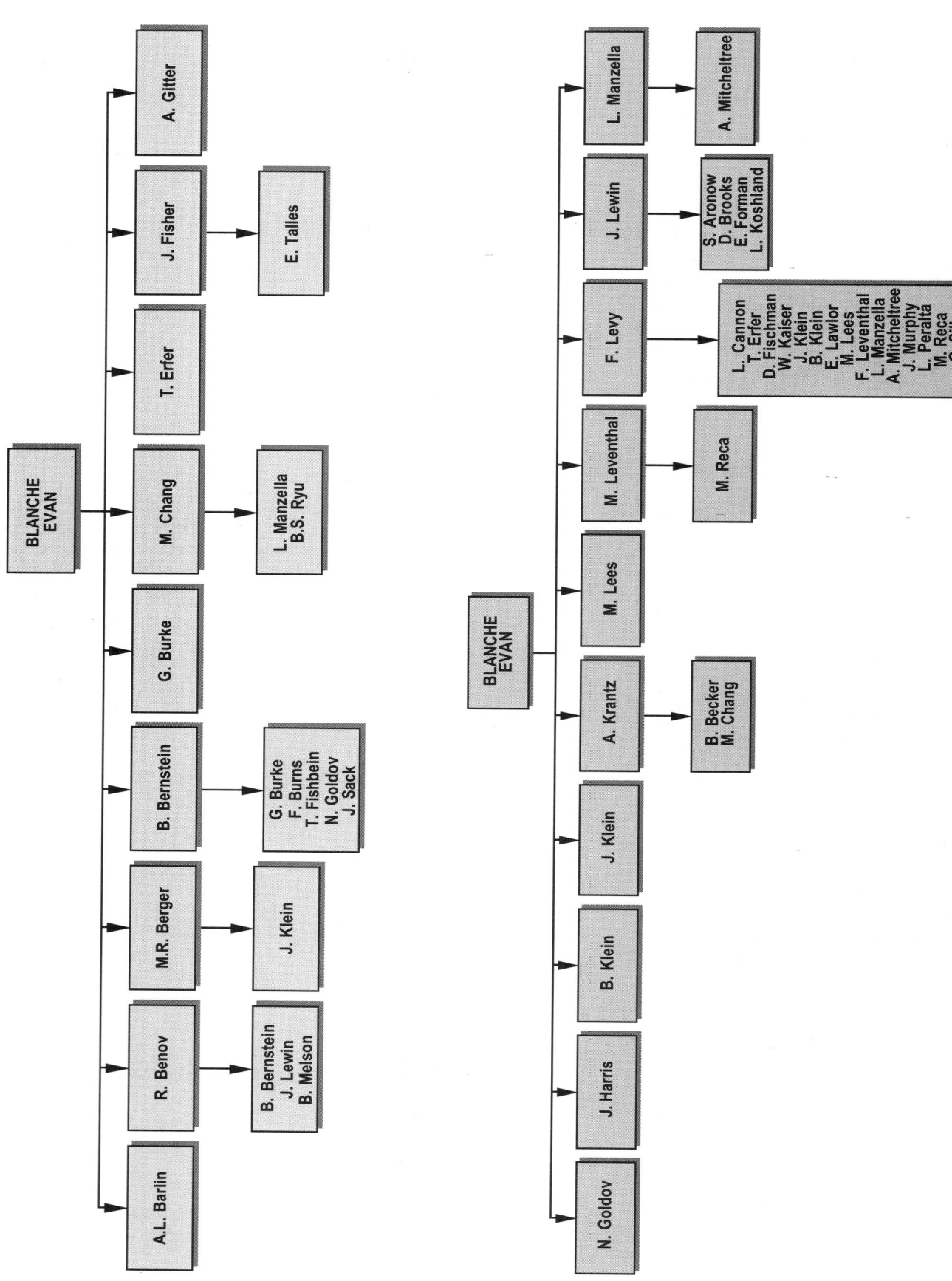

296 Dance Movement Therapy

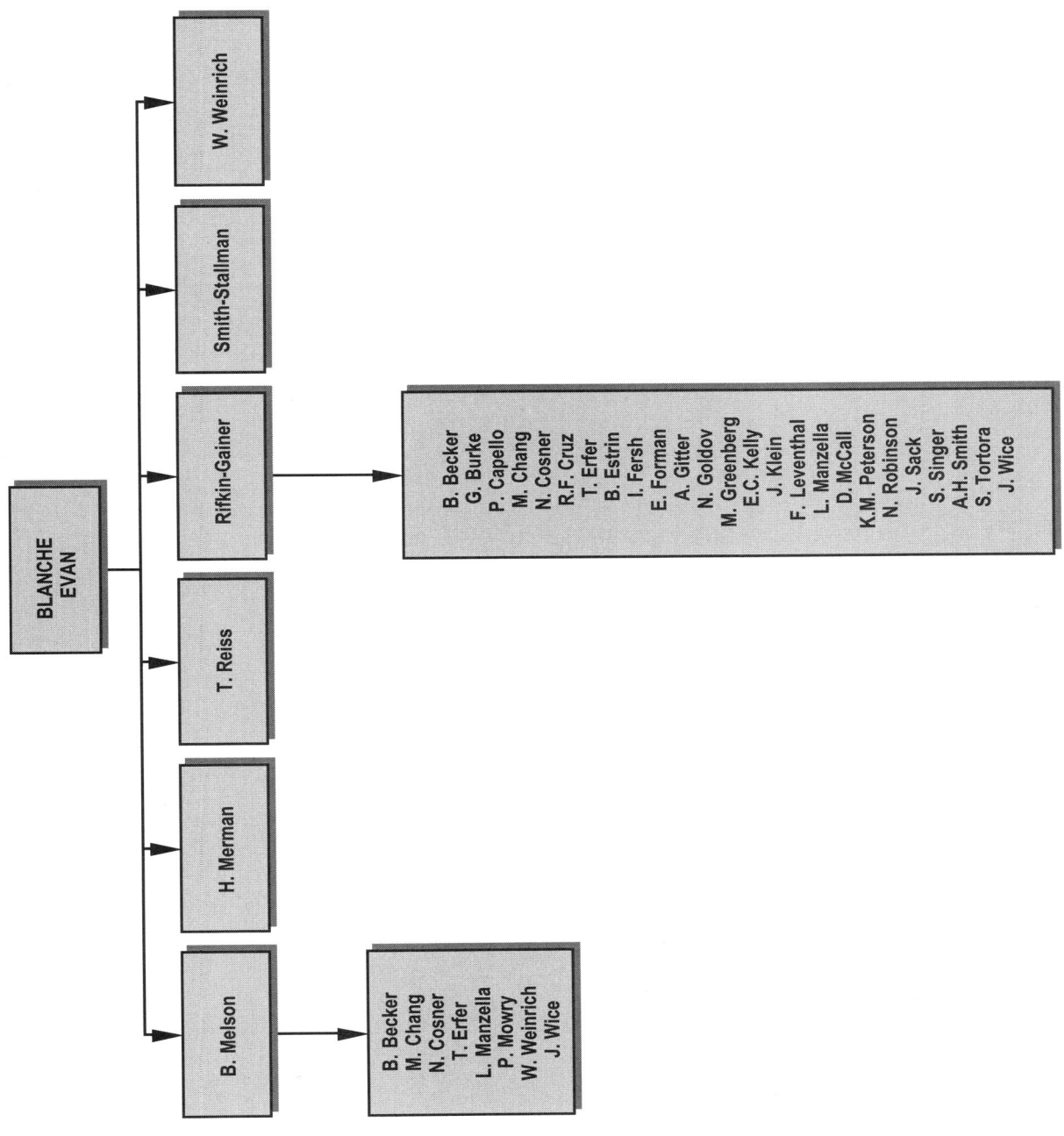

Dance Therapy Heritage Trees—The Spread of Influence of the Major Pioneers

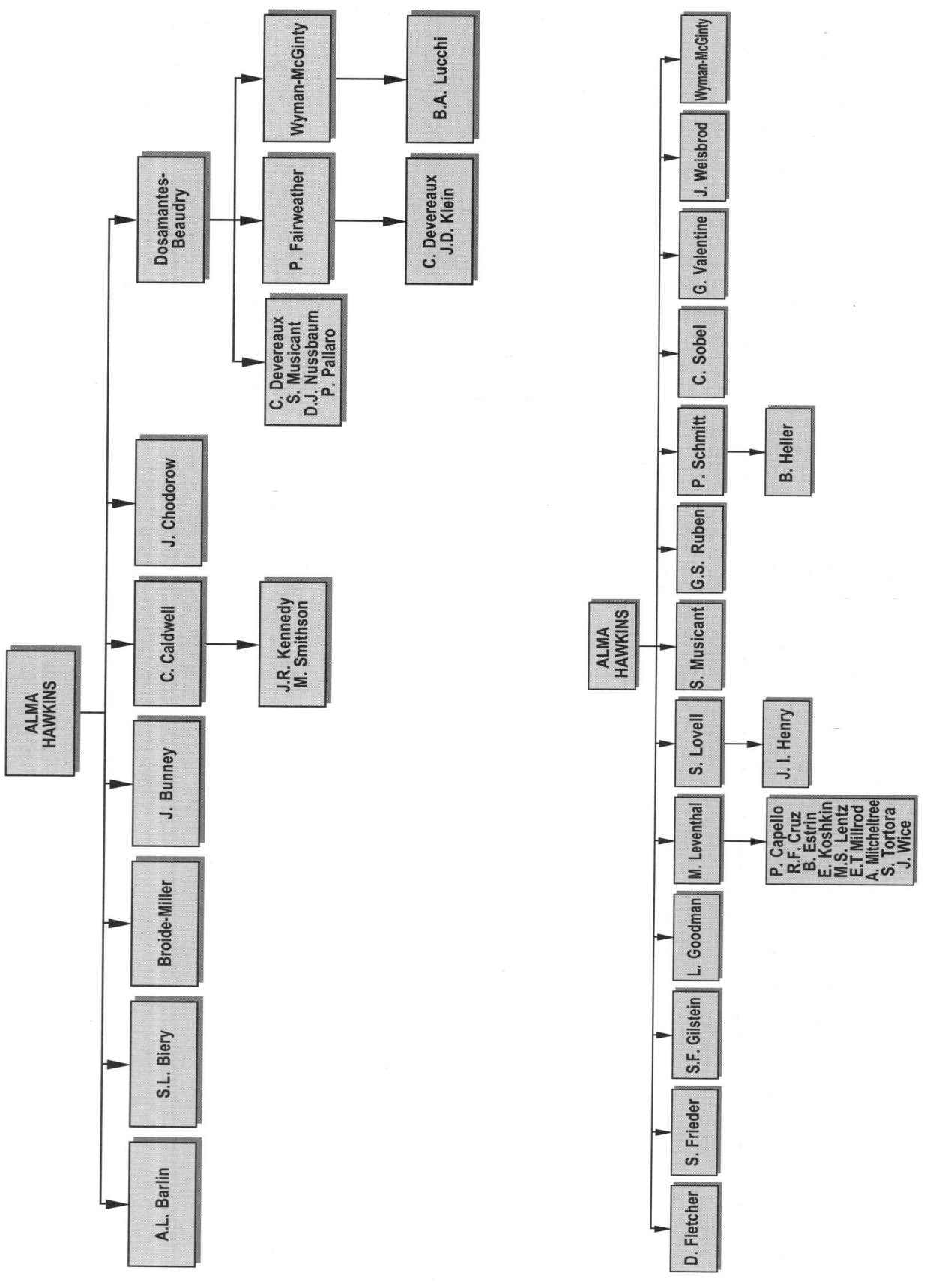

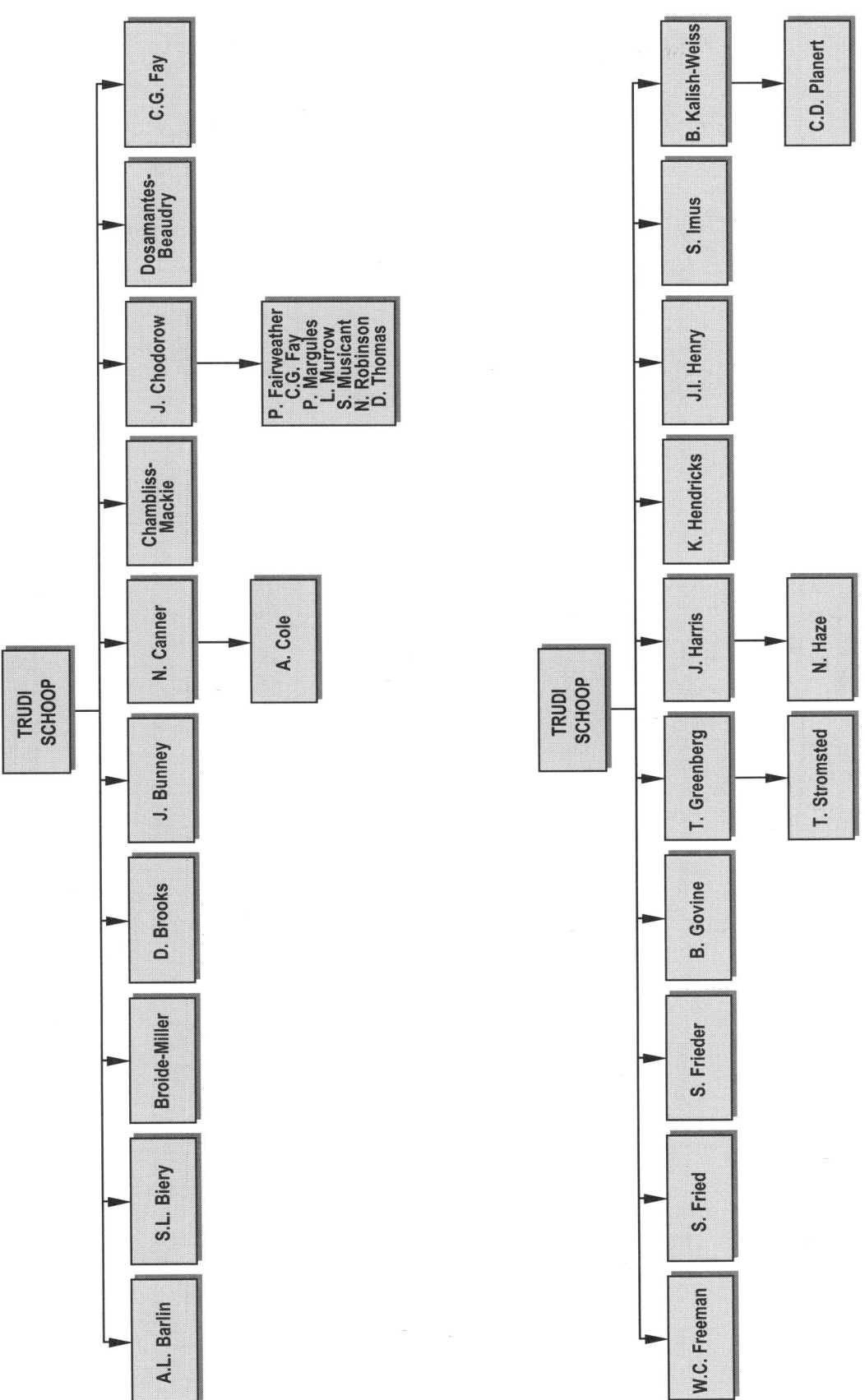

Dance Therapy Heritage Trees—The Spread of Influence of the Major Pioneers

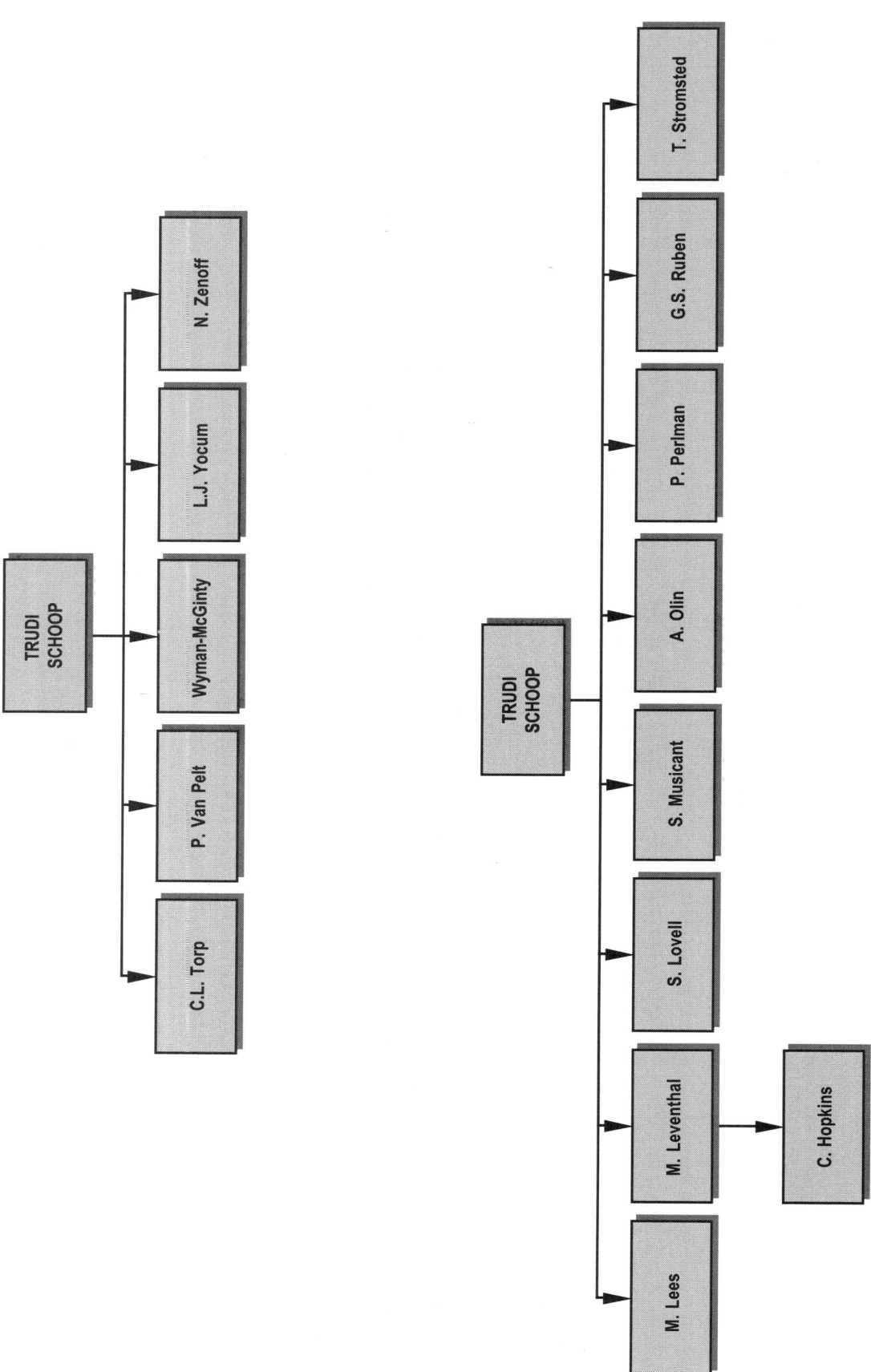

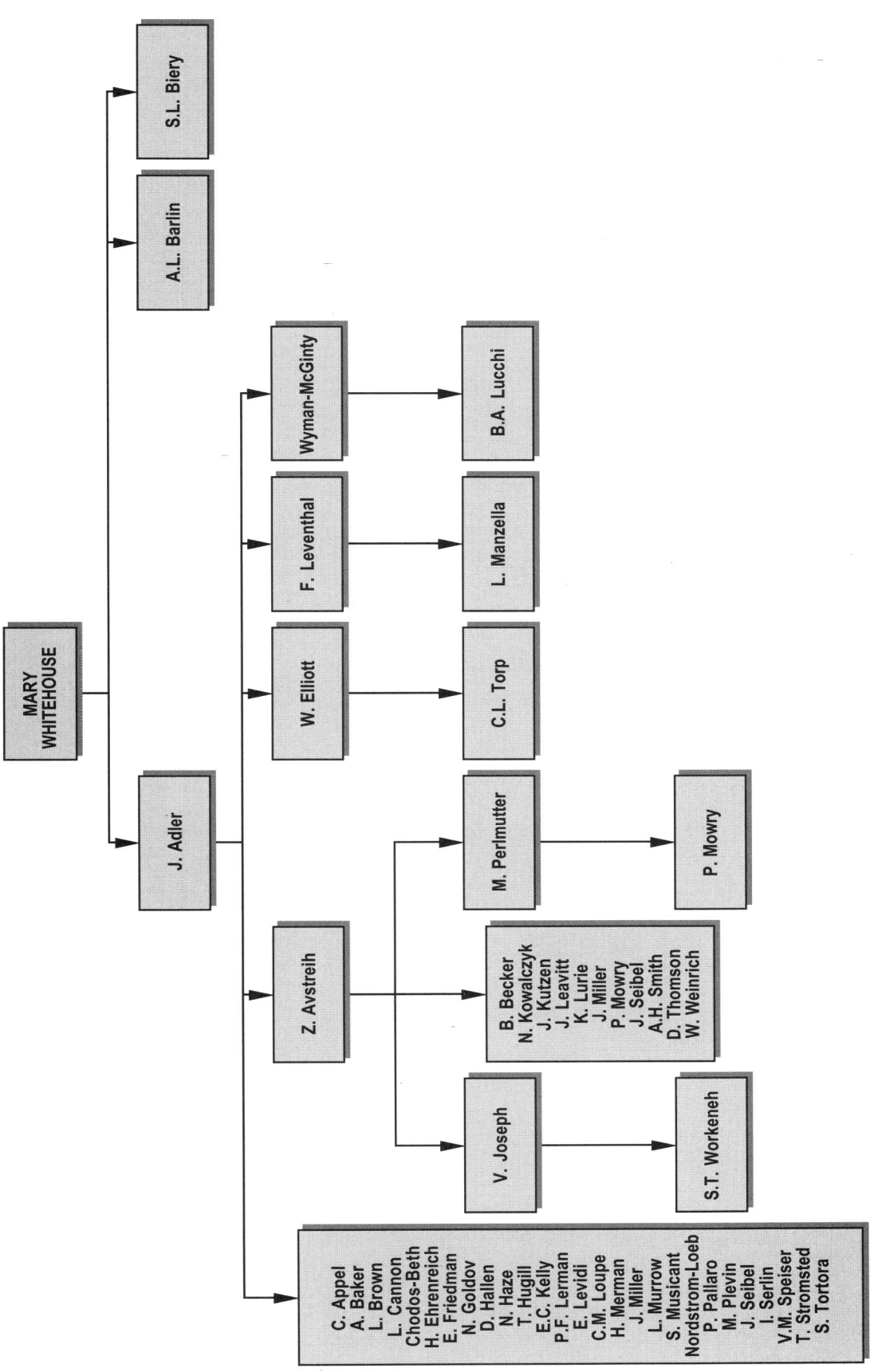

Dance Therapy Heritage Trees—The Spread of Influence of the Major Pioneers 301

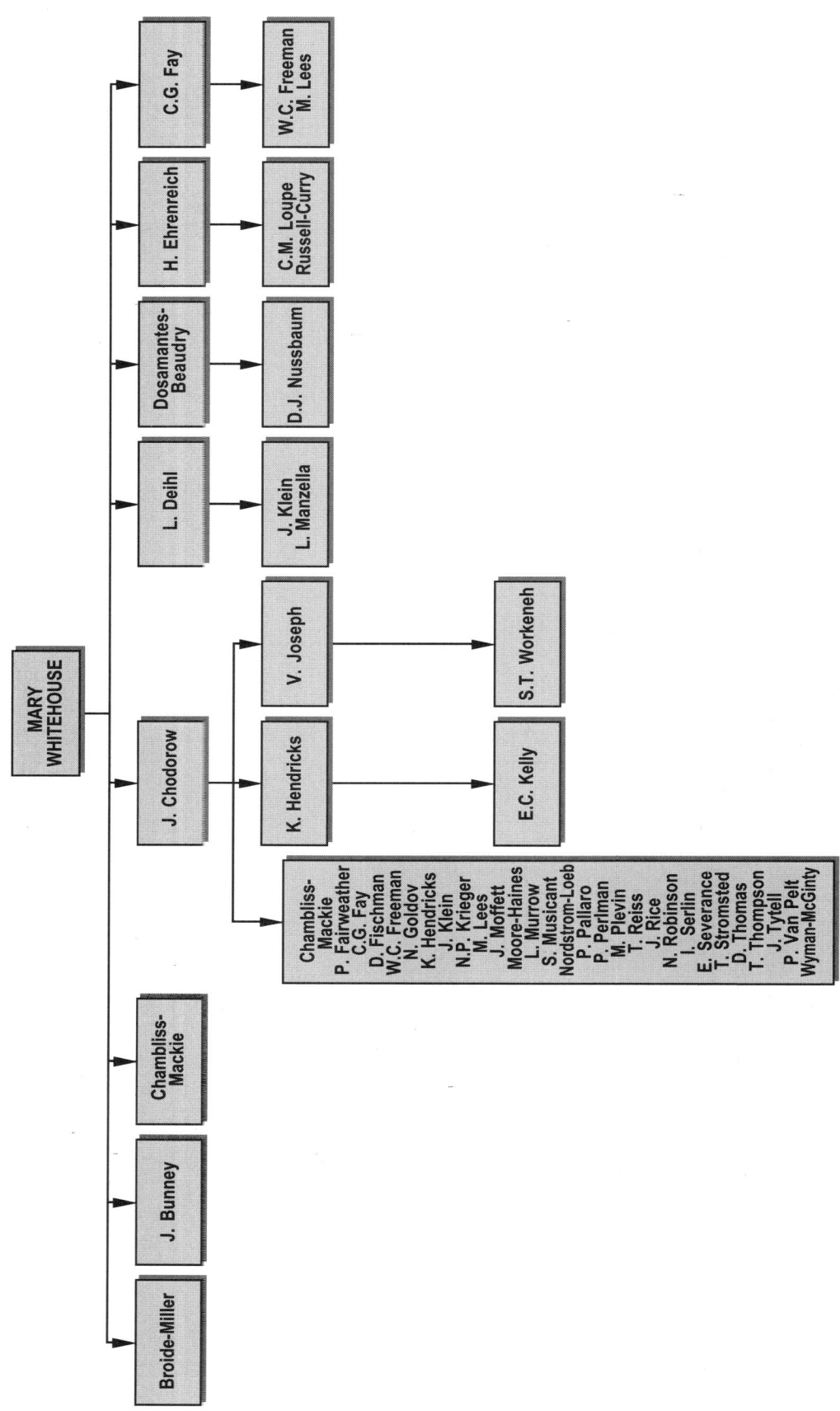

302 Dance Movement Therapy

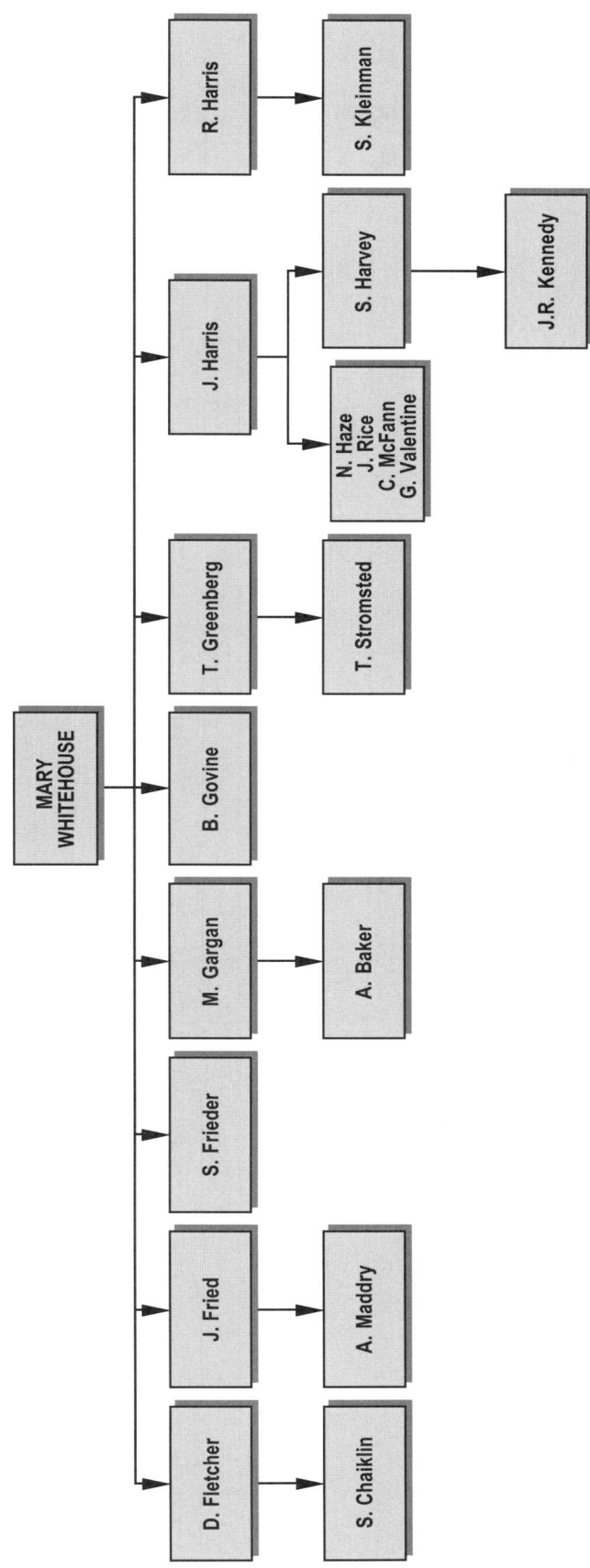

Dance Therapy Heritage Trees—The Spread of Influence of the Major Pioneers 303

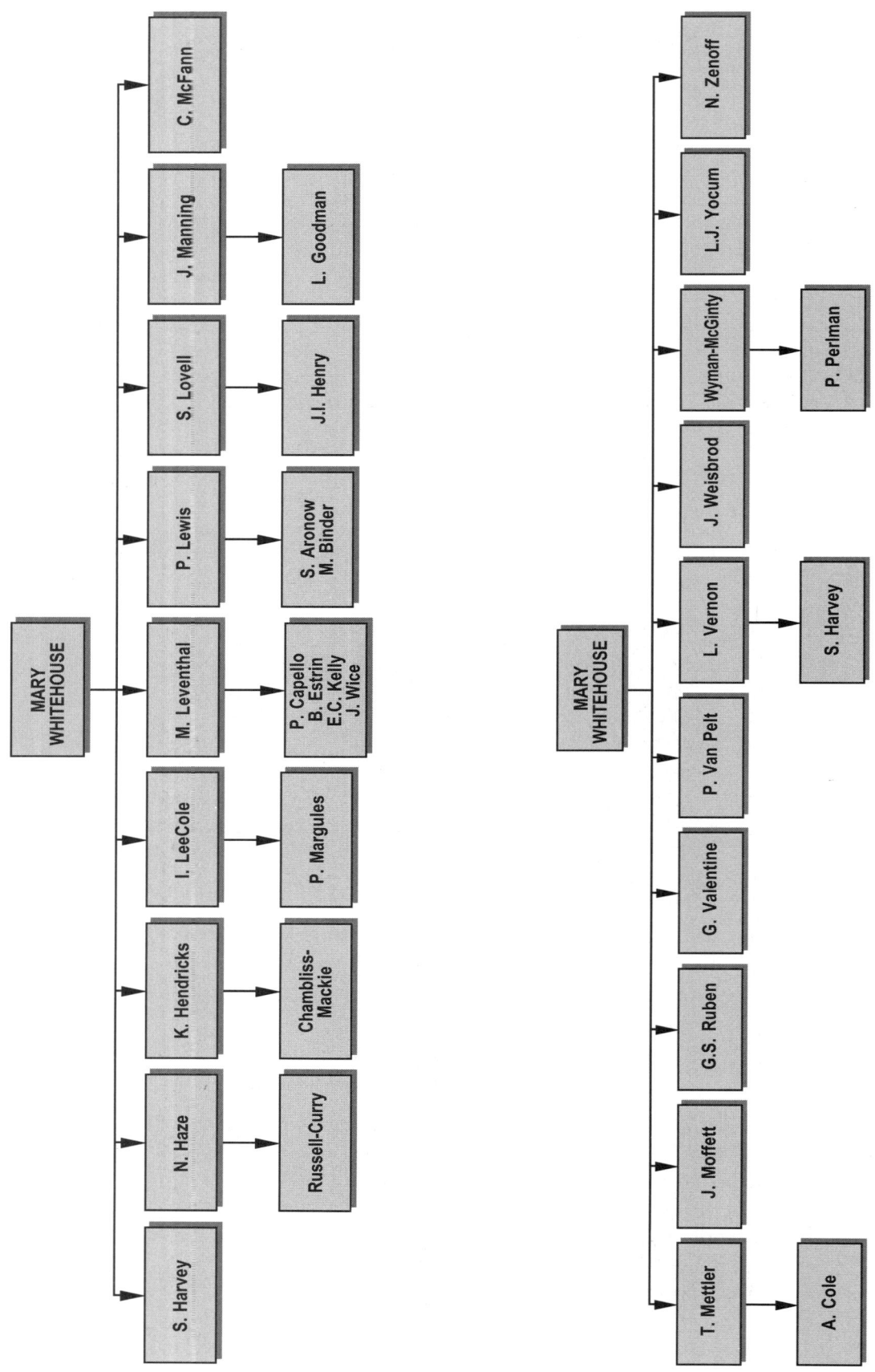

Heritage trees designed by Sheyi Ojofeitimi

304 Dance Movement Therapy

Concluding Remarks

Dance therapy began with a small group of pioneers whose work was limited to private dance studios and the back wards of mental hospitals. Built upon the foundations they laid, and shaped by a rich heritage of modern dance and psychoanalytic thought, today's dance therapists have achieved recognition within the mainstream of the mental health community. Nevertheless, dance therapy is still a relatively young field and, as practitioners, we need to remain open to innovative ideas and approaches.

Diversity is evident in the broad spectrum of theoretical and practical perspectives that are used in dance therapy today. While some dance therapists rely on traditional, psychoanalytic concepts, others engage their deep intuitive knowledge of movement and nonverbal communication with a greater emphasis on interactional methods. Still others stress the bodily-felt experience in the here and now. Many therapists attempt to integrate all of these while some are developing new theoretical constructs.

Our diversity is important. It keeps us true to our heritage as a creative art therapy. However, at times when I was working on this book, I found some of the language we use in the field to be confusing and unclearly defined. Words can describe and clarify, but they can also confuse and mystify a listener. This is one reason why dance therapists emphasize nonverbal expression to uncover the underlying meaning behind words and gestures.

A possible direction for the future might be to analyze the language of leading dance therapy theorists to see how they espouse new ideas and how these ideas compare to those of their peers. Consistency would be a potent tool for communication with allied professionals and with dance therapists from other countries.

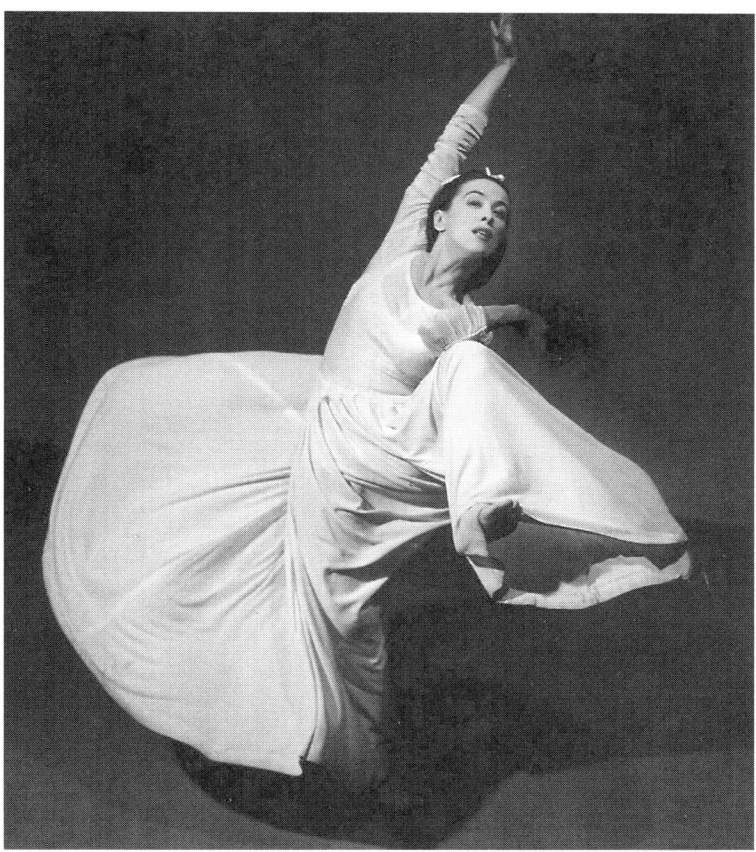

Martha Graham performing *Letter to the World*, 1940 (Photo courtesy Lloyd Morgan of the Barbara Morgan Archive)

We need to communicate the most basic truths about human expression in the simplest and most universal language.

We stand solidly on the shoulders of a small group of pioneers who preceded us in dance, dance therapy and psychology. Understanding our commonality provides a stronger basis to explain who we are in order to promote dance therapy as a cohesive profession that encompasses a broad scope of practice. This is especially important today since the field is rapidly expanding into different parts of the world.

Many dance therapists from the United States travel internationally, teaching and starting educational and mental health programs. Some bring dance therapy to countries that are war-torn or have experienced natural disasters and are aiding the survivors of these traumas. These professionals impact the lives of those they work with and, in turn, their own lives are profoundly changed.

It is inspiring to know that dance therapists are reaching so many parts of the world, overcoming the barriers of culture and language through movement, gesture and empathy. These therapists, pioneers in their own right, use their skills to communicate what we most believe in—the universality of body expression as conveyed through movement and the human need to be seen, heard and understood.

Every time a dance therapist faces a patient, he or she is confronted with the immediacy of nonverbal expression, stripping the veil of intellectualization. Through movement, the dance therapist unlocks the secrets stored in the body, the traumas as well as the joys, love as well as loss. The body remembers what the conscious mind forgets. The dance therapist receives this information and responds in the moment. "It is within this empathic and spontaneous dance between patient and therapist that healing occurs" (F. Levy, p.xii, 1995). In this sense, I believe that all dance therapists—past, present and future—are pioneers, navigating the unknown.

Perhaps it is a dream, but I like to think that dance, along with the study of movement and human emotion, can help us in the pursuit of world communication and peace. For us as dance therapists, it is a dream worth contemplating.

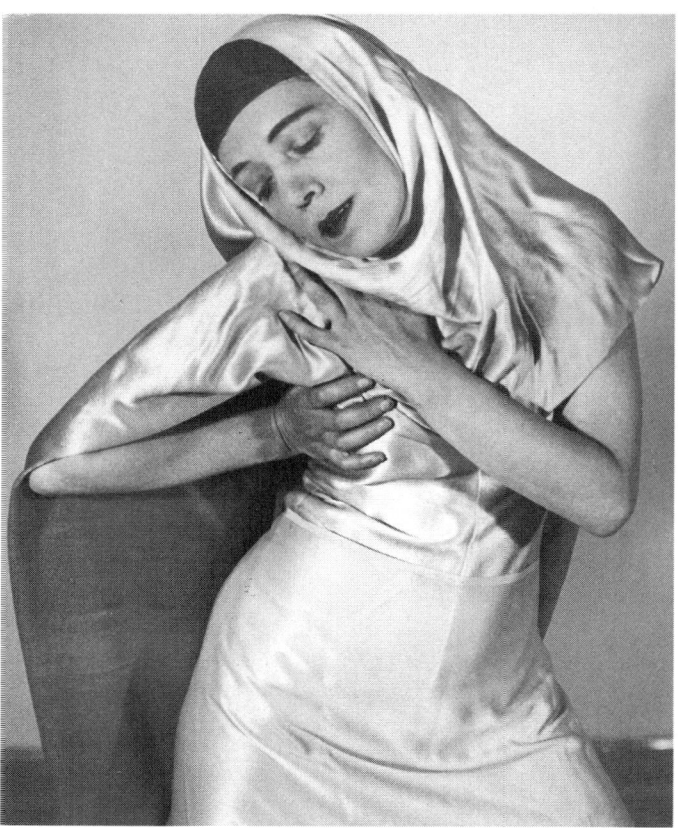

Mary Wigman in performance (Photo courtesy Jerome Robbins Dance Division, The New York Public Library for the Performing Arts)

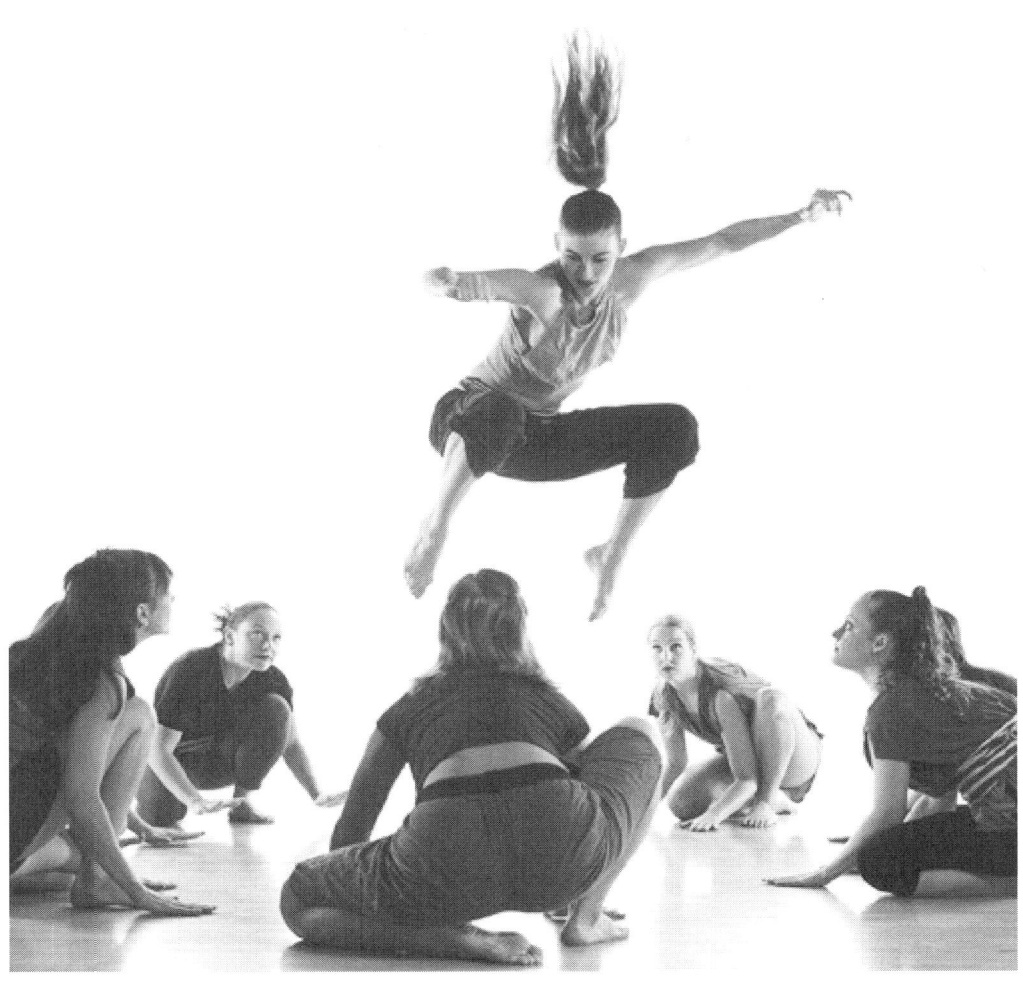

Full Circle—Young dancers and dance movement therapists around the world pioneer nonverbal communication. Dancers: Shawn Bowman-Hicks, Rhian Jaques, Kelly Swindell, Virginia Freeman, Katie Baker, Rai Anne Ivey (Photo courtesy Steve Clarke)

References*

Adler, A. (1927). *Understanding human nature.* New York: Greenberg Publishers.
Adler, J. (1968). The study of an autistic child. *Proceedings of the Third Annual Conference of the American Dance Therapy Association,* USA, 43-48.
Adler, J. (1985). *Who is the witness? A description of authentic movement.* Unpublished manuscript.
Adler, J. (Producer). (1989). *Still Looking?* [Motion Picture]. United States.
Adler, J. (2002). *Offering from the conscious body: The discipline of authentic movement.* Rochester, VT: Inner Traditions.
American Alliance for Health, Physical Education, Recreation & Dance. (1956). *Dance therapy study.* Reston, VA: Author.
American Dance Therapy Association. (1978). *American Dance Therapy Association Annual Report.* Columbia, MD: Author.
American Dance Therapy Association. (1979). *American Dance Therapy Association Annual Report.* Columbia, MD: Author.
American Psychiatric Association. (2000). *Diagnostic and statistical manual of mental disorders: DSM-IV TR.* Washington, DC: Author.
Amighi, J., Loman, S., Lewis, P., & Sossin, M. (1999). *The meaning of movement: Developmental, multicultural, and clinical perspectives as seen through the Kestenberg movement profile.* Newark, DE: Charles C. Thomas.
Ansbacher, H. L., & Ansbacher, R. R. (Eds.). (1956). *The individual psychology of Alfred Adler.* New York: Basic Books.
Arieti, S. (1974). *Interpretation of schizophrenia.* New York: Basic Books.
Avstreih, A. (1979, October). *The emerging self.* Unpublished paper presented at the Fourteenth Annual Conference of the American Dance Therapy Association, Philadelphia, PA.
Bartenieff, I. (1975). Dance therapy: A new profession or rediscovery of an ancient role of dance. In H. Chaiklin (Ed.), *Marian Chace: Her papers* (pp. 246-255). Columbia, MD: American Dance Therapy Association.
Bartenieff, I., & Davis, M. (1965). *Effort-shape analysis of movement: The unity of expression and function.* Unpublished monograph. Bronx, NY: Albert Einstein Colleges of Medicine. (Copies available from Dance Notation Bureau, 8 E. 12th St., New York: NY 10003).
Bartenieff, I., & Lewis, D. (1980). *Body movement: Coping with the environment.* New York: Gordan and Breach, Science Publishers.
Bartkey, C. (1980). *A comparison of the movement profiles of battered, ex-battered, and nonbattered women: A pilot study.* Unpublished master's thesis, Hahnemann Medical College, Philadelphia.
Bartlett, V. (Director). & Brock, N. (Producer). (1970). *Looking for me?* [Motion Picture]. United States.
Baum, E.Z. (1991). Movement therapy with multiple personality patients. *Dissociation,* 4(2), 99-104.
Baum, E.Z. (See Levy, F., 1995, pp. 88-89).
Beebe, B., Jaffe, J., Lachmann, F., Feldstein, S., Crown, C., & Jasnow, M. (2000). Systems models in development and psychoanalysis: The case of vocal rhythm coordination and attachment. *Infant Mental Health Journal,* 21(1-2), 99-122.
Bell, J. (1984). Family therapy in motion: Observing, assessing, and changing the family dance. In P. L. Bernstein (Ed.), *Theoretical approaches in dance-movement therapy, Vol. II.* Dubuque, IA: Kendall Hunt.
Bender, L. (1952). *Child psychiatric techniques.* Springfield, IL: C. C. Thomas.
Benov, R. (1991). *The collected works by and about Blanche Evan.* Available from Blanche Evan Dance Foundation, 146 Fifth Avenue, San Francisco, CA 94118.
Bernstein, B. (See Levy, F., 1995, pp. 41-42).
Bernstein, P. L. (1972). *Theory and methods in dance-movement therapy: A manual for therapists, students and educators.* Dubuque, IA: Kendall Hunt.

Bernstein, P. L. (1973). Recapitulation of ontogeny: A theoretical approach in dance movement therapy. *Proceedings of the Eighth Annual Conference of the American Therapy Association, USA*, 107-115.

Bernstein, P. L. (1975). *Therapeutic process movement as integration*. Columbia, MD: American Dance Therapy Association.

Bernstein, P. L. (1979). *Eight theoretical approaches in dance-movement therapy*. Dubuque, IA: W.C. Brown-Kendall Hunt.

Bernstein, P. L. (1979). The use of symbolism within a Gestalt movement therapy approach. In P.L. Bernstein (Ed.), *Eight theoretical approaches in dance-movement therapy* (pp. 111-130). Dubuque, IA: Kendall Hunt.

Bernstein, P. L. (1980). A mythologic quest: Jungian movement therapy with the psychosomatic client. *American Journal of Dance Therapy*, 3(2), 44-55.

Bernstein, P. L., & Loman, S. (1981). The Kestenberg movement profile. In D. Dulicai (Chair.), Laban-influenced movement profiles: A critical discussion of their reliability, validity and value to dance therapy. *Symposium American Dance Therapy Association*, Madison, WI.

Bernstein, P. L. & Singer, D. (Eds.) (1982). *The choreography of object relations*. Keene, NH: Antioch University.

Berrol, C. (2000). The spectrum of research options in dance/movement therapy. *American Journal of Dance Therapy*, 22(1), 29-46.

Berrol, C., & Katz, S. (1985). Dance movement therapy in the rehabilitation of individuals surviving severe head injuries. *AJDT*, 8, 46-66.

Berrol, C. F., Ooi, W. L., & Katz, S. S. (1997). Dance/movement therapy with older adults who have sustained neurological insult: A demonstration project. *American Journal of Dance Therapy*, 19(2), 135-160.

Birdwhistell, R. L. (1952). *Introduction to kinesics*. Louisville, KY: University of Louisville Press.

Birdwhistell, R. L. (1970). *Kinesics and context*. Philadelphia: University of Pennsylvania Press.

Blume, E. S. (1991). *Secret survivors: Uncovering incest and its aftereffects in women*. New York: Ballantine Books.

Boas, F. (1941-42). Psychological aspects in the practice of teaching dancing. *Journal of Aesthetics and Art Criticism*, 2, 3-20.

Boas, F. (1971). Origins of dance. *Proceedings of the Sixth Annual Conference of the American Dance Therapy Association*, USA, 75-78.

Boas, F. (1978). Creative dance. In M. N. Costonis (Ed.), *Therapy in motion*. Chicago: University of Illinois Press.

Bovard-Taylor, A. B., & Draganosky, J. E. (1979). Using personal space to develop alliance in dance therapy. *American Journal of Dance Therapy*, 3(1), 51-61.

Braun, B. G. (1986). *The treatment of multiple personality disorder*. Washington, DC: American Psychiatric Press.

Brown, L. M., & Gilligan, C. (1992). *Meeting at the crossroads: Women's psychology and girls' development*. Cambridge, MA: Harvard University Press.

Brownell, A. (Producer) & Freeman, W. C. (Producer). (1998). *A Time to Dance: The life and work of Norma Canner* [Motion Picture]. United States.

Brownmiller, S. (1975). *Against our will: Men, women, and rape*. New York: Simon and Schuster.

Canner, N. (1968). *. . . and a time to dance*. Boston, MA: Beacon Press.

Canner, N. (1980). Movement therapy with multi-handicapped children. In M. B. Leventhal (Ed.), *Movement and growth: Dance therapy for the special child* (pp. 53-56). New York: New York University.

Caplow, E. L., Harpaz, L., & Samberg, S. (1978). *Therapeutic dance/movement: Expressive activities for older adults*. New York: Human Science Press.

Chace, M., & Dyrud, J. (1968, October). Movement and personality. *Proceedings of the Third Annaul Conference of the American Dance Therapy Association*, 16-20.

Chaiklin, H. (1968). Research and the development of a profession. *Proceedings of the Third Annual Conference of the American Dance Therapy Association*, 64-74.

Chaiklin, H. (1975). *Marian Chace: Her papers*. Columbia, MD: American Dance Therapy Association.

Chaiklin, H. (1997). Research and the development of a profession revisited. *American Journal of Dance Therapy, 19*(2), 93-103.

Chaiklin, S. (1974). Curriculum development in dance therapy. In K. Mason (Ed.), *Focus on Dance VII: Dance Therapy*. Reston, VA: American Alliance for Health, Physical Education, Recreation and Dance.

Chaiklin, S. (1975). Dance therapy. In S. Arieti (Ed.), *American handbook of psychiatry*. New York: Basic Books.

Chaiklin S., & Schmais, C. (1979). The Chace approach to dance therapy. In P. L. Bernstein (Ed.), *Eight theoretical approaches to dance therapy* (p. 16). Dubuque, IA: Kendall-Hunt.

Chang, M. & Leventhal, F. (See F. Levy, 1995, p. 57).

Clarke, Steve. (2004). *Seeing while being seen: Dance photography and the creative process*. Reston, VA: National Dance Association.

Chodorow, J. (1991). *Dance therapy and depth psychology: The moving imagination*. London: Routledge.

Chodorow, J. (1997). *Jung on active imagination*. Two simultaneous editions. London: Routledge. Princeton, NJ: Princeton University Press.

Chodorow, J. (2004). *Active imagination: Healing from within*. College Station, TX: Texas A&M University Press.

Cohen, S., & Walco, G. (1999). Dance/Movement therapy for children with cancer. *Cancer Practice, 7*(1), 36.

Condon, W. S. (1963). *Synchrony units and the communication hierarchy*. Unpublished paper.

Condon, W. S. (1964). *Process in communication*. Unpublished paper. (Available from the author, School of Medicine, Western Psychiatric Institute and Clinic, 3811 O'Hara St., Pittsburgh, Pennsylvania 15213)

Condon, W. S. (1968). Linguistic-kinesic research and dance therapy. *Proceedings of the Third Annual Conference of the American Dance Therapy Association*, 21-42.

Condon, W. S., & Brosin, H. W. (1969). Micro linguistic-kinesic events in schizophrenic behavior. In D. V. Siva Sankar (Ed.), *Schizophrenia: Current concepts and research*. Hicksville, NY: PJD Publications.

Condon, W. S., & Ogston, W. D. (1966). Sound film analysis of normal and pathological behavior patterns. *Journal of Nervous and Mental Disease, 143*, 338-347.

Condon, W. S., & Ogston, W. D. (1967a). A method of studying animal behavior. *Journal of Auditory Research, 7*, 359-367.

Condon, W. S., & Ogston, W. D. (1967b). A segmentation of behavior. *Journal of Psychiatric Research, 5*, 221-235.

Condon, W. S., & Sander, L. W. (1974). Neonate movement is synchronized with adult speech: Interactional participation and language acquisition. *Science, 183*, 99-101.

Costonis, M. (1974). How I learned to wall-bounce and love it. *Proceedings of the Ninth Annual Conference of the American Dance Therapy Association*, 143-155.

Costonis, M. (Ed.). (1978). *Therapy in motion*. Chicago: University of Illinois Press.

Cruz, R. F., & Hervey, L. W. (2001). The American Dance Therapy Association research survey. *American Journal of Dance Therapy, 23*(2), 89-118.

Darwin, C. (1872). *The expression of the emotions in man and animals*. London: John Murray.

Davis, M. (1965). Effort/Shape analysis of movement: The unity of expression and function. Unpublished manuscript available from Dance Notation Bureau.

Davis, W. N. (2000, Fall). A word from the editor, W. N. Davis (Ed.). *The Renfrew Center Foundation Perspective, 6*(1), 1.

Davis, W. N., & Kleinman, S. (Ed). *Healing within relationships: The Renfrew Center perspectives in eating disorders recovery*. Manuscript in preparation.

Dell, C. (1970). *A primer for movement description: Using effort/shape and supplementary concepts*. New York: Dance Notation Bureau.

Dell, C. (1970). *Space harmony: Basic terms*. New York: Dance Notation Bureau.

Deutsch, F. (1922). Psychoanalyse and organkrankheiten. *Int. Z. Psa., 8*, n.p.

Deutsch, F. (1947). Analysis of postural behavior. *Psychoanalytic Quarterly, 16*, 195-213.

Deutsch, F. (1951). Thus speaks the body: IV, some psychosomatic aspects of the respiratory disorder: Asthma. *Acta Medica Orientalia, 10*, 67-86.

Deutsch, F. (1952). Analytic posturology. *Psychoanalytic Quarterly, 21*, 196-214.

Dosamantes-Alperson, E. D. (1974a). Carrying experiencing forward through authentic body movement. *Psychotherapy: Theory, research and practice*, 11(3), 211-214.

Dosamantes-Alperson, E. D. (1979b). The intrapsychic and interpersonal in movement psychotherapy. *American Journal of Dance Therapy*, 1, 20-31.

Downes, J. (1980). Movement therapy for the special child: Construct for the emerging self. In M. B. Leventhal (Ed.), *Movement and growth: Dance therapy for the special child* (pp. 13-17). New York: New York University.

Downes, J. (1982). The phenomenology of object relations in dance-movement therapy. In P. L. Bernstein & D. L. Singer (Eds.), *The choreography of object relations*. Keene, NH: Antioch New England Graduate School.

Dratman, M. L. (1967). Reorganization of psychic structures in autism: A study using body movement therapy. *Proceedings of the Second Annual Conference of the American Dance Therapy Association*, 39-45.

Dratman, M. L. (1971, June). *Reorganization of psychic structures in autism: A study using body movement therapy*. Paper presented at the meeting of the American Dance Movement Therapy Association, Columbia, MD.

Duggan, D. (1978). Goals and methods in dance therapy with severely multiply handicapped children. *American Journal of Dance Therapy*, 2(1), 31-34.

Duggan, D. (1995). The "4's": A dance therapy program for learning disabled adolescents. In F. J. Levy, J. P. Fried, & F. Leventhal (Eds.), *Dance and other expressive art therapies: When words are not enough*. New York: Routledge.

Dulicai, D. (1976). Dance therapy and its research. *Bulletin of the International Conference on Nonverbal Communication*, 16-18.

Dulicai, D. (1977). Nonverbal assessment of family systems: Clinical implications. *International Journal of Art Psychotherapy*, 6(2), 55-62.

Dulicai, D., & Rogers, S. B. (1980). The collaborative use of nonverbal assessment of family systems and practical clinical approaches. In M. B. Leventhal (Ed.), *Movement and growth: Dance therapy for the special child* (pp. 101-107). New York: New York University.

Erfer, T. (1995). Treating children with autism in a public school system. In F. Levy, J. P. Fried, & F. Leventhal (Eds.), *Dance and other expressive art therapies: When words are not enough*. New York: Routledge.

Erfer, T., & Ziv, A. (2002). Dance movement therapy with children in a short-term psychiatric setting. Unpublished manuscript.

Espenak, L. (1970). Movement diagnosis tests and the inherent laws governing their use in treatment: An aid in detecting the life style. *The Individual Psychologist*, 7(1), 8-13.

Espenak, L. (1972). Body-dynamics and dance in individual psychotherapy. In F. Donelan (Ed.), *American Dance Therapy Association Writings on body movement and communication. Monograph No. 2* (pp.111-127). Columbia, MD: American Dance Therapy Association.

Espenak, L. (1975, March). *A means of removing interpersonal barriers of the retarded*. Lecture at the Eighth Annual International Symposium, University of Seville, Spain.

Espenak, L. (1979). The Adlerian approach in dance therapy. In P. L. Bernstein (Ed.), *Eight theoretical approaches to dance therapy* (pp. 71-88). Dubuque, IA: Kendall-Hunt.

Evan, B. (1945-78). *Packet of pieces by and about Blanche Evan*. San Francisco, CA: Blanche Evan Foundation.

Evan, B. (1964). *The child's world: Its relation to dance pedagogy* (a collection of out-of-print articles). New York. (Available from the author at 9491/2 Marine, Boulder, Colorado 80302).

Fay, C. G. (1977). *Movement and fantasy: A dance therapy model based on the psychology of Carl C. Jung*. Unpublished master's thesis, Goddard College, Plainfield, VT.

Feldenkrais, M. (1972). *Awareness through movement*. New York: Harper & Row.

Feldenkrais, M. (1973). *Body and mature behavior: A study of anxiety, sex gravitation and learning*. New York: International Universities Press.

Fenichel, O. (1928/1953). Organ libidinization accompanying the defense against drives. *The collected papers of Otto Fenichel: First series*. New York: Norton.

Fenichel, O. (1934). *Outline of clinical psychoanalysis*. New York: The Psychoanalytic Quarterly Press and Norton.

Ferenczi, S. (1916). *Sex in psycho-analysis: Contributions to psycho-analysis*. (Jones, trans.). Boston: Richard G. Badger.

Fersh, I. (1980). Dance movement therapy: A holistic approach to working with the elderly. *American Journal of Dance Therapy*, 3(2), 33-43.

Finkelhor, D. & Browne, A. (1985, August). *A model for understanding: Treating the trauma of child sexual abuse*. Paper presented at the conference of the American Psychological Association, Los Angeles, CA.

Fisher, P. (1995). *More than movement for fit to frail older adults: Creative activities for body, mind and spirit*. Baltimore, MD: Health Professions Press.

Fletcher, D. (1979). Body experience within the therapeutic process: A psychodynamic orientation. In P. L. Bernstein (Ed.), *Eight theoretical approaches to dance therapy* (pp. 131-154). Dubuque, IA: Kendall Hunt.

Fonteyn, M. (1979). *The magic of dance*. New York: Alfred A. Knopf.

Freeman, W. C. (Producer). (1998). *You're okay right where you are: Expressive movement in education* [Motion Picture]. United States: Bushy Theatre.

Freeman, W. C. (See Brownell, A.).

Freud, A. (1965). *Normality and pathology in childhood: Assessment of development*. New York: International Universities Press.

Freud, S. (1905/1953). Three essays on the theory of sexuality. *The standard edition* (Vol. VII). London: Hogarth.

Freud, S. (1923/1955). The ego and the id. *The standard edition* (Vol. XIX). London: Hogarth.

Frost, M. (1984). Changing movement patterns and lifestyle in a blind, obsessive compulsive. *American Journal of Dance Therapy*, 7, 15-31.

Garnet, E. (1974). A movement therapy for older people. In K. Mason (Ed.), *Focus on dance VII: Dance therapy*. Reston, VA: American Alliance for Health, Physical Education, Recreation and Dance.

Gendlin, E. (1971). A theory of personality change. In A. Mahrer & L. Pearson (Eds.), *Creative developments in psychotherapy*. Cleveland, OH: Case Western Reserve University.

Genther, S. (1954). A place to begin. *Impulse*, 19-22.

Gil, E. (1988). *Treatment of adult survivors of childhood abuse*. Rockville, MD: Launch Press.

Gillman, I. (1980). An object-relations approach to the phenomenon of and treatment of battered women. *Psychiatry*, 43, 346-358.

Groninger, V. (1980, May 23). Dance therapist changes lives. *Daily Camera*, 17.

Harris, J. (1980, July). In memoriam: Maja Schade. *ADTA Newsletter*, 14(4), 1.

Harvey, S. (1995). Sandra: The case of an adopted sexually abused child. In F. Levy, J. P. Fried, & F. Leventhal (Eds.), *Dance and other expressive art therapies: When words are not enough*. New York: Routledge.

Hawkins, A. (1972). Dance therapy today-points of view and ways of working. *Proceedings of the Seventh Annual Conference of the American Dance Therapy Association*, 61-68.

Hervey, L. W. (2000). *Artistic inquiry in dance/movement therapy*. Springfield, IL: Charles C. Thomas.

Hood, C. (1959). The challenge of dance therapy. *Journal of Health, Physical Education, Recreation*, 17-18.

Huston, K. (1984). Ethical decisions in treating battered women. *Professional Psychology: Research and Practice*, 15(6), 822-832.

Hutchinson, M. G. (1985). *Transforming body image: Learning to love the body you have*. Freedom, CA: The Crossing Press.

Irwin, K. (1972). Dance as prevention of, therapy for, and recreation from the crisis of old age. In F. Donelan (Ed.), *A.D.T.A. Writings on body movement and communication. Monograph No. 2* (pp. 151-190). Columbia, MD: American Dance Therapy Association.

Jacobson, E. (1929). *Progressive relaxation*. Chicago: University of Chicago Press.

Johnson, D. & Sandel, S. (1977). Structural analysis of group movement sessions: Preliminary research. *American Journal of Dance Therapy*, 1(2), 32-36.

Johnson, D., Sandel, S., & Eicher, V. (1983). Structural aspects of group leadership styles. *American Journal of Dance Therapy*, 6, 17-30.

Johnson, D., Sandel, S., & Bruno, C. (1984). Effectiveness of different group structures for schizophrenic character disordered, and normal groups. *International Journal of Group Psychotherapy*, 34(3), 415-429.

Kalish, B. (1968). Body movement therapy for autistic children. *Proceedings of the Third Annual Conference of the American Dance Therapy Association*, 49-59.

Kalish, B. (1974). Developmental studies using the behavior rating instrument for autistic and other atypical children (BRIAAC). *Proceedings of the Ninth Annual Conference of the American Dance Therapy Association*, 131-138.

Kalish, B. (1976). Body movement scale for autistic and other atypical children (Doctoral dissertation, Bryn Mawr College, 1977). *Dissertation Abstracts International*, 37, 12. (UMI No. 77-06524)

Kalish-Weiss, B. (1982). *Clinical and objective assessment of a multi-handicapped child*. Unpublished manuscript.

Kanner, L. (1955). *Child psychiatry*. Springfield, IL: Charles C. Thomas.

Kelly, M. (1996). *My body my rules: The body esteem, sexual esteem connection*. Ithaca, NY: Planned Parenthood of Tompkins County.

Kendon, A. (1970). Movement coordination in social interaction: Some examples described. *Ada Psychologica*, 32, 100-125.

Kernberg, P., & Chazan, S. (1991). *Children with conduct disorders—A psychotherapy manual*. New York: Basic Books.

Kestenberg, J., & Sossin, M. (1979). *The role of movement patterns in development, Vol. 2*. New York: Dance Notation Bureau Press.

Klaus, H., & Kennell, J. H. (1976). *Maternal-infant bonding*. St. Louis, MO: Mosby.

Kleinman, S. (1977). *A circle of motion*. Unpublished master's thesis, Lone Mountain College, San Francisco.

Kleinman, S. (2002, October). Challenging body image distortions through the eyes of the body. *Proceedings of the 37th Annual Conference of the American Dance Therapy Association*.

Kleinman, S., & Hall, T. (2001, October). Challenging the illusion of control: Dance/Movement Therapy for clients with eating disorders. *Proceedings of the 36th Annual Conference of the American Dance Therapy Association*.

Kleinman S., & Hall, T. (manuscript in preparation). Dance/Movement therapy. In W. N. Davis & S. Kleinman (Eds.), *Healing within relationships: The Renfrew Center Perspective on eating disorders recovery*. Philadelphia: The Renfrew Center.

Kluft, R.P. (1983). *Childhood antecedents of multiple personality*. Washington DC: American Psychiatric Press.

Kluft, R. P. (1991). Multiple personality disorder. In A. Tasman & S. M. Goldfinger (Eds.), *American Psychiatric Press Review of Psychiatry* (pp. 161-188). Washington, DC: American Psychiatric Publishing.

Kohut, H. (1971). *The analysis of the self*. New York: International University Press.

Kornblum, R. *Moving towards peace: Violence prevention through movement*. Video.

Kornblum, R. (2003) *Disarming the playground: Violence prevention through movement and pro-social skills*. Oklahoma City, OK: Wood 'N' Barnes.

Kramer, E. (1971). *Art as therapy with children*. New York: Schocken Books.

Krout, M. H. (1931). A preliminary note on some obscure symbolic muscular responses of diagnostic value in the study of normal subjects. *American Journal of Psychiatry*, 8, 29-71.

Krout, M. H. (1937). Further studies in the relation of personality and gesture: A nosological analysis of autistic gestures. *Journal of Experimental Psychology*, 20, 279-287.

Kuppers, F. (1980). *A history of dance movement therapy*. Unpublished master's thesis, Immaculate Heart College.

Lamb, W. (1965). *Posture and gesture: An introduction to the study of physical behavior*. London: Gerald Duckworth & Company.

Lavender, J. (1977, Summer). Moving toward meaning. *Psychotherapy: Theory, Research and Practice*, 14(2), 123-133.

LeDoux, J.E. (1996). *The emotional brain: The mysterious underpinnings of emotional life*. New York: Simon & Schuster.

Lefco, H. (1974). *Dance therapy: Narrative case histories and therapy sessions with six patients*. Chicago: Nelson Hall.

Leventhal, M. (1999). *The quantum healing dance matrix: The dance therapy journey into change and healing*. National Congress of the Hungarian Psychiatric Association: Psychopathology of Expression Section: Published Proceedings, Budapest, Hungary.

Leventhal, M. B. (1980). Dance therapy as treatment of choice for the emotionally disturbed and learning disabled child. In Riordan and Pitt, (Eds.), *Dance for the handicapped*. Reston, VA: American Alliance for Health, Physical Education, Recreation and Dance.

Leventhal, M. (1981). *An overview of dance therapy for the special child*. Workshop presented at Laban Bartenieff Institute for Movement Studies, New York City.

Leventhal, M. B. (1984). An Interview with Alma Hawkins. *American Journal of Dance Therapy*, 7, 5-14.

Levy, F. (1979). Psychodramatic movement therapy: A sorting out process. *American Journal of Dance Therapy*, 3(1), 32-42.

Levy, F. (1988). *Dance movement therapy: A healing art*. Reston, VA: American Alliance for Health, Physical Education, and Dance.

Levy, F. (1995). Nameless: A case of multiplicity. In F. Levy, J. P. Fried, & F. Leventhal (Eds.), *Dance and other expressive art therapies: When words are not enough*. New York: Routledge.

Levy, F., Fried, J. P., & Leventhal, F. (Eds.). (1995). *Dance and other expressive art therapies: When words are not enough*. New York: Routledge.

Levy, S. (1950). Figure drawing as projective test. In L. E. Abt & L. Bellak (Eds.), *Projective psychology* (pp. 257-297). New York: Knopf.

Levy, S. (1958). Symbolism in animal drawings. In E. Hammer (Ed.), *Clinical application of projective drawings*. New York: C. C. Thomas.

Lewis, P. (1986). *Theoretical approaches in dance movement therapy, Vol. I and Vol. II*. Dubuque, IA: Kendall Hunt.

Lewis, P. (1993). *Creative transformation: The healing power of the arts*. Wilmette, IL: Chiron Publications.

Lewis, P. (1994). *The clinical interpretation of the Kestenberg movement profile*. Keene, NH: Antioch New England Provost Fund.

Lewis, P. (2000). *Alternate route training handbook in drama therapy*. Washington, DC: National Association for Drama Therapy.

Lewis, P. (2002). *Integrative holistic health, healing and transformation: A guide for holistic health practitioners, consultants, and administrators*. Springfield, IL: Charles C. Thomas Pub.

Lewis, P. & Johnson, D. (Eds.). (2000). *Current approaches in drama therapy*. Springfield, IL: Charles C. Thomas Pub.

Lewis, P. & Loman, S. (1990). *The Kestenberg movement profile: Its past, present applications and future directions*. Keene, NH: Antioch New England Graduate School.

Loman, S., & Brandt, R. (1992). *The body mind connection in human analysis*. Keene, NH: Antioch New England Graduate School.

Lowen, A. (1967). *The betrayal of the body*. New York: Macmillan.

Lowen, A. (1975). *Bioenergetics*. New York: Penguin Books.

Mackay, B. (1989). Drama therapy with female victims of abuse. *Arts in Psychotherapy*, 16, 293-300.

Mahler, M. (1968). *On human symbiosis and the vicissitudes of individuation*. New York: International Universities Press.

Malmo, R. B. (1950). Experimental studies of mental patients under stress. In M. L. Reymert (Ed.), *Feelings and emotions* (pp. 169-180). New York: McGraw-Hill.

Malmo, R. B., Boag, T. J., & Smith, A. A. (1957). Physiological study of personal interaction. *Psychosomatic Medicine*, 19, 105-119.

Malmo, R. B., Shagass, C., Belanger, D. J., & Smith, A. A. (1951). Motor control in psychiatric patients under experimental stress. *Journal of Abnormal and Social Psychology*, 46, 539-547.

Malmo, R. B., Smith, A. A., & Kohlmeyer, W. A. (1956). Motor manifestation of conflict in interview: A case study. *Journal of Abnormal and Social Psychology*, 52, 268-271.

Martin, G. J. (1977). *Supporting visually impaired students in the mainstream*. Reston, VA: The Council for Exceptional Children.

Martin, J. (1933/1972). *Modern dance*. New York: Dance Horizons.

Marcow, V. (1990). An interview with Norma Canner. *American Journal of Dance Therapy*, 12(2), 83-93.

Maslow, A. H. (1962). *Toward a psychology of being*. New York: D. van Nostrand Co.

Maslow, A. H. (1970). *Motivation and personality* (2nd ed.). New York: Harper & Row.

Maslow, A. H. (1978). *The farther reaches of human nature*. New York: Penguin Books.

Mazo, J. H. (1977). *Prime movers: The makers of modern dance in America*. New York: William Morrow and Co.

McNamara, J. (1989). *Tangled feelings*. Ossining, NY: Family Resources.

McNiff, S. (1998). *Art-based research*. Philadelphia: Jessica Kingsley.

Meerloo, J. (1960). *The dance*. New York: Chilton.

Moreno, J. L., & Z. T. Moreno. (1975a). *Psychodrama: Foundations of psychotherapy*. New York: Beacon House.

Moreno, Z. (1966). Psychodramatic rules, techniques and adjunctive methods. *Psychodrama and Group Psychotherapy Monographs* No. 41. Beacon, NY: Beacon House Inc.

Moss, S., Anolik, S. (1984). The use of skin temperature biofeedback to facilitate relaxation training for retarded adults: A pilot study. *American Journal of Dance Therapy*, 7, 49-57.

Murphy, J. M. (1979, October). The use of nonverbal and body movement techniques in working with families with infants. *Journal of Marital and Family Therapy*, 6, 1-66.

Naess, J. (1982). A developmental approach to the interactive process in dance/movement therapy. *American Journal of Dance Therapy*, 4(1), 25-41.

North, M. (1972). *Personality assessment through movement*. Boston: Plays, Inc.

Ornstein, R. (1972). *The psychology of consciousness*. San Francisco: W. H. Freeman Co.

Paley, A. N. (1988). Growing up in chaos: The dissociative response. *American Journal of Psychoanalysis*, 48, 72-83.

Pallaro, P. (ed.) (1999). *Authentic movement: Essays by Mary Starks Whitehouse, Janet Adler and Joan Chodorow*. London: Jessica Kingsley.

Perls, F. S. (1947). *Ego, hunger and aggression*. New York: Random House.

Perls, F. S. (1971). *Gestalt therapy verbatim*. New York: Bantam Books.

Perls, F. S. (1972). *In and out of the garbage pail*. New York: Bantam Books.

Pert, C.B. (1997). *Molecules of emotion: Why you feel the way you feel*. New York: Scribner.

Pesso, A. (1969). *Movement in psychotherapy: Psychomotor techniques in training*. New York: New York University.

Pesso, A. (1973). *Experience in action: A psychomotor psychology*. New York: New York University.

Putnam, F.W. (1989). *Diagnosis and treatment of multiple personality disorder*. New York: Guilford.

Reich, W. (1949). *Character analysis*. New York: Noonday Press.

Ressler, A. (manuscript in preparation). Body image. In W. N. Davis & S. Kleinman (Eds.), *Healing within relationships: The Renfrew Center perspectives on eating disorders recovery*. Philadelphia: The Renfrew Center.

Rifkin-Gainer, I., Bernstein, B., & Melson, B. (1984). Dance movement/word therapy: The methods of Blanche Evan. In P. L. Bernstein (Ed.), *Theoretical approaches in dance movement therapy, Vol. IL*. IA: Kendall Hunt.

Ritter, M., & Low, K.G. (1996). Effects of dance/movement therapy: A meta-analysis. *The Arts in Psychotherapy*, 25(3), 105-108.

Robbins, A. (Ed.) (1980). *Expressive therapy: A creative arts approach to depth oriented treatment*. New York: Human Sciences.

Rogers, C. R. (1951). *Client-centered therapy*. Boston: Houghton Mifflin.

Rogers, C. R. (1961). *On becoming a person*. Boston: Houghton Mifflin.

Rolf, I. P. (n.d.). Postural release: An exploration in structural dynamics. Unpublished manuscript.

Rosen, E. (1956). *Dance in psychotherapy*. Unpublished doctoral dissertation, Columbia Teachers College, New York.

Rosen, E. (1957). *Dance in psychotherapy*. New York: Teachers College Press, Columbia University.

Rounaville, B., Lifton N., & Bieber, M. (1979). The natural history of a psychotherapy group for battered women. *Psychiatry*, 42, 63-78.

Russell, R. W. (1970). The Wisconsin dance idea: Tribute from a movement therapist. *Impulse*, 68-70.

Ryan, J. (1989). Victim to victimizer: Rethinking victim treatment. *The Journal of Interpersonal Violence*, 4(3), 325-341.

Samuels, A. S. (1972). Movement change through dance therapy—A study. In F. Donelan (Ed.) *A.D.T.A. Writings on body movement and communication. Monograph No. 2* (pp. 50-77). Columbia, MD: American Dance Therapy Association.

Samuels, A. S. (1973). Dance therapy for geriatric patients. *Proceedings of the Eighth Annual Conference of the American Dance Therapy Association*, 27-30.

Sandel, S. A., Chaiklin, S., & Lohn, A. (Eds.). (1993). *Foundations of dance/movement therapy: The life and work of Marian Chace*. Columbia, MD: The Marian Chace Memorial Fund of the American Dance Therapy Association.

Sandel, S. L. (1973). Going down to dance. *Proceedings of the Eighth Annual Conference of the American Dance Therapy Association*, 1973, 15-23.

Sandel, S. L. (1978a). Movement therapy with geriatric patients in a convalescent home. *Hospital and Community Psychiatry*, 27(11), 738-741.

Sandel, S. L. (1978b). Reminiscence in movement therapy with the aged. *Art Psychotherapy*, 5(4), 217 221.

Sandel, S. L. (1980a). Countertransference stress in the treatment of schizophrenic patients. *American Journal of Dance Therapy*, 3(2), 20-32.

Sandel, S. L. (1980b). *Movement therapy with the elderly: An international approach*. Paper presented at Dance Movement Therapy Conference, East Meadow, New York.

Sandel, S. (1982). The process of individuation in dance-movement therapy with schizophrenic patients. *The Arts in Psychotherapy*, 9, 11-18.

Sandel, S., & Johnson D. (1983). Structure and process of the nascent group: Dance therapy with chronic patients. *The Arts in Psychotherapy*, 10, 131-140.

Sanders, L. (2000). Where are we going in the field of infant mental health? *Infant Mental Health Journal*, 21(1-2), 5-20.

Scheflen, A. E. (1965). Quasi-courtship behavior in psychotherapy. *Psychiatry*, 28, 245-257.

Scheflen, A. E. (1973). *Communicational structure: Analysis of a psychotherapy transaction*. Bloomington, IN: Indiana University.

Schilder, P. (1950). *The image and appearance of the human body*. New York: International Universities Press.

Schmais, C. (1974). Dance therapy in perspective. In K. Mason (Ed.), *Focus on dance VII: Dance therapy*. Reston, VA: American Alliance for Health, Physical Education, Recreation and Dance.

Schoop, T., & Mitchell, P. (1974). *Won't you join the dance?: A dancer's essay into the treatment of psychosis*. Palo Alto, CA: National Press Books.

Schoop, T. (1978). Motion & emotion. *American Journal of Dance Therapy*, 22(2), 91-101.

Schoop, T., & Mitchell, P. (1979). Reflections and projections: The Schoop approach to dance therapy. In P. L. Bernstein (Ed.), *Eight theoretical approaches to dance therapy* (pp. 31-50). Dubuque, IA: Kendall Hunt.

Scott, C. (1963). *Analysis of human motion: A textbook in kinesiology*. New York: Appleton-Century-Crofts.

Searles, H. F. (1961). Phases of patient therapist interaction in the psychotherapy of chronic schizophrenia. *British Journal of Medical Psychology*, 34, 169-193.

Siegel, E. (1972). The phantasy life of a Mongoloid: Movement therapy as a development tool. In F. Donelan (Ed.), *A.D.T.A. Writings on body movement and communication. Monograph No. of the American Dance Therapy Association* (pp. 103-110).

Siegel, E. (1974). Psychoanalytical thought and methodology in dance-movement therapy. In K. Mason (Ed.), *Focus on dance VII. Dance therapy*. Reston, VA: American Alliance for Health, Physical Education, Recreation and Dance.

Siegel, E. (1979). Psychoanalytically oriented dance-movement therapy—a treatment approach to the whole person. In P. L. Bernstein (Ed.), *Eight theoretical approaches in dance-movement therapy* (pp. 89 110). Dubuque, IA: Kendall Hunt.

Siegel, E. (1980). An introduction to psychoanalytically oriented dance movement therapy. In M. B. Leventhal (Ed.), *Movement and growth: Dance therapy for the special child* (pp. 23-28). New York: New York University.

Siegel, E. (1984). *The mirror of our selves: Dance-movement therapy and the psychoanalytical approach*. New York: Human Science Press.

Siegel, M., Brisman, J., & Weinshel, M. (1988). *Surviving an eating disorder: Strategies for family and friends*. New York: Harper Perennial.

Sigel, J. G. (1986). Keynote speech, National Conference.

Smallwood, J. C. (1974). Philosophy and methods of individual work. In K. Mason (Ed.), *Focus on Dance VII: Dance Therapy*. Reston, VA: American Alliance for Health, Physical Education, Recreation and Dance.

Smallwood, J. C. (1978). Dance therapy and the transcendent function. *Americal Journal of Dance Therapy*, 3, 16-23.

Sorell, W. (1969). *Hanya Holm: The biography of a dancer*. Middletown, CT: Wesleyan University.

Speck, R. (1964). Family therapy in the home. *Journal of Marriage and the Family*, 26, 72-76.

Spitz, R. (1965). *The first year of life*. New York: International Universities Press.

Stark, A. (1980). The evolution of professional training in the American Dance Therapy Association. *American Journal of Dance Therapy*, 3(2), 12-19.

Stark, A., & Lohn, A. (1993). The use of verbalization in dance/movement therapy. In S. Sandel, S. Chaiklin, & A. Lohn. (Eds.), *Foundations of dance/movement therapy: The life and work of Marian Chace* (pp. 130-131). Columbia, MD: The Marian Chace Memorial Foundation of the American Dance Therapy Association.

St. Clair, M. (2000) *Object relations and self psychology*. (3rd ed.). Stamford, CT: Brooks/Cole.

Steinberg, C. (Ed.). (1980). *The dance anthology*. New York: New American Library.

Stern, D. (1985). *The interpersonal world of the infant*. New York: Basic Books.

Sullivan, H. S. (1962). *Schizophrenia as a human process*. New York: Norton.

Summit, R. (1983). The child sexual abuse accommodation syndrome. *Child abuse and neglect*, 7, 177 193.

Sweigard, L. E. (1974). *Human movement potential: Its ideokinetic facilitation*. New York: Harper & Row.

Todd, M. E. (1937/1968). *The thinking body*. New York: Dance Horizons.

Todd, M. E. (1953). *The hidden you*. New York: Exposition Press.

Ullmann, L. (Ed.). (1971). *Rudolf Laban speaks about movement and dance*. Boston: Plays, Inc.

Victor, G. (1983). *The riddle of autism—A psychological analysis*. Lexington, MA: Lexington Books.

Walker, L. E. (1979). *The battered woman*. New York: Harper & Rowe.

Wallen, R. (1970). Gestalt therapy and Gestalt psychology. In J. Fagan & I. Shepherd (Eds.), *Gestalt therapy now* (pp. 8-13). Palo Alto, CA: Science and Behavior Books.

Wallock, S. (1977). *Dance-movement therapy: A survey of philosophy and practice*. Doctoral dissertation, United States International University. (University Microfilms No. 7907640).

Weiner, C., Jungels, W., & Jungels, G. (1973). Moving/making/me. *Proceedings of the Eighth Annual Conference of the American Dance Therapy Association*, 41-49.

Weisbrod, J. (1974). Body movement therapy and the visually impaired person. In K. Mason (Ed.), *Focus on dance VII: Dance therapy*. Reston, VA: American Alliance for Health, Physical Education, Recreation and Dance.

Weltman, M. (1986). Movement therapy with children who have been sexually abused. *American Journal of Dance Therapy*, 9, 47-66.

Whitehouse, M. (1963). *Physical movement and personality*. Paper presented at the meeting of the Analytic Psychology Club, Los Angeles.

Whitehouse, M. (1979). C.J. Jung and dance therapy: Two major principles. In P. L. Bernstein (Ed.), *Eight theoretical approaches to dance therapy* (pp. 751-70). Dubuque, IA: Kendall Hunt.

Winnicott, D. W. (1957). *Mother and child*. New York: Basic Books.

Winnicott, D. W. (1958). *Collected papers*. New York: Basic Books.

Winnicott, D. W. (1971). *Playing and reality*. New York: Penguin Books.

Wisher, P. (1974). Therapeutic values of dance therapy for the deaf. In K. Mason (Ed.), *Focus on dance VII: Dance therapy*. Reston, VA: American Alliance for Health, Physical Education, Recreation and Dance.

Wooten, B. (1959). Spotlight on the dance. *Journal of Health, Physical Education, Recreation*. 75-76.

Yalom, I. (1983). *Inpatient group psychotherapy*. New York: Basic Books.

Yalom, I. (1985). *The theory and practice of group psychotherapy* (3rd ed.). New York: Basic Books.

Zenoff, N. (1986). An interview with Joan Chodorow. *American Journal of Dance Therapy*, 9, 6-22.

Zerbe, K. (1995). *The body betrayed: A deeper understanding of women, eating disorders and treatment*. Carlsbad, CA: Guirse Books.

Zwerling, I. (1979). The creative arts therapies as psychotherapies: An address to the conference. (Under grant from the Maurice Falk Medical Fund.) *The Use of the Creative Arts in Therapy*, 2-7.

* References, medical/technical terminology and all other materials within this text represent the views of the author and do not necessarily reflect the position of the National Dance Association (NDA). The author's research, citations and reference structure herein do not completely follow NDA/AAHPERD publications guidelines. The author granted permission and provided all materials for publication. Copyright permission for any material that is not the original work of the author is the sole responsibility of the author and not the responsibility of NDA/AAHPERD. For queries, please contact the author directly.

All photography credits are found within the photographs' accompanying captions.

Index

A

AAHPERD's National Section on Dance 99
AAUW (American Association of University Women) report 187
Abreaction 137, 216
Abruptness 268
Academic standards 12
Academy of Registered Dance Therapists 127
Accelerando 92
Accessible Arts, Inc. 190, 237
"Accommodation syndrome" 197
Aching muscles 270
"Active imagination" 53-55, 58-60, 93, 148, 149
Active movement 94
Action mode 143, 144
Action-oriented psychotherapy 9, 106
Adaptive tasks for families 243
Adaptive/functional movement patterns 129
Adler, Alfred 3, 4, 6, 30, 32, 43, 44, 77
Adler, Janet 58, 140, 141, 147, 181, 192, 195, 262
ADTA (American Dance Therapy Association) 11, 12 19, 21, 84, 85, 105, 119, 129, 147, 152, 153, 162, 272
    alternate route 270-72
    Annual Conference in Rye, NY 263
    charter members 154
    Global Membership Services Subcommittee 263
    international growth 263-72
    International Hub of Task Force II 263
    International Panel of Dance Movement Therapists 263
    newsletter 283
    registry 264
    Research Subcommittee 275
ADTR 270
Adult psychiatric patients 84, 203-11
African dance 137, 277
Agenesis of the corpus callosum 183
Aggressive 97, 170, 210
Aggression 95
Aggressive drive 6, 44
Albert Einstein Medical Hospital College 113
Alcoholism 241
Alexander, F. Mathias 10
Alexander Technique 10
Alfred Adler Institute of Individual Psychology 29, 43
Alfred Adler Mental Hygiene Clinic 43
Alkmaar 271
Allergies 270
Alignment 241
Allport, Gordon Willard 193
Ambivalence 40, 219, 267

"Ambivalent symbiosis" 205
American Alliance for Health, Physical Education, Recreation and Dance—see AAHPERD
American Dance Therapy Association–see ADTA
"American Journal of Dance Therapy" 148
Amsterdam 271
Analytic concepts 94
Anger 39, 211, 216, 221
Animal fantasies 92
Animal projections 91
Annual American Dance Therapy Association Conference 138
Anolik, Stephen 249
Anorexia Nervosa 221, 223, 224
Antioch New England Graduate School 128, 129, 264
Aphasia 241
Appel, Cathy 178, 235-45, 262-72
Arendsen-Hein, Willem 271
Argentina 270, 271
Arieti, Silvano 169
Art therapy 91, 169-72, 175, 213, 214, 257, 258, 261, 269, 276, 305
Art Therapy Italiana (ATI) in Bologna 268
Artistic inquiry 275
Arts 73, 88, 166-71, 213, 215
Arts in Human Development in Quebec 269
Arts with the Handicapped Program of the Kansas State Department of Education 237
Asociación Argentina de Danzaterapia 271
Assimilation of dance therapy 279
Association for Dance Movement Therapy in the UK (ADMT) 263
    registry 264
Ataxia 238
Athens 267
Attunement (Kinesthetic empathy) 129
Auditory cues 257
Auras 241
Australia 267, 271
Auxiliary ego 174
Authentic movement 3, 53, 55, 56, 59, 75, 137, 141, 147, 151
Autism 136, 137, 147, 155, 255
Avstreih, Zoë 135, 138, 140, 156, 157

B

Baker, Katie 307
Ballet 1, 31, 61, 136, 137, 139, 277, 281
Ballroom dancing 95
Barkai, Yael 264
Barlowe, Jay 127
Barnard College 3

Bartenieff, Irmgard 2, 3, 11, 12, 106, 111, 113-18, 121, 123, 124, 126, 131, 152, 155, 156, 184, 192, 240, 253, 254, 283
   Heritage Tree 284-87
Bartenieff Fundamentals 113, 253
Bartkey, C. 219
BASK (Behavior, Affect, Sensation and Knowledge) 216
Battered women 218-20
Baum, Edith Z. 215, 216
Beardall, Nancy 181, 187, 188
Beebe, B. 184
Behavior Rating Instrument for Autistic and Other Atypical Children (BRIAAC) 193, 194
Behavioral psychology 279
Bell, Judith 255, 256
Bellevue Hospital 7, 29, 87, 89, 91, 94
Bender, Lauretta 7, 87, 89, 91, 94
Bennington College 73, 113
Benov, Ruth 217
Bergan, Norway 43
Berger, Miriam Roskin 121, 253, 261-63, 267, 271, 272
Berlin 262, 268
Berlin University 43
Bernstein, Bonnie 30, 213, 217, 218
Bernstein, Penny—see Lewis, Penny
Berrol, Cynthia 238-40, 275
Bieber, M. 219
Bioenergetic therapy 9, 279
Bio-Energy Field Lab in Malibu, CA 155
Birdwhistell, Ray 8, 254
Blanche Evan Method 217
Blind and visually impaired 240, 241, 256-58
Blythedale Hospital 113
BMS—see Body Movement Scale
Boas, Franz 87
Boas, Franziska 3, 7, 15, 85, 87-94, 163, 277, 281
Body action 21, 22
Body and mind 54
Body Awareness Techniques 101
Body-Dynamics 45
"Body experience" 144
Body image 6, 40, 46, 63, 90, 187, 191, 195, 196, 200, 211, 223, 224, 250, 256
Body language experts 253
Body movement 59
Body Movement Scale (BMS) 193, 255
Body movement theory of function and adaptability 193
Body musculature 32
Body-self 75

"Body therapy" 10
Bologna 268
Bonn 262, 268
Borderline personality disorder 205
Boston 235, 236
Boston University 236
Bowman-Hicks, Shawn 307
Bovard-Taylor, Alice 85, 206
Bradley, Karen 253
Brandt, Rose 129
Braun, B. G. 213, 216
Brazil 265
Breast cancer 273
Breathing 47, 75, 239, 241
Brecha 270
BRIAAC—see Behavior Rating Instrument
Brisman, J. 221
Broadening movement choices 219
Bronx State Hospital 114, 119-21, 254
Brooklyn 219
Brooklyn Museum 113
Brooklyn State Hospital 94
Brown, Crystal 78
Brown, Lyn Mikel 187
Brownell, Anne 190, 236, 237
Brownmiller, Susan 218
Bruno, C. 208
Buddhism 265
Buddhist monk's dance 272
Buelte, Arnhilt 127, 129
Bulimia Nervosa 221, 224
Bunney, Judith 261, 262, 271, 272
Bush, George 253

C

Calisthenics 229
Camarillo Hospital 61
Campbell, Robert Jean 8
Canada 265, 269, 270
Cancer 156, 241, 273
Canner, Norma 85, 178, 190, 199, 200, 235-38, 245, 257
Cannon, Lou 73
Capello, Patricia 262
Caplow-Lindner, E. L. 230
Capy, Mara 264
Case Studies
   Alice 70
   Amy 195
   Ana 193-95
   Ann 205
   Brenda 170-72
   Brianna 183

Celine 223
Chris 168-70
D. 239-41
Daniel 197
Dennis 245
David 167, 168, 170
Edward 197
Elly 166
Greg 243
"J" 124, 126
J. 241
Jay 206, 207
Jennifer 165
Joshua 184
Karen 172-74
Katharine 175
Kim 221
Lisa 224
Luke 68-70
"Marcia" 139
Maya 216, 217
Melissa 197, 198
Michael 244, 245
"Mr. C" 145, 146
"Mrs. G" 156
"Nameless" 213-16
Nick 204, 205
nine-year-old 250
"O" 45, 46
Pamela 37-40
Patty 245
R. 240
Rachel ("Nameless") 213-16
Randy 216
Richard 257, 258
Sandra 198, 199
Sara 224-26
Sarah and Susie 255, 256
seven-year-old 255
seventeen-year-old 254
"Sharon" 143
Tanya 224
Valerie 244
Vera 205
W. 241, 242
Catatonic schizophrenia 96
Catharsis 66, 137
Cathcart, Jane Wilson (formerly Downes) 154, 157, 181, 183-85
CBS News 258, 259
Center for Parents and Children in Long Island 128, 129
Center on Disability and Community Inclusion at the University of Vermont 190

Cerebral palsy 236
Chace, Marian 3, 4, 6, 9, 11, 12, 15, 19-22, 24-27, 43, 51, 67, 77-79, 84, 85, 92, 98, 119-21, 137, 138, 140, 146, 151-54, 157, 158, 163, 192, 203, 226, 229, 230, 236, 261
   Heritage Tree 288-94
Chace Foundation 275
Chace Technique 23-27, 119, 140, 141, 144, 162, 187, 230, 179
   warm-up 23-25
   theme development 23, 25
   closure 23, 26, 27
Chace's Therapeutic Movement Relationship 156
Chacian circle 189
Chaiklin, Sharon 19-21, 24-26, 151-53, 206, 207, 264, 265, 270
Chang, Meg 213, 218-20, 272
Characterization 65
"Chasing Away the Ghost" 199
Chazan, Saralea E. 191
Chestnut Lodge 21
Chi 241
Chicago 85
Child abuse 173
Child Development Research (CDR) 127
Child Life at Tomorrow's Children's Institute in New Jersey 242
Children and adolescents with disabilities 113, 181, 181-200, 207, 264, 268, 269
   Acute myelogenous leukemia (AML) 243
   ADHD 185
   anal fixation 250
   attachment disorder 185
   autism 185, 189, 192-96, 205, 244, 255
   domestic violence 185
   emotional abuse 213-16
   emotional disabilities 185, 188-92, 254
   foster care and adoption issues 185, 198
   hydrocephalus 243
   infants 256
   Japanese 265
   language handicapped 250
   learning disabilities 183, 185, 188-90, 240
   mental illness 183
   neglect 185
   physical abuse 39, 185
   physical disability 235
   psychosis 29, 244
   sexual abuse 185, 196-99, 271
   stem cell transplant 243
Children's Apperception Test 124
Chodorow, Joan 58, 140, 141, 147, 148, 262, 270, 284

Choreographing of emotions 78
Choreography of Object Relations 157, 184
Chronically ill and dying 241-43
Circle formation 95
Circle structure 26
Class, Stephanie 185
Classical Greek theater 2
Climenko, Johanna 210, 211, 271
Clinical Community Nursery School Program in Boston 236
Clinton, Bill 253
CNN 253
Coconut Creek, FL 222
Cognitive goal 230, 251
Cognitive Marker Work Sheet 226-27
Cognitive Markers 224-27
Cognitive Rehabilitation Program 240
Cohen, Susan 242, 243
Collateral sprouting 238
Collective unconscious 281
Colombia 271
Columbia College in Chicago 85
Columbia University Teachers College 3, 73, 94, 113
Community 117, 118
Community dance programs 263, 264
Complex in-depth improvisation 41
Components of movement 74
Concomitant psychic associations 37
Condon, William 8
Conscious "self" 55
Contact perception 138
Contrasting movement dynamics 37
Control 168, 170
Control of Dynamic Drive (Rhythm, Time Concepts) 47
Coordination (Body-Awareness and Locomotion) 47
Costa Rica 271
Costonis, Maureen 8, 87, 250
Council for Accreditation of Counseling and Related Education Programs 12
Countertransference 121, 208, 211, 220
"Creating a Peaceable School" 187
Creative and Movement Arts Psychotherapy Program in IDC's Mental Health Department in New York City 240
Creative dance 29, 30, 34, 35, 43, 84, 218, 277
 improvisation 41
 techniques 89
Creative dance movement 58
Creative expression 97
Creative imagery 46, 184, 214
Creative improvisational approach 43

Creative modern dance 87
Creative Movement training program 269
Creative movement 257
Creative movement-oriented evaluation methods 273, 275, 276
Creativity 73, 75
Crescendo 92
Cruz, Robyn Flaum 271, 275
Cunningham, Merce 84, 277
Czech Republic 261, 272

D

Dalcroze—see Jaques-Dalcroze, Emile 431
Dance and the Child International (DACI) 267
Dance and movement education 83, 84
Dance Department at the University of California 72
Dance/dramas 164
"Dance for communication" 19
Dance forms 98
Dance movement 30, 46, 68
Dance Movement Therapy (DMT) 47, 99, 109, 126, 129, 156, 157, 175, 177, 178, 220, 222-27, 237, 238, 242-45, 253-59, 263-72, 268, 278, 305, 306
 research 273, 275, 276
 skills 276
Dance Movement Therapy at California State University at Hayward 238
Dance Notation Bureau (DNB) 115, 119, 127
Dance technique 58
Dance Therapy Association of Australia Inc. (DTAA) 267
Dance Therapy Center 30
Dance Therapy Core Group at the Institute for the Arts and Human Development at Lesley College 237
Dance Therapy Heritage Trees 283-304
 Bartenieff, Irmgard 284-87
 Chace, Marian 288-94
 Evan, Blanche 296, 297
 Espenak, Liljan 295
 Hawkins, Alma 298
 Schoop, Trudi 299, 300
 Whitehouse, Mary 301-04
Dance Therapy Institute of Princeton 155
Dance Therapy Master's Program 128
Dance Therapy Master's Specialty 129
Dance Therapy Study 99
Dance Therapy Study Committee of the American Alliance Health, Physical Education, Recreation and Dance (AAHPERD), National Section on Dance 98

Darwin, Charles 8
Daschle, Tom 253
Davis, Martha 11, 114, 115, 119, 126, 253, 254
Davis, W. N. 221, 226
Day Hospital 113
D. C. Moore Gallery 162
Deaf and hearing impaired 258, 259
Deaver, George 113
Defensive mannerisms 69, 70
Definition of Dance Therapy 11
Degree of Dynamic Drive (Rhythm, Time Concepts) 47
Deihl, Linni 157
Dell, Cecily 110
Delsarte, François 2, 3
Delusions 68
Denishawn School of Dance 3, 19, 20, 278
Dependence versus independence 239
Depression 171
Destiné, Jean-Léon 139
Detachment 223
Destructive parental restrictions 172
Deutsch, F. 8
Developmental Center for Autistic Children in Philadelphia 255
Developmental disabilities 46, 85, 114, 116, 117, 206, 236, 249-51, 236, 249-51
Developmental psychology 279
Dewey, Thomas 83
Di George Syndrome 193
Diagnostic movement tests 47
Diabetes 241
Dickinson, Mildred 85
"Diminished effort" 115
Diminuendo 92
Direct question approach 99
Directive approach 77, 125
Directive roles 78
"Directness" 116
Disembodiment 222
Dissociation 216, 219
Dissociative Identity Disorder—see Multiple Personality Disorder
"Dissolution" 210
Distance perception 138
Distorted body image 144
Distortions in perception and experience 145
Disturbed/psychotic patients 147
DMT—see Dance Movement Therapy
Domestic violence 219, 271
Dosamantes-Alperson, Erma (also Dosamantes-Beaudry, Erma) 73, 141-44, 148
Doubling 174

Dragonosky, J. E. 206
Drama 65, 70, 163-65
Dramatic dance (see also movement drama) 95
Dramatic enactment 38
Dramatic movement expression 66, 77, 174
Dramatic play 92
Dratman, M. 193
Dream enactment 40
Dresden 43, 51
Dualism 1
Duggan, Diane 181, 188-90
Dulicai, Dianne 126, 177, 190, 254, 255, 262, 273
Dullemen, Sima Van 271
Duncan, Isadora 2, 10, 61, 277, 278
Duncan Centre Modern Dance Conservatory in Prague 272
Dunlap, Valerie 126
Dyads 37, 184, 239, 255
Dyrud, J. 226

E

Early childhood development theory 181
Early Childhood Intervention 236
Early childhood trauma 159
Early developmental experiences 156
Early modern dance 109
Early symbiotic phase 193
Eastern philosophies 8
Eating disorders 221-27, 269, 270
Eclectic approach 156
"Ed" 222
Education and Training for the International Dance Therapy Institute of Australia 267
Educational approach 64-66, 71
"Effort/shape"—see Laban Movement Analysis
Ego 6, 10, 32, 40, 46, 55, 71, 90, 118, 123, 124, 137, 147, 151, 193, 208, 249, 279
Eicher, V. 209
Elderly 229-31
    Japanese 265
Electric shock therapy 96
Electromagnetic field 241
Eliot Pearson School at Tufts University 236
Ellis, Havelock 2
Emotional abuse 213, 221
Emotional Catharsis 2
Emotional warm-up 37
Emotionally disturbed 117, 240
Empathic movement reflection 157
Empathic therapeutic relationship 276
Empathy 165, 200, 203, 244, 267, 306

Enactment 68
Energy 62, 71
Energy flow 257
Energy modulation 186
Erfer, Tina 181, 190-92, 195, 196
Erickson, Milton 253
Escobar, Teresa 269
Espenak, Liljan 3, 6, 11, 15, 43-46, 78, 79, 113, 135, 151, 152, 249, 265, 277
   Heritage Tree 295
Eubanks, Susan 12
European modern dance movement 113
Eurythmics 3, 43
Evaluation and Planning and Individualized Education (IEP) Teams 190
Evan, Blanche 6, 11, 15, 29, 32, 38-40, 45, 66, 77-79, 96, 138, 151, 152, 155, 163, 217, 267, 277
   Heritage Tree 296, 297
Evan's dance therapy methodology 41
Evan's System of Functional Technique 32-34
Exertion-recuperation 253
Exhibitionist 97
"Experiential movement psychotherapy" 141
"Experiential-educational approach" 256
Expression of conflict 61
Expression of Emotions in Man and Animals 8
Expressive improvisational dance 29
Expressive movement 44, 257
Expressive movement potential 24
Expressive Movement Project 190
Expressive Movement Project at Center on Disability and Community Inclusion at the University of Vermont 236
Expressive movement vocabulary 67
Expressive symbolic movement 258
Expressive therapies 84
Expressive Therapy Program at Lesley College 237
"External-interactional movement" 143

F
Facilitator 75
Faith 281
Families 254-56, 265, 268, 270, 280
"Family sculpting" 254
Family therapy 256
Fantasies 36, 64, 68, 69, 70, 91, 243, 250
Fay, Carolyn Grant 190
Feldenkrais, Moishe 10
Fenichel, Otto 8
Ferenczi, Sándor 8
Fersh, Isabel 230

Figure drawing 7, 91
Finkelhor, D. 197
FIRO—see Fundamental Interpersonal Relationship Orientation
First International Dance Therapy Congress 262
Fischer, Judith 85, 229, 230
Fischman, Diana 270
Fitch, Edna 84
Flamenco 137
Flax, Cece Ritter 131
Fletcher, Diane 141, 145, 146
Flow-adjustment 268
"Flow readiness" 156
Folk dances 95, 277, 281
Follow-the-leader 199
Fonteyn, Margot 2, 3
"Four B's of self-control" 186, 187
"4's" 189, 190
Fox Cable News 253
Fragmentation of the personality 215
France 61, 269
Frank, Mary 162
Frank, Zweike 271
Frazer, Sir James George 2
Free association 35, 36, 96, 98
Freedom of expression 183
Freeman, Virginia 307
Freeman, William C. 177, 181, 190, 236, 237, 273
Freud, Sigmund 4, 6, 30, 44, 77, 141, 193
Freud, Anna 127, 157
Fried, Judith 58, 188
Fried, SuEllen 190
Fromm-Reichmann, Frieda 153
Frost, Mary 257, 258
Function of dance 88
Functional Technique 39, 37 41, 45, 218
Fundamental Interpersonal Relationship Orientation (FIRO) 256

G
Gallaudet College in Washington, D. C. 258
Ganet Sigel, Jane 85, 270
Garnet, E. 229
Gendlin, Eugene 73, 141
Genther, Shirley 83, 84, 163
Geriatric patients 209, 210
Germany 43, 51, 61, 262, 267, 268, 271
Gestalt therapy 9, 84, 123, 155, 156, 279
Gesture 70, 306
Gil, E. 217
Gilligan, Carol 187
Gillman. I. 219

Goddard College 129 161
Govini, Rosa Maria 269
Graham, Martha 3, 4, 51, 58, 271, 277, 278, 305
Gray, Amber 262
Greece 267
Groninger, V. 30, 34
Gross motor coordinations 257
Group dance therapy 44, 189
    fantasy 70
    techniques 103, 207, 216
Group identity 209
Group Process 25, 26, 77
Group psychology 21, 79
Group rhythmic activity 67, 162
Group Rhythmic Movement Relationship 21-23
Group therapy 9, 22, 27, 97, 153, 166, 211, 208, 217, 229, 236, 239, 241
Growth model 75
Guided imagery 253
Guided movement experiences 75
"Guidelines for Graduate Therapy Programs" 12
Guilt 217, 218
Gunma, Japan 265

H
Hahnemann University 126, 264
Haitian dance 137, 189
Hall, Terese 177, 221-27, 254
Hallucinations 68
Hamburg 262
Hancock Center for Movement Arts and Therapy 185
Hanya Holm Dance Studio 113
Harpaz, L. 230
Harris, Joanna 84
Harrison, Barbara J. 155
Hartmann, Heinz 127
Harvard University 7, 187
Harvey, Steve 181, 193, 199
Hasegawa, Mikiko 266
Hasegawa, Tsunehito 266
Hasegawa Hospital, Tokyo 266, 267
Hawkins, Alma 9, 15, 73, 75-77, 141, 144, 151, 152, 155, 267, 277
    Heritage Tree 298
H'Doubler, Margaret 83, 84, 277
    dance curriculum 83
    movement 83
Heart disease 241
Hemiparesis 241
Hervey, Lenore Wadsworth 273, 275, 276

Hillside Hospital 94, 95, 97
Hitler, Adolf 113
Hochscule für Liebesubungen 43
Hoffman, Jay 20
"Holding environment" 129
Holistic approach 44
Holistic Health Society of Tokyo 265
Holm, Hanya 73, 87, 94, 277, 281
Holocaust survivors 271
Homosexual abuse 218, 219
Hood, C. 98
Hope, Stephanie 173
Horiuchi, Kumiko 266
Horizontal process 77
Horizontal stress 79
Hospitalized patients 51, 78, 98, 146
Hotel St. Elizabeth 20
Hruza, Thelma 84
Human behavior 8
Human movement potential 109
Humanistic movement 8, 9, 123
Humanistic psychology 76, 84
Humor 64, 268
Humphrey, Doris 3, 73, 277, 278
Hungary 265
Hunt, Valerie 73, 155, 193, 267
Hunter College 11, 119, 120, 138, 163, 265
Huston, K. 219
Hutchinson, M. G. 224
Hyperactivity/hypoactivity 22
"Hypnogogic images" 143
Hypnosis 253

I
"I am moved" 56, 57
"I move" 56, 57
Id 10, 71, 124, 151
Ideations 68
Identity of character 22
Idiosyncratic movement patterns 225-226
Image consultants 253
Imagery 24, 36, 47, 58, 75, 76, 138
"Imaginative responses" 144
Imitation 66
Improvisation 29, 30, 32-34, 36-38, 45, 46, 53, 58, 59, 63, 64, 68, 69, 71, 77, 79, 94, 98, 135, 138, 175, 176, 204, 206, 218, 219, 240, 250, 253, 256, 258, 277
Improvisational dance technique 3, 30, 204
Improvisation/enactment 32, 34, 35
Incest 218
Inclusion 256
Individual 9, 21, 77
Individualism 270, 271

In-depth movement 37
Inferiority feelings 44
Inhibition 170, 175
Inner dance 87
Inner fantasy 64, 68
Inner infant self 213-15
Inner Movement Group 241
Inner sensing 73, 75
Insomnia 270
Institute for Mental Retardation 43
Institute of Body, Mind and Spirituality at
    Lesley University 235
Institute of Movement Studies 115
Institute of Pennsylvania Hospital 216
"Instrument of Dance" 34
Insulin therapy 96
Integration 30
Integration of the "self" 40
Intellectual 97, 305
Interactional approach 22, 211
Interactional synchrony 8
Internal conflicts 61
Internal rhythm 67
"Internal-intrapsychic movement" 143
Internalized characters 164
International Center for the Disabled (ICD) in
    New York City 240-42
    Creative and Movement Arts Psycho-
      therapy Program 241
International Dance Council 267
International Dance/Movement Therapy
    Conference in Berlin 268
International Workshops in Argentina 270
Interpersonal Improvisational Dance-Drama
    and Intermodal Therapy 159
Interpersonal theory of personality 6
Interpretation of music 97
Intervention 57
Intuition 57
Invisible movement 55, 56
Irwin, K. 229
Isolation of body segments 33
Israel 237, 261, 264, 265
    department of education 265
    mental health organizations 265
Italy 61, 269, 271
Itou, Assuka 266
Ivey, Rai Anne 307
Iwai, Kunitoshi 266

J

J. P. Morgan Chase 178, 253
Jackson, Jesse 250
Jackson, Melissa 188

Jacobson, Edmund 10, 73, 74, 84
Jaques-Dalcroze, Emile 3, 29, 43
Japan 265-67
Japan Art Therapy Association 266
Japanese Dance Therapy Association 265, 266
Jaques, Rhian 307
Jazz dance 277
Jean Erdman Theatre of Dance 121
Jewish General Hospital 269
Jingu, Kyoko 265
Job interviews 253
Johnson, David 207-10
Joint Council for Mental Health Services
    Legislative Coalition 13
Jung, Carl 4, 6, 55, 77, 147, 149, 151, 236
Jungels, G. and Jungels, W. 250
Jungian dance therapy 268
Jungian Institute in Zurich 153
Jungian psychoanalysis 51, 53, 54, 60, 84, 94,
    140, 147, 156, 157, 280

K

Kabuki 265
Kaji, Miyuki 266
Kalish-Weiss, Beth 137, 181, 192-95, 268
Kanner, Leo 192
Kansas State Department of Education 190
Katz, Stephanie 238-40, 275
Kaylo, Janet 272
Kelly, Maureen 221
Kendon, Adam 8
Kennedy, Rebekah 142
Kennell, J. H. 256
Kephart, N. 84
Kernberg, Paulina F. 191
Kestenberg, Judith 111, 124, 127-29, 140, 157,
    158, 193, 205, 244, 254
Kestenberg Movement Profile (KMP) 127, 129,
    157, 244, 245, 268
Kestenberg's tension-flow system 127, 129,
    193
Khoda, Makiko 266
Kinesics 8
Kinesthetic Awareness 53, 54, 58, 84, 237
Kinesthetic empathy 24, 174, 182, 243
Kinesthetic input 142
Kinesthetic seeing 182
"Kinetic Translations" 255
Kinetography Laban (Labanotation) 110
Kings County Hospital 7
Klaus, H. 256
Klebanoff, Harriet 237
Klebanoff, Lewis 236
Kleinman, Susan 177, 221-27

Klopfer, Bruno 7
Kluft, Richard 213, 216
KMP—see Kestenberg Movement Profile
Koch, Nana 265
Kohut, Heinz 140, 160
Komori, Chiyoko 266
Korea 272
Korean Dance Therapy Association 272
Kornblum, Rena 181, 185-87
Krantz, Anne 29, 30, 32
Krout, Maurice H. 8
Kuppers, Frederica W. 84

L
Laban, Rudolf 3, 43, 61, 84, 98, 99, 109-11, 113, 115, 118, 119, 123, 125-27, 135, 152, 157, 184, 193, 265, 277, 283
Laban Centre 126
    in London 272
Laban Movement Analysis 99, 106, 109-11, 113, 114 119-21, 123, 124, 127, 131, 141, 151, 152, 157, 181, 193, 207, 253, 254, 256, 278
Labanalysis—see Laban Movement Analysis
Laban/Bartenieff Institute of Movement Studies 114, 15, 126, 131
Labanotation—see Kinetography Laban
Laban's effort system 109
Laban's Movement Choir 110
Lack of attention 238
Lack of initiative 238
Lamb, Warren 109, 111, 115, 119, 126, 127
Lamb's shape system 109
Larson, Bird 3, 4, 29, 34, 87
Laughman, Melissa 161, 162
Lavender, Joan 204, 205
Lefco, Helene 207
La Meri 29
Lesley College (Lesley University) 235, 237
Lethargic patients 95
Leventhal, Marcia 73-75, 155, 156, 158, 188, 213, 218-20, 261, 267, 268, 270
Levy, Diana 131
Levy, Fran 9, 155, 158 161, 163, 164, 167, 182, 188, 198, 199, 213-20, 270
Levy, Sidney 7, 91, 163, 167, 213-15, 216
Lewin, Joan Naess 205
Lewis, Dori 113, 115
Lewis, Penny 128, 129, 155-60, 184, 262, 268
Libido 44
Lieberman, Sandi 243-45
Licensure 12
Limited mobility 241, 242
Limón, José 277

Lipton, P. 94, 219
Little Meadows Early Childhood Center 183
LMA—see Laban Movement Analysis
Logan, Billie 85
Lohn, Ann 21, 154
Loman, Susan 128, 129, 262, 268-70
London 262
Lowen, Alexander 6, 9, 43, 44, 73
Lowenstromska Psychiatric Hospital, Sweden 261

M
McCall, Debra 269
Machida, Shoichi 265
Machover, Karen 7, 91
Mackay, B. 220
McNamara, J. 198
McNamara, Monica Meehan 131
McNiff, Sean 275
Mahler, Margaret 127, 138, 140, 157, 160, 184, 193, 205
Malmo, R. J. 8
Manhattan Children's Psychiatric Center 183
Manhattan State Hospital 84, 94, 96, 97
Manic patients 95
Manning, Jane 58
Marcow-Speiser, Vivien 235, 236, 237
Marcus, Hershey 127
Marian Chace Foundation 154
Martial arts 265
Martin, G. J. 257
Martin, John 3, 55
Masculinity 69, 70
Maslow, Abraham 8, 9, 21
Massachusetts 236, 237
Masters of Arts in Dance Therapy 11, 12
Matsuo, Toshiko 266
Matsuda, Yokoko 266
Mazo, Joseph H. 2
Medau, Hinrich 43
Mediator 60
Meditation 241
Meerloo, Joost Abraham Maurits 1
Meier, Ruth 271
Meir, Walli 126
Melson, Barbara 29, 30, 32, 33, 36
Memory loss 238
Memory traces 75
Mendota State Hospital 84
Mensendieck, Bess M. 29, 43, 84
Mental illness 117, 269
Merchant, Claude 89
"Messaging" 254
Mettler, Barbara 190, 235

Mexico 262
Michelle, Simone 126
Michigan Rehabilitation Center 238
Midwestern Dance Therapy Conference 85
Milan 269
Mime/pantomime 64, 70, 77, 277
Mind and body 265
Mind-body unification 31
Minnesota 85
Mirroring (empathic reflection) 22, 24, 138, 156, 184, 196, 199, 219, 243, 250
"Misplaced concreteness" 169
Mississippi 237
Mitchell, Peggy 61-71
Mitcheltree, Anne 273, 283
"Mitchel Tree"—see Mitcheltree, Anne
Miyagi, Tadashi 266
Mobilization and Functional Technique 217
"Model of traumagenicdynamics" 197
Modern dance 1, 31, 43, 87, 96, 137, 281
Modern dance movement 1, 58, 94, 277
Modes of consciousness 73
Modulation of emotion and behavior 210, 211
Momentum 257
Montreal Children's Hospital 269
Moreno, J. L. 9, 164, 166
Moreno, Z. T. 164, 174
Moss, Susan 249
Mother-child dyad 135, 140, 255
Mt. Sinai Hospital in New York 190
Movement
    analysis 109
    assessment 190
    behavior 192
    configurations 109
    dialogue 166, 305, 306
    directives 220
    interactional dialogue 138
    tasks 75
    techniques 95
    themes 39, 40, 58
    tools 66
    vocabulary 117
Movement Diagnostic Tests 45-47
    Body Image, 46
    Emotional Response (Spatial Relationships) 46, 47
    Degree of Dynamic Forces (Force Adjustment) 47
    Control of Dynamic Drive (Force Adjustment) 47
    Control of Dynamic Drive (Rhythm, Time Concepts) 47
    Coordination (Body-awareness and Locomotion) 47
    Endurance (Constancy) 47
    Physical Courage (Anxiety States) 47
Movement drama (see also dramatic dance) 84
Movement dynamics 257
Movement elicitation/dialogue movement 24
Movement enactments 69
Movement exploration 37
Movement facilitation 94
Movement factors 110
Movement fantasy 79
Movement improvisation 58, 59, 71
"Movement impulse" 117
Movement-in-depth 6, 51, 53
"Movement interview" 38
Movement modulation 211
Movement observation 38
Movement observation scale 207
Movement performances 63
Movement potential 117
Movement Psychodiagnostic assessment 253
Movement Range Sampler (MRS) 250
Movement reflection 216
Movement repertoire 37, 123
"Movement retainer" 127
Movement sequences 44, 125
Movement Signature Impressions (MSI) 181
Movement tantrum 64
Movement Therapist 253
Movement therapy—see dance movement therapy
Multicultural dance 277
Multimodal approach 30, 155, 161, 163, 164, 166, 174, 276
Multiple Personality Disorder (MPD) 213-17, 220
Multiple sclerosis 53, 56, 241
Multisensory experiences 257
Munich 268
Murphy, James 256
Murray, Henry 7, 91
Muscle awareness and coordination 239
Muscular balance 10
Muscular dystrophy 241
Muscular Dystrophy Association (MDA) 235
Muscular manipulation 6
Muscular massage 10
Muscular release 53
Musculature 22, 32, 40, 55
Musculature armoring 22
Music 19, 24, 46, 58, 92, 96, 103, 123, 138, 173, 183, 225, 241, 242, 249, 250, 257, 268, 272
"Music therapist" 19
"Music visualization" 19

N

"Nameless" 213-216
Naropa Institute 138
"Nascent groups" 209
National Board of Certified Counselors 12
National Child Research Center in Washington, D. C. 236, 237
National Institute of Mental Health 12, 120
National Italian DMT professional association 269
Natural Dance 3, 29
Natural Expressive Movement 3
Naumberg, Margaret 7, 91
Negative transference 171
Netherlands 261, 265, 271
Neumann, Erich 267
Neurogenic movement disorders 238
Neuropathology 240
Neuroplasticity 238
Neuropsychiatric Institute in Los Angeles 197
Neuropsychiatric Institute of UCLA 73, 197
Neurosis 29, 32, 136, 269
"Neurotic urban adult" 29, 32
Neutral expressive body rhythms 41
New Caledonia, South Pacific 272
New School for Social Research 29, 113
New York City 43, 85, 217, 266
New York City Public Schools 195, 250
New York Coalition of Creative Arts Therapy 13
New York Medical College 43, 44
New York University 7, 74, 113, 267, 269
    Dance Education program 188
    Graduate Dance Therapy Program 155
    Masters of Arts Program in Sweden 261
Newton (Mass.) Public Schools 187
Nikolais, Alwin 84, 141, 277
Noh 265
Nondirective approach 77
Nondirective roles 78
Nonverbal body cues 181
Nonverbal communication 5, 6, 8, 40, 77, 168, 182, 184, 192, 196, 198, 215, 237, 254-56, 268, 305, 306
Nonverbal dance of attunement and adjustment 244
Nonverbal facilitation 77
"Normal neurotic" 41
"Normalization" 244
North, Marion 123-26, 219, 254
Northport Hospital 7
Norway 43, 237
Noumea Dancers 272
Noverre 29

O

Oberum, Maria-Luise 262
Object relations theory 156, 205, 279
Occupational Therapy School at Tufts University 236
Oedipal feelings 169
Ohio 85
Ooi, Wee Lok 275
Openness 256
Operation Head Start 237
Opposing drive 61
Ornstein, Robert 73, 75
Ott, Corinne 262, 272

P

Pair interaction 208
Paley, A. N. 219
Pallaro, Patrizia 51
Palo Alto, CA 217
Paralysis 172, 238, 239
Paranoia 96
Parkinson's disease 241
Partial paralysis 40
"Participation mystique" 149
Passive movement 94
Patient reactions (Rosen's patterns) 94
Patient/therapist relationship (see also therapist/patient relationship) 203-07, 211, 220
Paulay, Forrestine 111, 115
Pediatric Oncology and Hematology 242, 243
Penfield, Kedzie 126
Peralta, Laura 270
Perception 193
Perceptual-motor disability 238
Perceptual-motor integration 195
Percussive instruments 91, 92
Perez de Villa, Mariano 270
Perkins School for the Blind 237
Perls, Frederick S. 9, 141, 157, 236
Perot, Ross 253
Personal unconscious 55
Personal space 206
Personal symbolism 59
Personality 65, 110, 135, 136
Personality Assessment through Movement 124
Peru 271
Pesso, Albert 9
Peterson, Jean 163
Pettigrew, Gaetan 78
Physical abuse 39, 213, 221
Physical and emotional mastery 251

Physical disabilities 117
Physical expression 40
Physical regression 90
Physical therapy 113, 240
Physical warm-up 33, 37
Pioneers in dance therapy 15-99, 283-304
    East Coast 19-41
    Midwest 83-85
    West Coast 51-79
Pittsburgh Child Guidance Center 158
Pittsburgh University Medical School 158
Planned movement formulation 64, 71
Plasticity 238
Play 24, 199, 208
Play-acting 250
Pleasure principle 44
Plevin, Marcia 269
Plouvier, Annemieke 271
Pohlmann, Anna 262
Polarity 53, 54, 74
Polio 113
Polish Dance Theatre 262
Polak, Frank 271
Polk, Elizabeth 3, 113, 277
"Positive memories" 214
Post traumatic stress disorder 268
Posture 65, 70
Postural attitudes 63
Potential movement expression 36, 115, 116
Pozen 262
Prague 262, 272
Prahna 241
Pratt Institute 138, 269
"Present moment" attitude 191
Primal selves 238
"Primary Illusion" 138
Princeton 155
Privacy 267
Professional standards 12
Projective technique 7, 35-37, 58, 94, 167
Props 36, 206, 219, 223, 237, 250
Prussian Board of Education 43
Psyche 30, 61
Psychoanalysis 99, 123, 270, 279, 280, 305
Psychoanalytic approach 135, 305
Psychoanalytic theory 4, 6, 43, 87, 106, 135, 123, 127, 254
Psychodrama 9, 155, 166, 167, 174, 279
Psychodramatic double 174
Psychodramatic movement therapy 84, 163
Psychodramatic techniques 84
Psychodynamics 175, 192
Psychology 5, 41, 43, 44, 98, 269, 278-80
Psychomotor development 127

Psychomotor events 59
Psychomotor free association 35, 93, 94
Psychomotor therapy 9, 44, 60, 249, 268
Psychomotor therapeutic interventions 22
Psychophysical integration 90
Psychosexual stages of development 157
Psychosynthesis 155
Psychotherapeutic modality 94
Psychotherapeutisches Institut für Tanztherapie 262
Psychotherapy 30, 43, 45, 94, 121, 131, 149, 155, 158, 269, 279
Psychotic-catatonic 96
Puppetry 6, 7, 91
Putnam, F. W. 213

Q
Qualitative aspects of movement 110
Quebec 269, 270

R
Rahmin, Nadirah 160, 173
Rape 218
Rational Emotional Therapy 84
Reca, Maralia 270
Receptive mode 142-44
Reed, Virginia 131, 178, 253
Regression 32, 40
Rehabilitation 235-45
Reich, Wilhelm 6, 9, 22, 77, 236
Relationship awareness 257
Relationship building 197
Relaxation 10, 45, 73-75, 84, 229, 239, 249, 250
Releasing superficial/excess tension 33
Religion 262
Reminiscences 229, 230
Renfrew Center in Philadelphia 222, 225
Repetition 66, 92, 93, 249, 250
Repressed drive 61
Repressed traumas 32, 55
Residential group homes 243-45
Residual tension 74
Ressler, Adrienne 223, 224
Restrained movement 270
Retardando 92
Rhythm 22, 33, 36, 103, 257
    therapeutic benefits 155, 183
Rhythm and repetition 64, 66, 67, 249-51
Rhythmic activity 9, 21-23
Rhythmic movement 25, 27, 95
Rifkin-Gainer, Iris 30, 32-34, 36
Right hemisphere of the brain 75
Ritual dance 2, 280

Robbins, Arthur 269
Robbins, Bonnie 131
Robbins, Esther 127
Rogers, Carl 8, 9, 21, 141
Rogers, S. B. 255
Role 208
Role-playing 24, 70, 91, 92, 164-66, 169, 174, 204, 257
Role-reversal 9, 166, 169, 174
Rolf, Ida 10
Rome 269
Rorschach test 7
Rosen, Elizabeth 11, 15, 84, 87, 94-98, 163, 203
Rotterdam Dance Academy 261, 271
Rousaville, B. 219
Royal College of Music, Sweden 261
Rugg, Harold 73
Russell, Rhoda Winter 3, 83, 84, 121
Russia 262
Ruttenberg, B. 193
Ryan, J. 198
Ryu, Boon Soon 272

S

Sack, Joanabbey 269, 270
St. Clair, Michael 160
St. Denis, Ruth 2, 5, 19, 278
St. Elizabeth's Hospital 9, 19, 20, 119, 153
Samberg, S. 230
Samuels, Arlynne—see Stark, Arlynne
Sandel, Susan 12, 20. 177, 203, 204-11, 229, 230, 273
Sanders, L. 184
Sands Point Movement Study Group 127
Schade, Maja 83, 84
Scheflin, Albert 8, 254
Schilder, Paul 6, 7, 89, 90, 94, 191
Schizophrenia 6, 21, 90, 169, 170, 203-07, 209, 210, 211, 236
Schmais, Claire 2, 11, 12, 20, 21, 94, 114, 119, 120, 138, 192, 254
Schoop, Trudi 3, 11, 15, 61, 62, 64, 66-71, 78, 79, 141, 144, 147. 148, 151, 152, 163, 203
   Heritage Tree 299, 300
Schutz, William 256
Sculpting 239
Seabury, B. J. 237
Searles, Harold 205
"Self" 55, 56, 191, 196
Self-concept 219
Self-conscious 97
"Self-directed process oriented sessions" 197
Self-directed responses 76

Self-esteem 63, 197, 210, 219, 221, 229, 251, 257
Self-expression 93, 211, 251
Self-image 217
Self-observation 71, 120
Self-realization 26
Self-synchrony 8
Seminar Kibbutzim in Tel Aviv 264
Sensitization to and mobilization of potential body action 36, 37
Sensorimotor activities 195
Sensory impairment 238
Sensory input 142
"Sensory integration" 196
Seoul 272
Separation/individuation 138, 193, 205, 206
Serlin, Ilene 273
Severe head injury 238-41
Severely disabled patients 243-45
"Sex Ed" 197, 198
Sexual abuse 213, 217, 221, 271
Sexual drive 44
Sexual identity 40, 171, 197
Sexuality 44, 169
"Shadow movements" 143
Shamanic healing 272
Sharing 174
Shawn, Ted 1, 5, 19, 278
Shock therapy 207
Show dancing 1
Sibling rivalry 44
Sickle cell anemia 241
Siegel, Elaine 135-38, 140, 250, 262
Siegel, M. 221
Sigel, Jane Ganet 85, 270
Sign language 258
"Significant others" 164
Silberman, Linni—see Linni Deihl
Simple movement techniques 97
Siroka, Robert 163
Sixth Annual Conference of the American Dance Therapy Association 87
Skeletal alignment 10
Skyros, Greece 267
Social feelings 44
Social/emotional relationship 181
Socialization 251
Societal taboos 61
"Sociometric choice" 166, 174
Soma 30, 61
Somatic approach 230
Somatic countertransference 158, 159
Somatic reality 40
Soodak, Martha 127

Sorell, Walter 94
Sourkova, Radana 262, 272
South America 271
Southern Methodist University in Dallas 269
Space 37, 205, 206, 208, 256, 257
Spain 271
Spatial designs 117
Spatial relationships 46
Specific movement factor 115
Specific physical exercises 9
Speck, R. 256
Spiritual goal 230
Spirituality 280, 281
Spitz, R. 140, 205
Split-body exaggeration 66
SPMI (seriously and persistently mentally ill) 271
Spontaneous movement 59, 64
Stanislovsky 29, 235
Stark (Samuels), Arlynne 11, 12, 206, 207, 229
Steinberg, Cobbett 2
Stern, Daniel 184
Stockholm 261
Storytelling 91
"Stress model of behavior" 253
Strokes 270
Structural Analysis of Movement Sessions (SAMS) 207-10
Structure 188, 189, 191, 192, 200
Structured dance experience 98
Structured Movement Sequences 45
Structured therapeutic movement exercises 84, 156
Study of natural human movement 2
Sullivan, Harry Stack 6, 21, 77, 141, 153, 236
Summit, R. 197
Superego 10, 90, 124, 137, 151
Supportive closure 26
Suppressive adaptive patterns 29
Survey of dance therapists 277-81
Sweden 237, 261, 267
Swedish Expressive Arts Therapy Program 261
Sweigard, Lulu 10
Swindell, Kelly 139, 307
Swindell, Zoë 139
Swinging the body 33
Switzerland 61, 237, 262
Symbolic dialogue 169
Symbolic expression 220
Symbolic realization 214
Symbolism 7, 21, 22, 47, 70, 91
System of notation 109
Systems theory 280

T

TBI Movement Psychotherapy Group 240
Taiwan 262
Task 208
Teacher-therapist 90
Teitlebaum, P. 193
Tempo 37, 39
Tension flow 244, 245
Thematic Apperception Test 7, 91
Thematic movement explorations 63
Theme development 26, 239
Theme-oriented movement pattern 26
Themes 47
Theory and practice 277-79
Theory of active imagination 6
Theory of dance therapy 77
Theoretical model of dance psychology 53
Therapeutic Movement Relationship 21, 22, 27, 77, 78, 121, 136, 157-58, 162
Therapeutic process 92, 131
Therapeutic Recovery Program in Southfield, MI 239
Therapeutic relationship/Intuition 53, 57, 58, 156
Therapeutic role-playing 9
Therapist as mediator 57
Therapist/patient relationship (see also patient/therapist relationship) 203-07, 211, 220
"Third force" 9
Thomas, Deborah 83
Thomas, Tamara 160, 173
Tinos, Greece 267
Todd, Mabel E. 10
Tokyo 265, 266
Toledo State Hospitals 236
Tortora, Suzi 181-84
Total movement profile 116
Totenbier, Sally 190, 263, 264
"Touch attunement" 244
Touching 229, 237, 243, 244
Training 120, 271, 280
"Transcendent function" 147
Transference 135, 136, 204, 208, 211, 251
Transformational experiences 280
"Transitional space" 138
Transpersonal energy 241, 279, 280
Traumatic Brain Injury (TBI) 238-41
Trautmann-Voight, Sabine 262, 268
Tremors 238
Tropea, Elise Billock 177, 190, 273
Trust 197, 245
Tug-of-war 199
Turtle Bay Music School 21, 43, 119, 192

U

Uchida, Elli 266
UCLA 155
Ulcers 270
Ullmann, Lisa 109
Umea University, Sweden 261
Unconscious, The 3, 4, 10, 51, 56, 60, 79
Unconscious emotions 55
Unconscious material 37
Unconventional movement exploration 240
Unified physical state 66
United Cerebral Palsy (UCP) 235
United Kingdom 43, 262-64, 271
    registry 264
    school system 264
Unity of body, mind and spirit 1
Universality of movement 262
Universally associated action 66
University College of Dance, Sweden 261
University of California, Los Angeles—see UCLA
University of Haifa 264
University of London's Goldsmiths College 126
University of Vermont 190
University of Wisconsin 83, 84
Unstructured environment 58
"UR experience" 61
Urban adult 40

V

Veleweland 271
Verbal and nonverbal communication 21, 249, 250
Verbal communication 75, 198
Verbal intervention 267
Verbal narration 25, 27
Verbal facilitation 36, 77
Verbal free association 135
Verbal groups 44
Verbal psychotherapy 51, 278, 280
Verbal sessions 258
Verbalization 26, 32, 7, 65, 103, 145, 172, 211, 240, 280
    versus somatization 135
Vertical process 77
Vertical stress 79
Veteran's Administration Mental Hygiene Service 7
Viola 29
Violence prevention 185-87
Violence Prevention through Movement program 186
Virginia 237
Visualization 9
"Vocal attunement" 244
Vocal expression 93
Voyeuristic 97

W

Walco, G. A. 243
Walker, Lenore E. 219
Wallen, R. 142
Wallock, Susan 75, 51, 53-55, 59, 61, 65, 71
Wapner, Amy 266, 267
War trauma survivors 262
Warm-up 32, 36, 58, 101
Washington, D. C. 19
"Ways of Seeing" program 181
Weidman, Charles 3
Weight 37
Weiner, C. 250
Weinshel, M. 221
Weisbrod, Joanne 73, 256, 256
Weltman, Marsha 181, 197, 198
White, Elissa Queyquep 11, 12, 29, 114, 119, 120, 131, 139, 192, 254
Whitehouse, Mary 3, 4, 6, 11, 15, 51-60, 73, 77, 78, 84, 93, 94, 137, 141, 144, 147, 148, 151-53, 155, 267, 277
    Heritage Tree 303, 304
Whitehousian approach 141, 161, 279
Wiener, Carole 190
Wiesenthal 61
Wigman, Mary 3, 7, 43, 53, 55, 73, 84, 87, 88, 94, 113, 151, 235, 277, 281, 306
Wigman Conservatory 43
Wigman School 43, 51
Wigmanian improvisational approach 60, 161
Willard Parker Hospital 113
Winnicott, D.W. 127, 138, 140, 159, 160, 184
Wisher, Peter 258, 259
Withdrawn 97
Witnessing 182
"Witness/mover relationship" 140, 147
Wittig, Joan 13
Wollman, Adolf 7, 91
Wooten, B. 99
Work therapy 30
Wright Oral School of the Deaf 43

Y

Yahata, Yoh 265
Yalom, Irvin 191
Yoga 229, 241, 253
YMCA 236

Yusa, Yasuichiro 266
YWCA 43

Z
Zacharias, Jody 126
Zenoff, Nisha 55, 58, 59, 148
Zerbe, Kathryn J. 224, 226
Ziv, Anat 190-92
Zwerling, Israel 113, 114, 119

Note: Names, words and topics identified above were submitted and approved by the author. Not all individuals within the Heritage Trees are noted here (please consult the Heritage Trees for the complete listing).